Third Edition

The
Sectional Anatomy
Learning System

CONCEPTS

Third Edition

The Sectional Anatomy
Learning System

CONCEPTS

Edith J. Applegate, MS

Professor of Science and Mathematics
Kettering College of Medical Arts
Kettering, Ohio

SAUNDERS

ELSEVIER

SAUNDERS
ELSEVIER

11830 Westline Industrial Drive
St. Louis, Missouri 63146

THE SECTIONAL ANATOMY LEARNING SYSTEM: CONCEPTS, ED 3   ISBN 978-1-4160-5013-1
Volume 1 PN 9996049264

Library of Congress Cataloging-in-Publication Data
Applegate, Edith J.
The sectional anatomy learning system / Edith J. Applegate. — Ed. 3.
    p. ; cm.
Includes bibliographical references and index.
ISBN-13: 978-1-4160-5013-1 (2 v. set, pbk. : alk. paper)
ISBN-13: 978-9996049262 (v. 1, pbk. : alk. paper)
ISBN-10: 9996049264 (v. 1, pbk. : alk. paper)
ISBN-13: 978-9996048364 (v. 2, pbk. : alk. paper)
[etc.]
1. Anatomy, Surgical and topographical. 2. Diagnostic imaging. I. Title.
    [DNLM: 1. Anatomy, Cross-Sectional. 2. Diagnostic Imaging. QS 4
A648s 2010]
    QM531.A65 2010
    611—dc22

2008046638

Vice President and Publisher: Andrew Allen
Publisher: Jeane Olson
Associate Developmental Editor: Luke Held
Publishing Services Manager: Julie Eddy
Senior Project Manager: Celeste Clingan
Design Direction: Paula Catalano

Printed in the United States

Last digit is the print number: 9 8 7 6

Dedicated to the three favorite men in my life:
Stan, Dave, and Doug

Reviewers

Mary Susan Helene Crowley, BScApl, M.Ed., MRT
Professor
The Michener Institute for Applied Health Sciences
Toronto, Ontario, Canada

Marianna C. Desmond BS, RDMS, RT(R)
Clinical Coordinator, DMS Program
Triton College
River Grove, Illinois

Frances Gilman, MS, RT(R)(CT)(MS)(CV) ARRT
Chair, Department of Radiologic Sciences
Thomas Jefferson University
Philadelphia, Pennsylvania

Parsha Y. Hobsnon, MP.A, RT(R)
Radiography Program
Passaic County Community College
Patterson, New Jersey

M. Diane Newham, MS, RT(R)(M)(CT)(QM)
Associate Professor
Weber State University
Ogden, Utah

Leslie Elona Rosenkoetter, MS, RT(R)(CT)(MR)
Assistant Professor
Boise State University
Boise, Idaho

Robert John Slothus, BS, MS, ARRT (RT(R))
Director and Associate Professor of Radiography
Pennsylvania College of Technology
Williamsport, Pennsylvania

Patricia Sperry, BS, RT(R)(CT)
Radiology Program Director
Mills-Peninsula Health Services
Burlingame, California

Susan Raatz Stephenson, MaEd, RDMS, RUT, RT(R)(C)
Adjunct Faculty
George Washington University
Belleville Community College
Washington, District of Columbia

Patricia A. Tew, MS, RT(R)(CT)
Radiography Program Director
University of Missouri
Columbia, Missouri

Renee Tossell, PhD, RT(R)(M)(CV)
Instructional Faculty and Clinical Coordinator
Pima Community College
Tucson, Arizona

Bill Whiteside, BA, MRT(T)
Professor, Radiation Therapy
Medical Radiation Sciences
The Michener Institute for Applied Health Sciences
Toronto, Ontario, Canada
Lecturer
Medical Radiation Sciences, Department of Radiation
    Oncology
University of Toronto
Toronto, Ontario, Canada

Preface

The Sectional Anatomy Learning System was created for teachers and students of anatomy in the diagnostic imaging sciences. It consists of two components: Concepts and Applications. Used together, these textbooks provide a tool for an understanding of anatomy in three dimensions that is essential for success in careers involving any of the imaging modalities. A thorough comprehension of anatomy from a sectional perspective greatly enhances the understanding of gross anatomy. Students should be able to observe a transverse, sagittal, or coronal section and mentally reconstruct the three-dimensional relationships of that area. Conversely, given a gross dissection of a region, students should be able to visualize the appearance and the relationships in the planar sections.

Work on the first edition of this project actually began in 1980 when I was asked to develop a collegiate course in sectional anatomy for radiography and sonography students at Kettering College of Medical Arts, a division of Kettering Health Network in Dayton, Ohio. At the time no student textbooks were available, no aids to guide teachers, and only a few atlases available for the physician. I had no choice but to create materials for student and classroom use. Needless to say, the first few years saw a steep learning curve and numerous improvements in response to student input. In addition to the classroom, those original materials were used for seminars and continuing education events sponsored by the Association of Educators in Imaging and Radiologic Sciences, Inc. (AEIRS), Ohio Society of Radiologic Technologists (OSRT), Michigan Society of Radiologic Technologists (MSRT), and American Society of Radiologic Technologists (ASRT). In response to requests from people who attended these events, the first edition of The Sectional Anatomy was published in 1991 and became available for widespread classroom use. It was, and still is, a textbook for sectional anatomy, not a discourse on technology. In response to comments and suggestions from users, the third edition of The Sectional Anatomy Learning System continues to show improvements and enhancements over the previous two editions.

The Sectional Anatomy Learning System is designed for radiography students and for those involved with the technologies of computed tomography, magnetic resonance imaging, sonography, and other modalities. It is also valuable to practicing clinicians who want to improve their skills and expertise through continuing education. Numerous educators use The Sectional Anatomy Learning System for online and distance learning courses. Because each chapter is self-contained, The Sectional Anatomy Learning System is a flexible mechanism for a continuing education series. Basic anatomy and physiology—at least one semester and preferably two—is necessary for background information and terminology.

Organization

The Sectional Anatomy Learning System textbook, Concepts, is designed for use with its companion workbook, Applications. The common focus of both books is "anatomical relationships." In other words, the emphasis is on the relationship of one organ to another, one blood vessel to another, a blood vessel to a nerve, or one body part to another. Understanding these relationships is essential if one is to truly understand sectional anatomy rather than engage in a rote memorization process, which rarely is beneficial because no two bodies are exactly alike.

The Concepts textbook presents information in a descriptive manner with numerous labeled illustrations, both line drawings and diagnostic images, to reinforce the relationships that are described. The Applications workbook is a collection of drawings and diagnostic images of transverse, sagittal, and coronal sections for students to label. Coloring exercises are included to help users see the relationships of important structures and follow them through several levels. Each illustration is accompanied by questions that reinforce the information.

Both Concepts and Applications are divided into eight chapters. Chapter 1 introduces basic concepts and terminology. Subsequent chapters each deal with a specific region of the body as follows:

- Chapter 2—Thorax
- Chapter 3—Abdomen
- Chapter 4—Male and female pelvis
- Chapter 5—Head
- Chapter 6—Vertebral column, spinal cord and neck
- Chapter 7—Upper extremity
- Chapter 8—Lower extremity

Each chapter may be used as a self-contained unit for a series of mini courses, or the books may be used in their entirety for a complete quarter or semester course. Instructors may select topics as the allotted class time permits, and they may choose the sequence in which to study each chapter. Previous editions started with the head, but numerous users suggested that the thorax would be a better starting point because it is more familiar to more students.

A distinctive feature of the *Sectional Anatomy Learning System* is the line drawings, which are derived from real cadaver specimens. The line drawings in the "Sectional Anatomy" portion of each chapter in both *Concepts* and *Applications* are made from actual cadaver specimens. They are not idealized or computer generated, and thus illustrate the variations that occur in real life. The photographs of the cadaver slices may be accessed online on Evolve. Using the photographs will aid in labeling the drawings in *Applications* and will reinforce the relationships to be learned.

Chapter Organization

After the first introductory chapter, each chapter in *Concepts* contains the following features:

- Outline
- Objectives
- Key Terms, Structures and Features to be Identified
- Anatomical Review
- Sectional Anatomy
- Working with Images
- Important Anatomical Relationships
- Bulleted Chapter Summary
- Review Questions
- Chapter Quiz

The objectives and the list of key terms help instructors and students know what to look for and what should be learned in each chapter. They are an introduction to what should be expected in the narrative. The first part of the narrative in each chapter is an overview of the anatomy of the region to provide a common starting point for all students in the class. It reviews and refreshes the terminology appropriate to the region so students can concentrate on the anatomical relationships of structures rather than becoming frustrated with anatomy and terminology.

The sectional anatomy of the region is presented after the review of gross anatomy and terminology. Sectional anatomy is discussed first in the transverse plane and then in the sagittal and coronal planes. Each level of section is illustrated by a labeled line drawing. Selected section discussions also contain labeled diagnostic images for additional reinforcement.

A new feature in the third edition is a section called "Working with Images." This portion of the chapter contains radiographs, computed tomography images, magnetic resonance images, and sonograms. Each image is accompanied by a description that indicates which structures should be identified. A few key items are labeled on the image and the remaining structures can be identified from the description and knowledge of relationships learned in the chapter.

Each chapter concludes with a chapter summary, a series of review questions, and a quiz. Pertinent chapters also contain pathology boxes. These boxes provide concise information about the common pathologies that may be encountered by the imaging professional. The summary relates to the objectives at the beginning of the chapter and serves as a quick reinforcement of the objectives. The review questions also relate to the objectives and chapter summary. In general, there is at least one question pertaining to each of the objectives at the beginning of the chapter. Instructors may wish to assign the review questions as homework or use them as test questions. Students may use the chapter quiz as a self-test to check their comprehension of the chapter. Answers to the review and quiz questions are available online on Evolve.

Concepts concludes with:

- **Suggested Readings.** A brief list of additional resources for interested readers.
- **Glossary.** Definitions of key terms and structures discussed in the book.
- **Combining forms.** Some of the more commonly used word roots and combining forms are listed with their definitions and examples of their uses to build words.
- **Eponyms.** Commonly used eponyms are identified with their corresponding anatomical names.
- **Quick Check Answers.** Answers to the new Quick Check questions are provided in the back of the book to allow students to quickly gauge their understanding of key material.

New to this Edition

- **More diagnostic images.** Over 150 new images with key anatomical structures labeled, including three-dimensional reconstructions, are included in the third edition of *Concepts*. Approximately 375 total labeled illustrations—line drawings and diagnostic images— throughout *Concepts* help imaging students and practitioners see and remember sectional anatomy.
- **Quick Check questions.** These are questions inserted after every few paragraphs in *Concepts* to evaluate learning and aid comprehension of the preceding discussions. The answers are given at the back of the book for instant feedback.
- **Working With Images section.** This portion of each chapter uses images from various imaging modalities, including three-dimensional reconstructions. Many of these are also included in *Applications*. This gives the student practice in looking at images from the various modalities and also reinforces the anatomical relationships that are present.
- **Important Anatomical Relationships section.** The emphasis in *The Sectional Anatomy Learning System* is on anatomical relationships rather than memorizing a given image or specimen. When the focus is on these relationships, the variations in individuals are less of a problem. Near the end of each chapter, a list of the important anatomical relationships is provided for that region. These are cross-referenced to figures within the chapter that illustrate the relationship.

- **List of key terms and structures.** Important terms and structures, bolded in previous editions, are now also compiled into lists at the beginning of the *Concepts* chapters to highlight the anatomical identifications that are necessary in the region under consideration.
- **Chapter summary.** The chapter summary reiterates the important information related to the objectives, providing a quick review.

Ancillaries

The following ancillaries are available for students and instructors online on Evolve at http://evolve.elsevier.com/Applegate/SAlearning/

For the Student

- Cadaver photographs from which the line drawings were made. These are cross referenced with the relevant figures in *Concepts* and *Applications*.
- Answers to Review Questions in *Concepts*.
- Answers to Chapter Quizzes in *Concepts*.
- Answers to labeling exercises in *Applications*.
- Answers to Chapter Recall in *Applications*.
- Weblinks to relevant imaging websites.

For the Instructor

In addition to access to the student resources listed above, instructors can access the following resources:

- Chapter objectives.
- Detailed chapter outlines.
- Key terms, structures and features to be identified. These are listed and defined for easy reference.
- Important anatomical relationships, which are cross-referenced to figures in *Concepts* and *Applications*.
- Test bank with over 950 questions and answers, in ExamView and rtf formats.

To gain maximum benefit from the learning experience provided by *The Sectional Anatomy Learning System: Concepts and Applications*, students are encouraged to:

- Review the basic gross anatomy in *Concepts*.
- Complete the anatomy review exercises in *Applications*.

- Answer the anatomy review Quick Check questions in *Concepts*.
- Study the sectional anatomy portion of the chapter in *Concepts*.
- Complete the sectional anatomy labeling exercises in *Applications* by correlating the line drawings in the book with the cadaver sections on the Evolve website.
- Complete the coloring exercises and answer the questions for each sectional anatomy line drawing in *Applications*.
- Study the working with images portion of the chapter in *Concepts*.
- Apply what has been learned by labeling the images in *Applications*.
- Answer the questions for each image in *Applications*.
- Review the chapter by answering the Review Questions in *Concepts*.
- Test yourself with the Chapter Quiz in *Concepts* and the Chapter Recall in *Applications*.

Author's Final Note

I have used some form of these materials for the last 25 years in a variety of ways from a semester course in the college classroom to a half-day seminar, from a continuing education series for technologists to a week-long workshop for teachers. *The Sectional Anatomy Learning System* is flexible enough to be used in a variety of venues. It is my intent that *The Sectional Anatomy Learning System* will serve as a comprehensive and effective teaching and learning package. The most benefit will be gained from using the two components, *Concepts* and *Applications*, with the photographs of the cadaver slices that are available on the Evolve website. The more than 150 new computed tomography, magnetic resonance, and ultrasound images that have been added to the books will enhance the learning experience and make it more meaningful. There is always more to learn and many different teaching methods. You can help improve this package with your comments. I welcome any suggestions you have to offer.

Acknowledgments

Writing a textbook requires the expertise, cooperation, collaboration, and encouragement of many people. This third edition of *The Sectional Anatomy Learning System* is no exception.

Although I am officially retired from classroom teaching, the Administration of Kettering College of Medical Arts (KCMA), a division of Kettering Health Network in Dayton, Ohio, generously provides me with office space and computer support. For this I am truly grateful.

Numerous individuals at Kettering College of Medical Arts and Kettering Medical Center (KMC), another division of Kettering Health Network, graciously worked with me to obtain the images for this book. These include:

Michele Bean RT, (KMC), Supervisor Diagnostic Radiology

Larry Beneke MSEd. Administration, ARRT (R) (CT), (KCMA), Professor and Program Director, Radiologic Sciences and Imaging

Roy Coggeshall RT, (KMC) Supervisor CT/interventional Radiology

Jay Coleman RT, (KMC), 3D Technologist

Joyce Grube MS, RDMS, (KCMA), Associate Professor and Program Director, Medical Sonography

Rob Hoover MA, RT, (KCMA), Associate Professor Radiologic Sciences and Imaging, Clinical and Didactic Instructor

Tom Kracus RT, (KMC) 3D Imaging Specialist

Beth Maxwell BS, RDCS, RDMS, RVT, (KCMA), Assistant Professor Medical Sonography

Margo Miller BS, RDMS, RVT, RT, (KMC), Supervisor Ultrasound

Amanda Nolan BS, RT, (KMC), Lead Technologist CT

Merle Peterson MS, RT, CRA, (KMC), Medical Imaging Director

Cathy Swick RT, MR(R), (KMC), Supervisor MRI

Melanie Willsey BS, RDMS, RVT, (KMC), Ultrasound Technologist

The assistance of these individuals adds a great deal to the learning experience provided by the third edition of *The Sectional Anatomy Learning System.* Many of these are former students of mine and I am proud of them. I thank them for their time and expertise.

The editorial and production staff at Elsevier, St. Louis, has been outstanding. Somehow they have taken my efforts and, through miracles only they can perform, transformed them into something usable. For this I am grateful.

The reviewers who read through the first draft offered comments, suggestions and corrections. Their critique improved the quality and accuracy of this third edition and I value their expertise.

My students, with their probing quest for knowledge, have been a driving force behind my efforts. They have been a source of enthusiasm and inspiration. Numerous colleagues and friends have prodded me with their interest and encouragement. Although many miles away, my sons, Dave and Doug, have encouraged me with their phone calls and enthusiasm. My husband and best friend for 50 years has been a constant source of love, encouragement, reassurance, strength, and patience.

To each one who has touched my life and helped me grow personally, professionally, and spiritually, I offer my deepest gratitude. To all I say a big *THANK YOU!*

Contents

CHAPTER ONE

Introduction to Sectional Anatomy | 1

**Comparison of Traditional Anatomy
and Sectional Anatomy**
Body Planes
Directional Terms

Body Cavities
Membranes of the Body Cavities
Regional Terminology
Important Anatomical Relationships

OBJECTIVES

Upon completion of this chapter, the student should be able to do the following:
- Identify the transverse, sagittal, midsagittal, parasagittal, and frontal planes.
- Describe the anatomical position.
- Use correct directional terms to describe the relative position of one body part to another.
- Describe the location, subdivisions, and contents of the dorsal body cavity and the ventral body cavity.
- Name and identify the nine abdominopelvic regions.
- Distinguish between connective tissue membranes and epithelial membranes and give two examples of each type.
- Describe the location of mucous membranes and serous membranes.
- Distinguish between the visceral and parietal layers of serous membranes.
- State the specific locations of the parietal and visceral layers of the pleura, pericardium, and peritoneum.
- Use correct regional terms to refer to specific areas of the body.

Key Terms, Structures, and Features to Be Identified and/or Described

Abdominal cavity
Abdominopelvic cavity
Anatomical position
Antebrachial region
Antecubital region
Anterior
Appendicular skeleton
Axial plane
Axial skeleton
Axillary region
Brachial region
Buccal region
Carpal region
Caudad
Cephalad
Cephalic region
Cervical region
Connective tissue membrane
Coronal plane
Costal region
Cranial cavity
Cranial region
Crural region
Cubital region
Deep

Distal
Dorsal body cavity
Epigastric region
Epithelial membrane
Femoral region
Frontal plane
Gluteal region
Hypochondriac region
Hypogastric region
Iliac region
Inferior
Inguinal region
Lateral
Leg region
Lumbar region
Mammary region
Medial
Mediastinum
Meninges
Midsagittal plane
Mucosae
Mucous membrane
Occipital region
Ophthalmic region
Oral region

Otic region
Parasagittal plane
Parietal serosa
Pectoral region
Pelvic cavity
Pelvic region
Pericardial cavity
Pericardium
Perineal region
Peritoneum
Plantar region
Pleura
Pleural cavity
Popliteal region
Posterior
Proximal
Sacral region
Sagittal plane
Serosa
Serous membrane
Spinal cavity
Sternal region
Superficial
Superior
Synovial membrane

Thigh
Thoracic cavity
Thoracic region

Transverse plane
Umbilical region
Ventral body cavity

Vertebral region
Visceral serosa

Comparison of Traditional Anatomy and Sectional Anatomy

In typical anatomy and physiology courses, the emphasis is on studying body systems. For example, you learn the entire skeletal system before moving on to the muscular system. You study all the organs of the digestive system, their location, structure, and how they relate to each other functionally. In sectional anatomy, you study regions instead of systems, and the focus is on the anatomical relationships of all structures within a given region, such as the thorax or abdomen. The traditional approach to anatomy is to study an entire organ. In sectional anatomy, the anatomy is viewed on what is commonly called a *slice* of the body. In other words, imagine the body (or organ) as a thinly sliced loaf of raisin bread. Each slice of bread has a different appearance because of the different number and positions of the raisins.

Visualization of an entire organ may require several sequential slices. Returning to the analogy of the raisin bread, finding all the pieces of a single raisin may require looking at several sequential slices, because the raisins have been sliced along with the bread. The same is true for visualizing slices of the body. By studying the anatomical relationships in sequential slices, you develop a more thorough understanding of anatomy. Sophisticated imaging equipment can take the information from the slices and create a three-dimensional (3D) image.

For orientation of a transverse (axial) slice, when viewing either the inferior of a cadaveric slice or a real image, imagine that the patient is supine and you are standing at the person's feet looking up into the patient's body. This means that your right is the patient's left. Fig. 1-1 shows a transverse CT image through the abdomen that illustrates this orientation. The right lobe of the liver, inferior vena cava, and caudate lobe of the liver are on the patient's right side, but they are on the

left side of the image. The left lobe of the liver, the stomach, the spleen, and the left kidney are on the patient's left side, but they are on the right side of the image. The aorta is slightly to the left of midline. Correct orientation is critical to proper identification of structures.

Now, a couple of cautionary notes for learning sectional anatomy:

1. A given organ varies in appearance at different levels in the same individual. Fig. 1-2 shows images of the liver at three different levels. Notice the changes in appearance at the different levels.
2. Attempting to memorize images likely will lead to mistakes, because no two images are the same. Every individual is different, and even images of the same individual taken at the same level differ because of breathing and involuntary movements. The key is understanding, not memorization.

Before you begin the study of sectional anatomy, it may be profitable to review some of the terminology and concepts you learned in gross anatomy or anatomy and physiology. This can help get you back into the "anatomy" mode and provide a common foundation for the class. The introductory material includes body planes, directional terms, body cavities, membranes of the body cavities, and regional terminology.

Body Planes

To visualize the spatial relationships of internal body parts, the body is sectioned, or cut, along a flat surface, or plane. The ability to interpret sections in various planes is becoming increasingly important in the clinical sciences, especially in the imaging sciences. The three most commonly used planes are the transverse (axial), sagittal, and frontal (coronal)

FIG. 1-1. Orientation of body slices—a transverse CT image through the abdomen.

FIG. 1-2. Appearance of the liver at three different levels. **A**, T10 level. **B**, T11 level. **C**, T12 level. In each of these scans, the liver is the structure on the left side (patient's right). At T10 **(A)** it appears large and uniform. At T11 **(B)** it shows lobes, and at T12 **(C)** it is much smaller.

planes, which are at right angles to each other (Fig. 1-3). By analyzing body parts in all three planes, you develop an understanding of the anatomical relationships within the body.

Transverse (axial) planes, or horizontal planes, cut across the body horizontally from right to left and divide the body into superior and inferior portions. Sections cut along transverse planes are sometimes called *cross sections*.

Sagittal planes are vertical planes that cut through the body from superior to inferior and divide the body into right and left portions. These vertical planes are also called *longitudinal planes*. The specific sagittal plane that passes through the midline is the **midsagittal plane,** or median plane, which divides the body into right and left halves. All other sagittal planes are **parasagittal planes.**

Frontal planes, like sagittal planes, are vertical planes. They are at right angles to the sagittal and transverse planes and divide the body into anterior and posterior portions. Frontal planes are also called **coronal planes.**

QUICK CHECK

1.1 Name the two vertical planes that are at right angles to each other.

1.2 What is another name for the horizontal plane, or cross section?

Directional Terms

If directional terms are to be meaningful, there must be some point of reference with which to start. In the body, the point of reference is the **anatomical position.** In this position, the body is standing erect, the face is forward, and the arms are at the sides with the palms and toes directed forward. Fig. 1-4 illustrates the body in anatomical position.

The following directional terms are used to describe the relative position of one body part to another. Note that the two items in each pair of terms are opposites.

- **Superior** means that a part is above another portion, or closer to the head.
  Inferior means that a part is below another part, or closer to the feet.
- **Anterior** (or *ventral*) means toward the front surface.
  Posterior (or *dorsal*) means that a part is toward the back.
- **Medial** means toward or nearer the midline of the body.
  Lateral means toward or nearer the side, away from the midline.
- **Proximal** means that a part is closer to a point of attachment, or closer to the trunk of the body, than another part.
  Distal is the opposite of proximal; it means that a part is farther away from a point of attachment than another part.

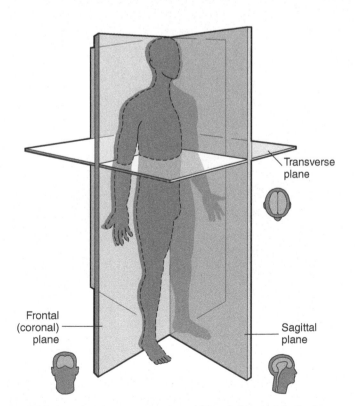

FIG. 1-3. Transverse, sagittal, and frontal planes of the body.

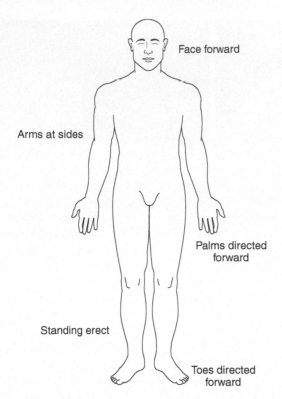

Face forward

Arms at sides

Palms directed
forward

Standing erect

Toes directed
forward

FIG. 1-4. Anatomical position.

- **Superficial** means that a part is located on or near the surface.
  Deep is the opposite of superficial; it means that a part is away from the surface.
- **Cephalad** means toward the head, or superior.
  Caudad means toward the inferior.

QUICK CHECK

1.3 What is the opposite of proximal?
1.4 What directional term describes the nose relative to the mouth?

Body Cavities

The two large, enclosed spaces within the axial portion of the body that contain the internal organs are called *closed body cavities*. In addition to the closed body cavities, there are several smaller, open body cavities, such as the oral cavity, nasal cavity, and orbital cavity. These open to the exterior of the body.

The smaller of the two closed cavities is the **dorsal body cavity.** This cavity is subdivided into the **cranial cavity,** which contains the brain, and the **spinal cavity,** which contains the spinal cord. The cranial and spinal cavities are continuous with each other at the foramen magnum.

The larger and more anterior of the two closed body cavities is the **ventral body cavity.** This cavity contains the group of internal organs commonly called the *viscera* or *visceral organs*. The ventral body cavity is subdivided by

the diaphragm into a smaller, superior **thoracic cavity** and a larger, inferior **abdominopelvic cavity.** The thoracic cavity is further subdivided into the right and left **pleural cavities** and the **mediastinum.** The pleural cavities contain the lungs, and the mediastinum, which is between the two pleural cavities, contains the **pericardial cavity,** which encloses the heart. The mediastinum also contains the esophagus, trachea, and great vessels.

Although no partition divides it, the abdominopelvic cavity often is subdivided into the **abdominal cavity** and the **pelvic cavity.** The abdominal cavity is more superior and contains the stomach, liver, spleen, intestines, and other organs. The inferior part, the pelvic cavity, contains the urinary bladder, rectum, and reproductive organs. The closed body cavities are illustrated in Fig. 1-5.

QUICK CHECK

1.5 What are the two subdivisions of the dorsal body cavity?
1.6 Name the thoracic cavity that is between the two pleural cavities and contains the heart, esophagus, and trachea.

To help describe the location of body parts or the location of pain, health care professionals frequently use imaginary lines to divide the abdominopelvic cavity into regions. One method uses a vertical plane through the midline and a horizontal plane that passes through the umbilicus. This divides the abdominopelvic cavity into four quadrants, illustrated in Fig. 1-6.

Cranial
cavity

Dorsal
cavity

Thoracic
cavity

Spinal
cavity

Ventral
cavity

Abdominopelvic
cavity

Abdominal
cavity

Pelvic
cavity

FIG. 1-5. The two major closed cavities of the body.

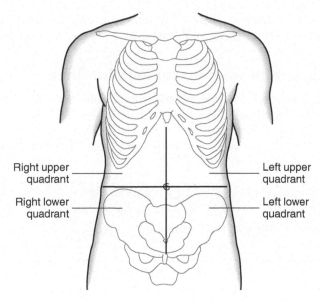

FIG. 1-6. The abdominopelvic quadrants.

Another method uses two parasagittal planes and two transverse planes to divide the abdominopelvic cavity into nine regions, illustrated in Fig. 1-7. The three central regions, from superior to inferior, are the **epigastric region,** the **umbilical region,** and the **hypogastric region.** To the right and left of these central regions, from superior to inferior, are the **hypochondriac regions,** the **lumbar regions,** and the **inguinal (iliac) regions.**

QUICK CHECK

1.7 What is the point on the surface of the body where the vertical and horizontal planes intersect to form the four quadrants?

1.8 Name the three abdominopelvic regions in the middle vertical column from superior to inferior.

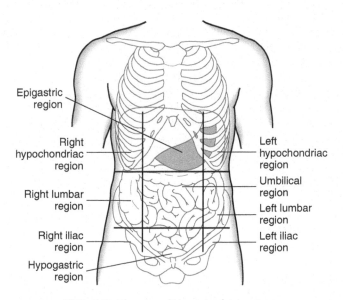

FIG. 1-7. The nine abdominopelvic regions.

Membranes of the Body Cavities

The membranes of the body cavities are thin sheets of tissue that line the cavities, cover the organs in the cavities, and line the cavities in hollow organs. Two structural types of membranes are associated with body cavities: connective tissue membranes and epithelial membranes.

Connective tissue membranes contain only connective tissue. The membranes of the dorsal body cavity and the joints are this type of membrane. The connective tissue membranes that cover the brain and spinal cord in the dorsal body cavity are called **meninges.** There are three layers of meninges: the outer dura mater, the middle arachnoid, and the inner pia mater. The meninges protect the vital structures in the dorsal cavity. The connective tissue membranes that line the joint cavities are **synovial membranes.** They secrete fluid for lubrication within the joint.

Epithelial membranes consist of epithelial tissue attached to connective tissue. The epithelial membranes that line the open cavities, such as the nasal cavity and the entire digestive tract, are **mucous membranes,** or **mucosae.** They are so named because they secrete mucus for lubrication and protection. The epithelial membranes that line the ventral body cavity and cover the organs in the cavity are very thin, double-layered **serous membranes,** or **serosa.** The portion of the serous membrane that lines the cavity wall is the parietal layer, or **parietal serosa.** It folds in on itself to form the **visceral serosa,** which covers the organs in the cavity. Serous membranes secrete a serous fluid that lubricates the surfaces of the membranes to allow the organs to move without friction.

Serous membranes have specific names according to their location. The membrane that lines the walls of the thoracic cavity is the **parietal pleura,** and the membrane that covers the lungs is the **visceral pleura.** The **parietal pericardium** lines the pericardial cavity, and the **visceral pericardium** covers the heart. In the abdominopelvic cavity, the serous membrane is called **peritoneum;** the **parietal peritoneum** lines the wall of the cavity, and the **visceral peritoneum** covers the organs. Fig. 1-8 illustrates the membranes of the body cavities.

QUICK CHECK

1.9 What is the name of the connective tissue membrane found in the dorsal body cavity?

1.10 What serous membrane is found in the mediastinum?

1.11 What specific serous membrane covers the outside of the stomach?

Regional Terminology

The body is divided into axial and appendicular portions. The axial part makes up the main axis of the body and consists of the head, neck, and trunk. The appendicular portion consists of the appendages, or limbs, that are attached to the

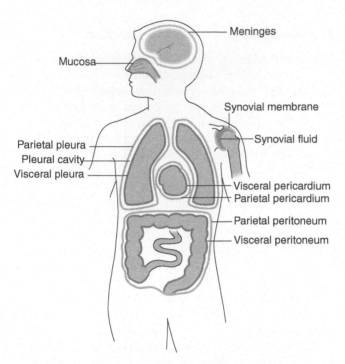

FIG. 1-8. The membranes of the body cavities. (From Applegate E: *The anatomy and physiology learning system,* ed 3, St Louis, 2006, Elsevier/Saunders.)

main axis. Regional terms that refer to specific parts or areas of the body are listed in Table 1-1 and illustrated in Fig. 1-9.

Important Anatomical Relationships

- The transverse, sagittal, and frontal planes are commonly used to visualize anatomical relationships (see Fig. 1-3).
- In anatomical position, the body is erect, face forward, arms at the sides, and palms and toes directed forward (see Fig. 1-4).

QUICK CHECK
1.12 Does the femoral region belong to the axial or the appendicular portion of the body?
1.13 Do the cephalic and costal regions belong to the axial or the appendicular portion of the body?

- *Superior* and *inferior*, *anterior* and *posterior*, *ventral* and *dorsal*, *medial* and *lateral*, *proximal* and *distal*, *superficial* and *deep*, and *cephalad* and *caudad* are terms used to describe relative positions in the body. The directions in each pair of terms are opposites (see pp. 3-4).
- The dorsal and ventral body cavities are closed body cavities. The dorsal body cavity is divided into the

TABLE 1-1   Terms for Specific Body Regions

Term	Body Region	Term	Body Region
Abdominal	Portion of the trunk below the diaphragm; between the thorax and pelvis	Mammary	Breast
		Occipital	Lower portion of the back of the head
Antebrachial	Region between the elbow and the wrist; forearm; cubital region	Ophthalmic	Eyes
		Oral	Mouth
Antecubital	Space in front of the elbow	Otic	Ears
Axillary	Armpit area	Pectoral	Chest region
Brachial	Arm; proximal portion of the upper limb	Pedal	Foot
		Pelvic	Inferior region of the abdominopelvic cavity; lower portion of the trunk
Buccal	Region of the cheek		
Carpal	Wrist		
Cephalic	Head	Perineal	Region between the anus and pubic symphysis; includes the region of the external reproductive organs
Cervical	Neck region		
Costal	Ribs		
Cranial	Skull		
Cubital	Antebrachial	Plantar	Sole of the foot
Cutaneous	Skin	Popliteal	Area behind the knee
Femoral	Thigh; the part of the lower extremity between the hip and the knee	Sacral	Posterior region between the hipbones
Frontal	Forehead	Sternal	Anterior midline of the thorax
Gluteal	Buttock region	Tarsal	Ankle and instep of the foot
Inguinal	Depressed region between the abdomen and the thigh; groin	Thoracic	Chest; part of the trunk inferior to the neck and superior to the diaphragm
Leg	Portion of the lower extremity between the knee and the foot; also called the crural region		
		Umbilical	Navel; middle region of the abdomen
Lumbar	Region of the lower back and side between the lowest rib and the pelvis	Vertebral	Pertaining to the spinal column; back-bone

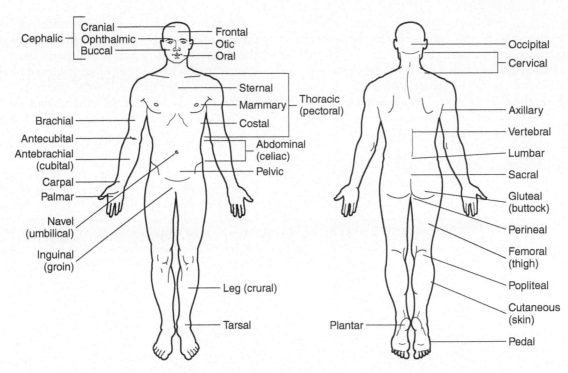

FIG. 1-9. Regional terms that refer to specific parts or areas of the body.

cranial cavity and the spinal cavity. The ventral body cavity is divided into the thoracic cavity and the abdominopelvic cavity (see Fig. 1-5).

- Horizontal and vertical planes through the umbilicus divide the abdominopelvic cavity into four quadrants (see Fig. 1-6).
- Two parasagittal planes and two transverse planes divide the abdominopelvic cavity into nine regions (see Fig. 1-7).
- Meninges and synovial membranes are connective tissue membranes (see Fig. 1-8).
- Mucous membranes and serous membranes are epithelial membranes (see Fig. 1-8).
- Serous membranes have visceral and parietal layers (see Fig. 1-8).
- The body is divided into axial and appendicular portions (see page 6).
- Regional terms refer to specific parts or areas of the body (see Fig. 1-9).

Summary

- A transverse plane is a horizontal, or axial, plane that divides a part into superior and inferior portions; a sagittal plane is a vertical plane that divides a part into right and left portions; a midsagittal plane is a specific sagittal plane that divides a part into right and left halves, and a parasagittal plane is any other sagittal plane; a frontal (coronal) plane is a vertical plane that divides a part into anterior and posterior portions.
- In anatomical position, the body is erect, face forward, arms at the sides, and palms and toes forward.

- *Superior* and *inferior, anterior* and *posterior, ventral* and *dorsal, medial* and *lateral, proximal* and *distal, superficial* and *deep,* and *cephalad* and *caudad* are terms used to describe relative positions in the body.
- The dorsal and ventral body cavities are closed body cavities; this means that they are not open to the external environment.
- The dorsal body cavity is divided into the cranial cavity, which contains the brain, and the spinal cavity, which contains the spinal cord.
- The ventral body cavity is larger than the dorsal cavity. It is divided into the thoracic cavity (above the diaphragm) and the abdominopelvic cavity (below the diaphragm). The thoracic cavity contains the heart and lungs. The abdominopelvic cavity is further divided into the abdominal cavity and the pelvic cavity, but no physical partition separates them.
- Two parasagittal planes and two transverse planes divide the abdominopelvic cavity into nine regions. From superior to inferior, the central regions are the epigastric region, the umbilical region, and the hypogastric region. Laterally, from superior to inferior, the regions are the right and left hypogastric regions, the right and left lumbar regions, and the right and left inguinal (iliac) regions.
- Connective tissue membranes contain only connective tissue. The meninges in the dorsal body cavity and the synovial membranes of the joints are this type of membrane.
- Epithelial membranes consist of epithelial tissue attached to connective tissue. The membranes in the ventral body cavity and the open cavities are this type of membrane. The epithelial membranes of the ventral

body cavity are called *serous membranes*, or *serosa*. The epithelial membranes of the open cavities are called *mucous membranes*, or *mucosae*.

- Serous membranes always consist of two layers, a visceral layer and a parietal layer. The parietal layer of a serous membrane lines the closed cavity. The visceral layer covers the organs within the cavity. A small amount of fluid between the two layers provides lubrication.
- The visceral pericardium is the outermost layer of the heart; the parietal pericardium lines the pericardial cavity. The visceral pleura is intimately attached to the outer surface of the lung, and the parietal pleura lines the thoracic wall. The visceral peritoneum covers the organs in the abdominopelvic cavity, and the parietal peritoneum lines the wall of the cavity.
- In the clinical setting, regional terms are used to refer to specific areas of the body.

• REVIEW QUESTIONS •

1. Define these terms: transverse plane, sagittal plane, and frontal plane.
2. What is the difference between a sagittal plane, a midsagittal plane, and a parasagittal plane?
3. What are the five conditions of a body in anatomical position?
4. Define each of the following pairs of directional terms and use each term in a sentence that describes the relative position of two body parts:
   a. Superior/inferior
   b. Anterior/posterior
   c. Medial/lateral
   d. Proximal/distal
   e. Superficial/deep
5. Indicate whether each of the following is a part of the dorsal body cavity or a part of the ventral body cavity:
   a. Thoracic cavity
   b. Spinal cavity
   c. Abdominal cavity
   d. Cranial cavity
   e. Mediastinum
6. Name the three abdominopelvic regions in the middle horizontal row of the nine regions.
7. Name the three abdominopelvic regions in the middle vertical row of the nine regions.
8. What is the difference between connective tissue membranes and epithelial membranes with respect to structure and location?
9. What specific layer of serous membrane covers the organs in the abdominopelvic cavity?
10. What regional term refers to each of the following?
    a. Armpit area
    b. Neck region
    c. Ears
    d. Sole of the foot
    e. Area behind the knee

• CHAPTER QUIZ •

Name the Following:

1. The specific plane that divides the body into right and left halves
2. The vertical plane that is not a sagittal plane
3. The directional term that means toward or nearer the midline of the body
4. The dorsal body cavity that contains the brain
5. The most central of the nine abdominopelvic regions
6. The abdominopelvic region that contains most of the stomach
7. The serous membrane that lines the abdominopelvic cavity and covers the organs in the cavity
8. The specific layer of serous membrane that covers the heart
9. The regional term that refers to the ribs
10. The regional term that refers to the wrist

True/False:

1. The plane that divides the body into anterior and posterior portions is a horizontal plane.
2. A frontal plane is the same as a coronal plane.
3. The brachial region is proximal to the carpal region.
4. The oral region is inferior to the ophthalmic region.
5. The mediastinum is a part of the dorsal body cavity.
6. Two divisions of the ventral body cavity are the thoracic cavity and the abdominopelvic cavity.
7. The parietal pleura covers the lungs.
8. The right hypochondriac region contains most of the liver.
9. The leg is also called the crural region.
10. The cephalic region refers to the lower portion of the back of the head.

Answers to the Review Questions and Chapter Quiz questions can be found at http://evolve.elsevier.com/Applegate/SAlearning/

CHAPTER TWO

The Thorax

Anatomical Review of the Thorax
  Osseous Components
  Muscular Components
  Thoracic Cavity
  Heart
  Other Structures Associated with the Thoracic
    Region

Sectional Anatomy of the Thorax
  Transverse Sections
  Sagittal Sections
  Coronal Sections
Working with Images of the Thorax
Important Anatomical Relationships
  in the Thorax

OBJECTIVES

Upon completion of this chapter, the student should be able to do the following:

- Identify and describe the bones that form the thoracic cage.
- State the vertebral level of the jugular notch, sternal angle, and xiphisternal junction.
- State the boundaries of the superior and inferior thoracic apertures.
- List three muscles that form thoracic boundaries.
- Identify muscles associated with the pectoral, back, and shoulder regions.
- Describe the pleura and pleural cavities.
- Compare the features of the right and left lungs.
- List the divisions of the mediastinum and the contents of each region.
- Describe the pericardial sac, pericardium, and pericardial cavity.
- Describe the three layers of the heart wall.
- Define and state the location of the apex, base, surfaces, and borders of the heart.
- Discuss the features and relationships of the chambers and valves of the heart.
- Compare the right and left coronary arteries with respect to origin, branches, location, and regions they supply.
- Describe the venous drainage of the heart.
- Trace the pathway of a stimulus through the conduction system of the heart.
- Identify the great vessels associated with the heart by describing the location and relationships of each vessel.
- Trace the flow of blood through the heart from the right atrium to the ascending aorta.
- Discuss the location and relationships of the thymus, trachea, esophagus, azygos vein, and hemiazygos vein.
- State the origin and location of the brachial plexus and name five nerves that emerge from the plexus.
- Describe the structure of the female breast.
- Name four groups of lymph nodes involved in lymphatic drainage of the breast.
- Identify the skeletal components, muscles, blood vessels, and viscera of the thorax in transverse, sagittal, and coronal sections.

Key Terms, Structures, and Features to Be Identified and/or Described

Aortic semilunar valve
Ascending aorta
Azygos vein
Bicuspid (mitral) valve
Brachial plexus
Brachiocephalic artery
Carina
Chordae tendineae

Clavicle
Common carotid arteries
Coronary sinus
Cricoid cartilage
Descending aorta
Esophagus
Inferior vena cava
Interatrial septum

Intercostal muscles
Internal carotid arteries
Internal jugular veins
Interventricular septum
Left atrium
Left ventricle
Papillary muscle
Pectinate muscle

Pericardium
Pulmonary semilunar valve
Pulmonary trunk
R & L brachiocephalic veins
R & L coronary arteries
R & L lungs
R & L mainstem bronchi

R & L pulmonary arteries
R & L pulmonary veins
R & L subclavian arteries
R & L subclavian veins
Ribs
Right atrium
Right ventricle

Superior vena cava
Thoracic duct
Trachea
Tricuspid valve
Vertebral arteries

Anatomical Review of the Thorax

The terms *thorax* and *chest* are used synonymously to refer to the region between the neck and the abdomen. The **superior thoracic aperture,** or thoracic inlet, is rather small and oblique in position. It separates the thorax from the root of the neck. The most superior portion of the aperture is situated posteriorly and slopes inferiorly in the anterior direction. It is bounded posteriorly by the first thoracic vertebra, laterally by the first pair of ribs and costal cartilages, and anteriorly by the manubrium of the sternum. The **inferior thoracic aperture,** or thoracic outlet, is bounded posteriorly by the twelfth thoracic vertebra and anteriorly by the xiphisternal junction. The lateral margins of the thoracic outlet are formed by the twelfth rib and the sloping cartilage of the costal margin. The diaphragm covers the inferior thoracic aperture and separates the thoracic cavity from the abdominal cavity. The musculoskeletal wall of the thorax protects the heart and lungs, which are located in the thoracic cavity.

QUICK CHECK
2.1 What is the posterior boundary of the superior thoracic aperture?
2.2 What covers the inferior thoracic aperture to separate the thoracic cavity from the abdominal cavity?

Osseous Components

The skeleton of the thorax is formed by the **sternum** anteriorly, the **12 thoracic vertebrae** posteriorly, and the **ribs with their costal cartilages** laterally. These bones form a thoracic cage that serves as an attachment for muscles and protects the vital viscera the cage encloses. The osseous components of the thorax are illustrated in Fig. 2-1.

Sternum. The **sternum** is an elongated, flat bone in the anterior midline of the thorax. Anteriorly, it is covered only by skin, superficial fascia, and periosteum. It consists of three parts: the **manubrium,** the **body,** and the **xiphoid process.** The manubrium is the most superior of the three parts. Its upper border is indented by a midline **jugular notch,** sometimes called the *suprasternal notch,* which is easily palpable. The jugular notch is at the level of the disc between the second and third thoracic vertebrae. **Clavicular notches,** located at the superolateral margins of the manubrium on either side of the jugular notch, form articulating surfaces for the clavicle.

FIG. 2-1. Osseous components of the thorax.

Inferiorly, the manubrium is joined to the body of the sternum by fibrocartilage and ligaments. The manubrium and body of the sternum do not articulate in a straight line. Instead, their line of junction projects forward, forming the **sternal angle** (angle of Louis). This reliable landmark generally is 5 cm below the jugular notch and locates the sternal end of the second rib. It also marks the level of the intervertebral disc between the fourth and fifth thoracic vertebrae. The trachea bifurcates into the two bronchi and the aortic arch begins at the level of the sternal angle. The body, forming the bulk of the sternum, articulates with second through seventh costal cartilages.

The smallest and most inferior part of the sternum is the xiphoid process. It consists of hyaline cartilage in youth but gradually ossifies during adulthood, so that by 40 years of age, it generally is bony in nature and is fused with the body of the sternum at the xiphisternal junction. The xiphisternal junction generally is at the level of the ninth thoracic vertebra.

QUICK CHECK
2.3 What anatomical landmark is located at the junction of the manubrium and the body of the sternum?
2.4 What easily palpable anatomical landmark is along the superior margin of the manubrium?
2.5 Which ribs articulate with the body of the sternum via costal cartilage?

Ribs. The lateral boundaries of the chest are formed by the **12 pairs** of ribs. These flat, elongated, curved, and slightly twisted bones, along with their costal cartilages, extend from the thoracic vertebrae posteriorly to the sternum anteriorly. The ribs make up the major portion of the thoracic skeleton. The first seven ribs are considered **vertebrosternal ribs,** or true ribs, because they articulate directly with the sternum by way of their costal cartilages. The remaining five pairs are called *false ribs.* The costal cartilage of the eighth, ninth, and tenth ribs (the first three pairs of false ribs) is attached to the cartilage of the preceding rib rather than directly to the sternum. These are called **vertebrochondral ribs.** The last two pairs of false ribs are **vertebral ribs,** or floating ribs, because they have no anterior attachment to the sternum. The costal cartilages of the vertebrochondral ribs join such that their inferior edges form a continuous **costal margin.** As the costal margins diverge from the xiphisternal junction, they delineate the **infrasternal angle,** or **costal arch.**

FIG. 2-2. Features of the thoracic vertebrae.

QUICK CHECK

2.6   Which ribs are classified as vertebrochondral ribs?

2.7   What forms the infrasternal angle?

Thoracic Vertebrae. The posterior median skeleton of the thoracic cage is formed by the **12 thoracic vertebrae.** Features of these vertebrae that are specifically related to the thorax include **facets** on the transverse processes and vertebral bodies for articulation with the ribs and the long **spinous processes.** Features of the thoracic vertebrae are illustrated in Fig. 2-2. When the vertebral column is flexed, the most prominent spinous process usually is that of the seventh cervical vertebra, although sometimes the first thoracic spinous process may be just as evident. When the arms are at the sides, a line drawn through the tip of the third thoracic spinous process indicates the level of the base of the scapular spine. The inferior angle of the scapula is at the same level as the middle of the seventh thoracic spinous process. The position of these landmarks changes when the arms are raised.

QUICK CHECK

2.8   On what two portions of the thoracic vertebrae are the facets for the ribs located?

2.9   How many thoracic vertebrae are there?

Muscular Components

Muscles of the Thoracic Wall. Numerous muscles are attached to the skeleton of the thorax. Most of these are muscles that move the pectoral girdle or are associated with the shoulder joint. This section discusses only the muscles that form a part of the thoracic boundary and are associated with a change in the intrathoracic volume during breathing. Increasing the volume of the thoracic cavity reduces the

pressure and permits inspiration. Conversely, reducing the volume increases the pressure and forces air out of the lungs during expiration. To increase intrathoracic volume, the boundaries of the thoracic cavity may increase in three different dimensions: vertically, transversely, and anteroposteriorly. Elastic recoil of the lungs and the weight of the thoracic wall primarily account for the decrease in each dimension during expiration. The muscles of the thoracic wall are illustrated in Fig. 2-3 and summarized in Table 2-1.

Diaphragm. The **diaphragm** covers the thoracic outlet, forming a muscular, movable partition between the thoracic and abdominal cavities. Contraction of the diaphragm enlarges the thoracic cavity in the vertical dimension during inspiration. Because the diaphragm is visualized to a greater extent in abdominal sections than in thoracic sections, it is described in greater detail in the Chapter 3.

Intercostal Muscles. Three layers of **intercostal muscles** fill the spaces between the ribs. These are the external, internal, and innermost intercostal muscles, all of which receive motor impulses from the intercostal nerves. The **external intercostal muscles** arise from the lower border of one rib and insert on the upper limit of the next rib below. The fibers are directed inferiorly and anteriorly. The **internal intercostal muscles** occupy the intercostal spaces deep to the external intercostals. Also originating from the lower border of one rib and inserting on the upper limit of the next one below, the fibers are directed inferiorly and posteriorly, at right angles to the external intercostal fibers. The **innermost intercostal muscles** appear similar to the internal intercostals but are separated from them by a neurovascular bundle containing an intercostal nerve, artery, and vein.

Levator Costarum Muscles. Twelve fan-shaped **levator costarum muscles** originate on the transverse processes of the thoracic vertebrae and insert on the rib immediately below. These are visualized on transverse sections as extending from the vertebral column to a rib. The action of the levator costarum muscles increases both the transverse and anteroposterior dimensions.

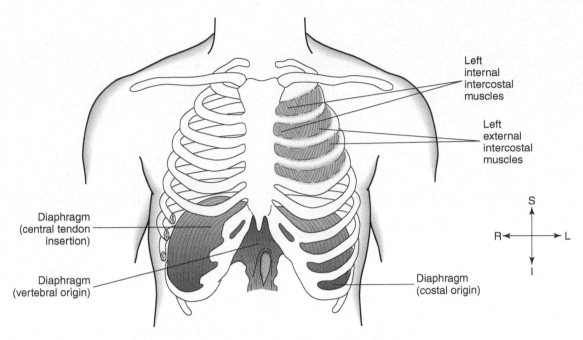

FIG. 2-3. Muscles of the thoracic wall.

QUICK CHECK

2.10 What muscles fill the spaces between the ribs?

2.11 What muscles extend from the vertebral column to the ribs?

Muscles of the Pectoral Region. Numerous muscles span the back and pectoral regions of the thorax but are functionally associated with the upper extremity. Many of these muscles anchor the arm to the trunk, as well as function in movement. Sections of the thorax also show the humerus and bones of the pectoral girdle. The **pectoral girdle** consists of the **clavicle,** or collar bone, anteriorly and the **scapula,** or shoulder blade, posteriorly. Because these skeletal and muscle components are clearly evident on thoracic sections, they are included here. (A more thorough discussion of the upper extremity and its associated articulations is presented in Chapter 7.)

The pectoral region is located on the anterior thoracic wall. Four muscles are associated with this region. These muscles help attach the upper limb to the thoracic skeleton. All are associated with movements of the arm either by acting directly on the humerus or by acting on the bones of the pectoral girdle. These muscles are summarized in Table 2-2 and are illustrated in Fig. 2-4.

Pectoralis Major Muscles. The **pectoralis major muscle** is a large, fan-shaped muscle covering the anterior chest wall. From an extensive origin on the clavicle, sternum, and ribs, the muscle fibers converge to insert on the humerus. Near its insertion, this muscle forms the anterior wall of the axilla, the region of the armpit or junction of the arm and thorax.

Pectoralis Minor Muscles. The **pectoralis minor muscle** is a smaller muscle that is deep to the pectoralis major muscle. The origin of the pectoralis minor muscle, from ribs three, four, and five, is much less extensive than the

TABLE 2-1   Muscles of the Thoracic Wall

Muscle	Origin	Insertion	Action	Innervation
Diaphragm	Interior body wall	Central tendon of diaphragm	Enlarges the thoracic cavity during inspiration	Phrenic nerve
External intercostal	Inferior border of rib above	Superior border of rib below	Assists in inspiration; synergists of diaphragm	Intercostal nerves
Internal intercostal	Inferior border of rib above	Superior border of rib below	Assists in expiration; antagonistic to external intercostals	Intercostal nerves
Innermost intercostal	Internal surface of rib above	Internal surface of rib below	Assists in expiration; antagonistic to external intercostals	Intercostal nerves
Levator costarum	Transverse processes of thoracic vertebrae	Ribs, close to the tubercle of rib below the vertebra from which it originates	Elevates the ribs	Dorsal branch of thoracic nerves

TABLE 2-2   Muscles of the Pectoral Region

Muscle	Origin	Insertion	Action	Innervation
Pectoralis major	Clavicle, sternum, and costal cartilages of ribs	Humerus	Adduct and medially rotate humerus	Pectoral nerves
Pectoralis minor	Third to fifth ribs	Coracoid process of the scapula	Pull scapula inferiorly	Pectoral nerves
Subclavius	First rib	Clavicle	Stabilize clavicle during shoulder movement	Subclavius nerve
Serratus anterior	First eight ribs	Scapula	Stabilize scapula; also rotate scapula	Thoracic nerve

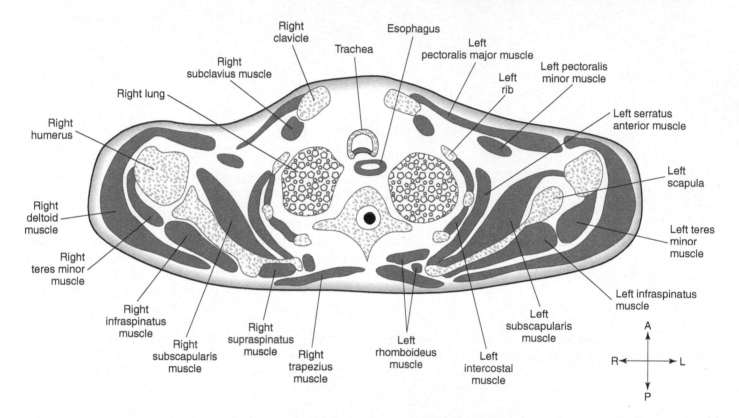

FIG. 2-4. Muscles of the pectoral region, back, and shoulder.

origin of the pectoralis major muscle. The pectoralis minor muscle inserts on the coracoid process of the scapula.

Subclavius Muscle.   A small **subclavius muscle** lies deep to the clavicle. It extends from its origin on the first rib to the posterior surface of the middle portion of the clavicle. It appears to stabilize the clavicle during shoulder movement. It also affords some protection for the subclavian vessels when the clavicle is fractured. It is mentioned because it usually is seen in sections of this region.

Serratus Anterior Muscle.   The **serratus anterior muscle** is associated with the pectoralis muscles in the axilla. The fan-shaped serratus anterior muscle originates from the first eight ribs and then passes posteriorly to insert on the medial border of the scapula. As it runs its course from ribs to scapula, the muscle is adjacent to the wall of the thorax. The serratus anterior muscle primarily acts with other

muscles to stabilize the scapula so that it can be used as a fixed point in producing movement of the humerus.

QUICK CHECK

2.12   What skeletal components form the pectoral girdle?

2.13   What is the most superficial muscle of the pectoral region of the thorax?

Muscles of the Back and Shoulder Region.   The muscles of the back and shoulder region may be divided into three groups: superficial back muscles, deep back muscles, and muscles associated with the scapula. Several of these muscles are illustrated in Fig. 2-4, and they are summarized in Table 2-3.

TABLE 2-3   Muscles of the Back and Shoulder Region

Muscle	Origin	Insertion	Action	Innervation
Superficial Back Muscles				
Trapezius	Occipital bone to T12 vertebra	Clavicle and scapula	Adduct, elevate, and rotate scapula; also extend the head	Accessory nerve
Latissimus dorsi	Thoracic and lumbar vertebrae; crest of ilium	Humerus	Adduct and medially rotate humerus	Thoracodorsal
Deep Back Muscles				
Levator scapulae	Cervical vertebrae	Scapula	Elevate scapula	Dorsal scapular
Rhomboideus major and minor	Cervical and thoracic vertebrae	Scapula	Adduct scapula	Dorsal scapular
Serratus anterior	First eight ribs	Scapula	Stabilize scapula; also rotate scapula	Thoracic nerve
Muscles in Scapular Region				
Supraspinatus	Supraspinous fossa of scapula	Humerus	Abduct humerus	Suprascapular nerve
Infraspinatus	Infraspinous fossa of scapula	Humerus	Laterally rotate humerus	Suprascapular nerve
Subscapularis	Subscapular fossa	Humerus	Medially rotate humerus	Subscapular nerve
Deltoid	Clavicle and scapula	Humerus	Abduct humerus	Axillary nerve
Teres major	Margin of scapula	Humerus	Adduct arm	Subscapular nerve
Teres minor	Margin of scapula	Humerus	Laterally rotate arm	Axillary nerve

Superficial Back Muscles. The **trapezius muscle** and the latissimus dorsi muscle are the two superficial muscles of the back and shoulder region. The origin of the trapezius muscle extends from the occipital bone to the spinous process of the twelfth thoracic vertebra. It inserts on both the clavicle and scapula. Weakness of the trapezius muscle or damage to the accessory nerve that innervates the muscle results in a drooping shoulder.

The extensive latissimus dorsi muscle originates from the spinous processes of the vertebrae from the seventh thoracic vertebra down through the sacrum. Some fibers also arise from the crest of the ilium. From this broad origin, the muscle fibers converge into a tendon that inserts in the intertubercular groove of the humerus.

Deep Back Muscles. Three relatively thin, straplike muscles lie deep to the trapezius. The **levator scapulae muscle, rhomboideus minor muscle,** and **rhomboideus major muscle** all originate on the vertebral column and insert on the medial border of the scapula. These muscles act on the scapula to stabilize and control its position during active motion of the humerus. A fourth muscle, the **serratus anterior muscle,** lies deep to the latissimus dorsi. This muscle was described previously with the pectoralis muscles because of its association with them in the axilla.

Muscles in the Scapular Region. Six muscles are described in the scapular region. All of these muscles pass from wthe scapula to the humerus and act on the shoulder joint. The **supraspinatus muscle** fills the supraspinous fossa of the scapula superior to the spine, and the **infraspinatus muscle** lies in the infraspinous fossa inferior to the spine of the

scapula. The **subscapularis muscle** occupies the subscapular fossa on the costal surface of the scapula. The **deltoid muscle** is superficial and covers the shoulder. This muscle forms the lateral mass and rounded contour of the shoulder. In addition to origins on the spine and acromion of the scapula, the deltoid also has a portion originating on the clavicle. The insertion is on the humerus. The **teres major muscle** is an oval muscle running from the inferior angle of the scapula to the intertubercular groove of the humerus, where it inserts with the tendon of the latissimus dorsi muscle. Along with the latissimus dorsi muscle, it forms a portion of the posterior wall of the axilla. Located superior to the teres major muscle, the **teres minor muscle** frequently is inseparable from the infraspinatus muscle. The supraspinatus, infraspinatus, subscapularis, and teres minor muscles all reinforce the fibrous capsule of the shoulder joint. These muscles, together with the fibrous capsule, are collectively referred to as the **rotator cuff** of the shoulder joint. The rotator cuff holds the head of the humerus in the glenoid cavity of the scapula, thus protecting and stabilizing the joint.

Several of the muscles associated with the back and shoulder are illustrated in Fig. 2-4. For further detail, refer to Chapter 7.

QUICK CHECK

2.14   Name two superficial back muscles.
2.15   What is the superficial muscle over the shoulder?
2.16   What four muscles form the rotator cuff of the shoulder?

Thoracic Cavity

The thoracic cavity, enclosed within the bones and muscles described previously, is divided into three major divisions. The **right** and **left pleural cavities,** filled with the lungs, occupy the lateral regions. The **mediastinum** is the central region between the two pleural cavities. It contains the heart and other structures such as the trachea, esophagus, thymus gland, and great vessels.

Pleural Cavities.   The two pleural cavities are completely closed and separated from each other. They are lined by a serous membrane called the **pleura.** The pleura is essentially a continuous sheet in each cavity; however, for descriptive purposes, it is divided into the **visceral layer** and the **parietal layer.** You can visualize this as a balloon indented by your fist. The balloon is a single sheet of material, but when you stick your fist into it, you have two layers, the outside, or parietal, layer and the layer next to your hand, the visceral layer. The **visceral pleura** is intimately adherent to the lung, covering its entire surface and continuing deeply into its fissures. The **parietal pleura** lines the thoracic wall and is divided into four regions, as illustrated in Fig. 2-5. The **costal parietal pleura** is applied to the ribs, costal cartilages, intercostal muscles, and sternum. The **diaphragmatic parietal pleura** is fused with the diaphragm and is continuous with the **mediastinal parietal pleura,** which is adjacent to the mediastinum. The **cervical parietal pleura** projects into the thoracic inlet to cover the apex of the lung.

The space between the parietal and visceral pleural layers is the **pleural cavity,** or **pleural space.** In reality, this is a **potential space** filled with only a capillary layer of serous lubricating fluid. This fluid reduces friction to allow the two surfaces to glide easily over each other during respiratory movements. The visceral pleura is insensitive to pain, but the parietal layer is very sensitive.

The most inferior portion of the pleural space is located in the posterolateral region where the diaphragm attaches to the ribs. This space is called the **costodiaphragmatic recess.** Fluid tends to accumulate in this space when a person is in an erect position.

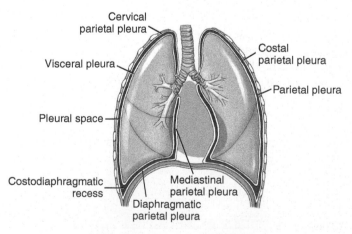

Cervical parietal pleura

Visceral pleura

Pleural space

Costodiaphragmatic recess

Costal parietal pleura

Parietal pleura

Mediastinal parietal pleura

Diaphragmatic parietal pleura

FIG. 2-5. The pleura of the lung.

QUICK CHECK

2.17   What are the three major divisions of the thoracic cavity?

2.18   All serous membranes have two layers. Which layer of the pleura is attached to the lung and is insensitive to pain?

2.19   What substance is found between the visceral and parietal layers of the pleura and what is its purpose?

Lungs.   Each lung is an elongated structure shaped roughly like a half cone. The apex, or cervical dome, lies posterior to the middle third of the clavicle. It extends slightly above the first rib to project through the superior thoracic aperture. The slightly concave medial (mediastinal) surface has an opening, called the **hilus,** where the bronchi, blood vessels, lymph vessels, and nerves enter and leave the lung. The structures that traverse the hilus are collectively called the **root** of the lung. Each lung is freely movable within its own pleural cavity except at the root or hilus, where it is attached. The right and left lungs are separated from each other by the mediastinum. The base of each lung is concave as it conforms to the dome of the diaphragm. The right lung, although shorter because of the volume of the liver on that side, is wider and has a greater volume than the left lung. The heart makes an indentation, called the **cardiac notch,** in the left lung. Each lung is partially transected by an **oblique fissure** that separates the lung into **superior** and **inferior lobes.** The right lung is further subdivided by the **horizontal fissure** to form a wedge-shaped **middle lobe.** Within the lung each primary bronchus divides into secondary bronchi, two on the left side and three on the right side, providing a secondary bronchus for each lobe of the lung. Each secondary bronchus further divides into tertiary segmental bronchi that supply specific regions. A tertiary segmental bronchus with the specific sector of lung it supplies is called a **bronchopulmonary segment.**

Pulmonary arteries transport deoxygenated blood from the heart to the lungs, where carbon dioxide diffuses into the alveoli and ultimately is exhaled. At the same time, oxygen diffuses from the alveoli into the blood. This freshly oxygenated blood is returned to the left atrium of the heart by the pulmonary veins. In general, the blood in the pulmonary arteries and veins does not provide for the vascular needs of the lung parenchyma. **Bronchial arteries,** which are branches of the descending thoracic aorta, supply blood for the nutrition and maintenance of the lung tissue. **Bronchial veins** drain the parenchyma of the lung. On the right side, these vessels terminate in the azygos vein. On the left side, the bronchial veins drain into either the **intercostal veins** or the **hemiazygos vein.**

Afferent vessels of the **tracheobronchial lymph nodes** drain lymph from the lungs and bronchi. The tracheobronchial lymph nodes are divided into five groups: **pulmonary lymph nodes** in the substance of the lungs;

bronchopulmonary lymph nodes in the hilus of each lung; **inferior tracheobronchial lymph nodes** and **superior tracheobronchial lymph nodes** at the tracheal bifurcation, in the region of the carina; and the **paratracheal lymph nodes** on each side of the trachea. Lymph vessels leaving these nodes join with efferent vessels of other nodes to form right and left bronchomediastinal trunks. These trunks may drain into the right lymphatic duct on the right side and the thoracic duct on the left, or they may open independently into the junction of the subclavian vein and internal jugular vein on the respective side. Pollutants from the air enter the tracheobronchial lymph nodes. These nodes usually are affected in tuberculosis and carcinoma of the lung.

QUICK CHECK

2.20   What is the collective term for the structures that traverse the hilus of the lung?
2.21   Which lung (a) has greater volume; (b) has a cardiac notch; (c) is shorter and wider; (d) has a horizontal fissure?

Mediastinum.   The lungs and pleura occupy the lateral portions of the thoracic cavity. All other thoracic structures are crowded into a central space called the *mediastinum*. The mediastinum is divided into four regions, as illustrated in Fig. 2-6.

Superior Mediastinum.   The **superior mediastinum** is the area above the fibrous pericardium. It is separated from the inferior mediastinum by a line that passes from the sternal angle to the intervertebral disc between the fourth and fifth thoracic vertebrae. It contains all the structures passing between the neck and the thorax, the aortic arch with its branches, the brachiocephalic veins, the superior vena cava, the thymus, the trachea, the esophagus, and the vagus and phrenic nerves.

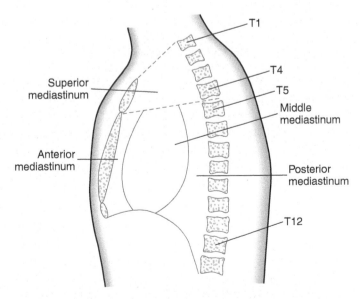

FIG. 2-6. The four regions of the mediastinum.

Inferior Mediastinum.   The **inferior mediastinum** is divided into the anterior, middle, and posterior mediastina.
Anterior Mediastinum.   The **anterior mediastinum** is a limited area anterior to the pericardium and posterior to the sternum, between the sternal angle and the diaphragm. At the sternal angle it is continuous with the superior mediastinum. It contains connective tissue with some fat, lymph nodes, and a portion of the thymus.
Middle Mediastinum.   The **middle mediastinum,** which is centrally located and limited by the fibrous pericardium, contains the heart and the roots of the ascending aorta, the pulmonary artery, the superior and inferior venae cavae, and the four pulmonary veins.
Posterior Mediastinum.   The **posterior mediastinum** is posterior to the pericardium and inferior to the fourth thoracic vertebra. The diaphragm limits the posterior mediastinum inferiorly. Between the two parietal pleurae of the lungs and anterior to the vertebrae, the posterior mediastinum contains the descending thoracic aorta, azygos and hemiazygos veins, thoracic duct, and esophgus.

QUICK CHECK

2.22   An imaginary line between what two structures separates the mediastinum into superior and inferior portions?
2.23   What vital structure is located in the middle mediastinum?

Heart

The heart is a hollow, muscular organ enclosed in a fibroserous sac in the middle mediastinum. Shaped somewhat like a cone, the heart lies obliquely in the chest, with two thirds of its mass to the left of the median plane and one third to the right. About the size of a clenched fist, the heart weighs approximately 250 to 300 g. Superficial relationships include an apex, base, three surfaces, and four borders.

Pericardium.   A fibroserous sac, the pericardium, surrounds the heart and proximal portions of the great vessels that enter and leave the heart. There are essentially two types of pericardium, fibrous and serous. The external, strong **fibrous pericardium** is composed of tough fibrous connective tissue. Superiorly, the fibrous pericardium blends with the tunica externa, the fibrous connective tissue outer layer of the great vessels. Inferiorly, the fibrous layer fuses with the central tendon of the diaphragm, and respiratory movements thus influence the movement of the pericardial sac. In the anterior midline the fibrous pericardium is attached to the posterior surface of the sternum by a strong **sternopericardial ligament.**

The double-layered **serous pericardium** is composed of a thin, transparent serous membrane. The outer, or parietal, layer of serous pericardium, sometimes called **parietal pericardium,** forms a smooth, moist lining for the fibrous pericardium. The fibrous and parietal serous pericardia are closely adherent and difficult to separate, and together they make up the pericardial sac. The inner, or visceral, layer of serous pericardium covers the cardiac muscle of the heart wall. Because it forms the outer layer of the heart wall, the visceral serous pericardium often is called **epicardium.**

The two layers of serous pericardium, parietal and visceral, form a continuous closed sac around the heart in the same way that the pleura surrounds the lungs. Between the parietal and visceral pericardia is a potential space, the **pericardial cavity,** which contains a small amount of serous fluid that is distributed as a capillary film on the opposing surfaces. The lubricating action of this fluid keeps the surfaces moist and reduces friction so that the surfaces glide easily over each other during heart movements.

Heart Wall.   The heart wall consists of three layers. The outermost layer is the **epicardium,** which is the visceral layer of serous pericardium. Heart muscle, called *cardiac muscle*, makes up the middle layer, the **myocardium.** This layer makes up the bulk of the heart wall and is the layer that contracts to perform the pumping action of the heart. The thickness of the myocardium in the heart wall varies. The harder a particular chamber has to work to pump blood, the thicker the wall. The atria have relatively thin walls because they are primarily "receiving" chambers rather than "pumping" chambers. Ventricles have thick walls because they forcefully eject blood from the heart. In an adult, the left ventricle has the thickest wall because it pumps blood into systemic circulation throughout the body. The **endocardium** is the innermost layer. This is a thin, smooth layer of simple squamous epithelium called the *endothelium*. The endothelial lining of the heart also covers the heart valves and is continuous with the endothelial lining of the blood vessels.

Superficial Features of the Heart.   Superficial features of the heart include an apex, base, three surfaces, and four borders. The **apex,** formed entirely by the left ventricle, points downward and to the left. Located in the fifth intercostal space, at the level of the eighth thoracic vertebra, it is the most inferior region of the heart, and it is to the left of midline. These positions vary and depend on the phase of respiration.

The **base** of the heart is the broad superior portion of the heart that is opposite the apex. This means that the base projects superiorly, posteriorly, and to the right. It extends between the fifth and eighth thoracic vertebrae. The two atria are the primary components of the base, and the posteriorly positioned left atrium is the predominate portion of the base. The ascending aorta, pulmonary trunk, and superior vena cava emerge from the base. The base sometimes is referred to as the **posterior surface.**

In addition to the posterior surface, or base, the heart has two other surfaces. The anterior **sternocostal surface** is created primarily by the right atrium and right ventricle, although the left auricular appendage and left ventricle contribute a small portion. The two ventricles resting on the diaphragm comprise the **diaphragmatic surface.**

The right atrium, in line with the superior and inferior venae cavae, forms the **right border.** The **left border** is more convex and is outlined by the left ventricle. The right ventricle, with a small contribution from the left ventricle near the apex, forms the horizontal **inferior border.** The **superior border,** where the great vessels enter and leave the heart, is formed by both atria.

QUICK CHECK

2.24   Which projects more to the left, the apex or the base of the heart?

2.25   What chamber of the heart forms the apex?

Chambers and Valves.   The heart is divided into four chambers: the right and left atria, and the right and left ventricles. On the surface a groove that encircles the heart separates the atria from the ventricles. This is the coronary sulcus, or atrioventricular sulcus. Similarly, an interventricular sulcus marks the division between the right and left ventricles.

Valves.   A system of valves is required to keep blood flowing through the heart in the appropriate direction. The heart has two basic types of valves. Both types consist of cusps, or flaps of fibrous tissue covered with endothelium. **Semilunar valves** are found at the exit ports of the ventricles. **Atrioventricular valves** function as inflow valves where the blood flows from the atria into the ventricles.

Semilunar valves consist of three cusps that balloon out from the vessel wall to prevent backflow of blood from the aorta and pulmonary trunk into the ventricles. When the ventricles contract, the increased pressure forces the valve cusps flat against the vessel wall, opening the valve to allow ejection of blood. After contraction, as ventricular pressure decreases, the cusps are caught in a passive backflow and balloon out from the walls to close the orifice. This prevents blood from flowing backward into the ventricles.

Atrioventricular valves are so named because they are located between the atria and ventricles. The atria have thin walls, do not contract strongly, and generate relatively little pressure. Consequently, the atrioventricular valves must open easily to allow blood to flow from the atria into the ventricles. These valves have thin cusps that move readily in the current of flowing blood. Stringlike structures called chordae tendineae attach the cusps to projections of myocardium called papillary muscles. When pressure in the ventricles increases because of contraction, these valves are forced back over the opening to prevent blood from going back into the atria. The papillary muscles contract with the ventricles, which creates a tension on the valve cusps and prevents them from protruding back into the atria. The valves of the heart are illustrated in Fig. 2-7.

Right Atrium.   The most right-sided portion of the heart is the **right atrium.** This thin-walled chamber

Ventricles relaxed—
blood flows from atria,
opens atrioventricular
valves

Ventricles contract—
blood leaves ventricles,
opens semilunar valves

Tricuspid valve

Bicuspid valve

Aortic
semilunar valve

Opening for
coronary artery

Pulmonary
semilunar valve

FIG. 2-7. Valves of the heart.

receives venous blood from the coronary and systemic circulations. Openings into this chamber include the **superior** and **inferior venae cavae,** which return venous blood from systemic circulation, and the opening of the coronary sinus, which returns blood from the circulation that supplies blood to the heart wall.

The smooth-walled posterior region of the right atrium, where the venae cavae enter, is called the **sinus venarum.** Anteriorly, the atrial wall is roughened by muscular ridges called pectinate muscle. A small muscular pouch, the **auricle,** projects toward the left from the right atrium and covers the root of the aorta. The posterior wall of the right atrium is formed by the interatrial septum, the partition between the right and left atria. In fetal circulation, the interatrial septum has an opening, called the **foramen ovale.** The foramen ovale allows blood to pass directly from the right atrium into the left atrium, bypassing pulmonary circulation. After birth, higher pressure on the left side of the heart pushes a flap of tissue across the opening to close it. After a time the foramen is sealed off, but a depression, the **fossa ovalis,** remains. The left or medial wall of the right atrium contains the right atrioventricular valve. This valve has three cusps and is called the **tricuspid valve.** The tricuspid valve has a vertical orientation and is posterior and slightly to the right of the sternum at the level of the fourth intercostal space between the fourth and fifth ribs.

Right Ventricle. The triangular-shaped right ventricle forms a major portion of the sternocostal, or anterior, surface of the heart. This chamber receives blood from the right atrium through the tricuspid valve and ejects the blood into the pulmonary trunk for oxygenation in the lungs. A pulmonary semilunar valve is located at the outflow from the right ventricle into the pulmonary trunk. An average surface projection places this valve at the third costal cartilage on the left side of the sternum. The upper anterior portion of the right ventricle, around the origin of the pulmonary trunk, is the smooth-walled **conus arteriosus.** The remainder of the right ventricular wall is roughened by muscular ridges called **trabeculae carneae** and projections called **papillary muscles.** Stringlike **chordae tendineae** extend from the three papillary muscles to the cusps of the right atrioventricular, or tricuspid, valve to prevent inversion of the valve when ventricular pressure increases.

Left Atrium. The **left atrium** is the most posterior structure of the heart. It forms most of the base of the heart and consists of the atrium proper and its auricular appendage. The wall of the left atrium is slightly thicker than the right atrium, and its interior is smooth except for a few pectinate muscles in the auricle. Four **pulmonary veins,** two on each side, return oxygenated blood to the heart from the lungs and enter the left atrium at its superolateral aspect. The anterior wall of the left atrium is formed by the left atrioventricular valve. This valve has two cusps and is called the **bicuspid,** or **mitral, valve.** The mitral valve is the one most often affected by disease, especially rheumatic fever. The surface projection of the bicuspid, or mitral, valve is at the level of the fourth costal cartilage on the left side of the sternum.

Left Ventricle. From the left atrium, blood enters the left ventricle through the bicuspid, or mitral, valve. In an adult, the left ventricle has much thicker walls than the right ventricle because it must work harder to pump blood throughout the body via the systemic circulation. Most of the internal surface of the left ventricle is covered with the muscular ridges of trabeculae carneae, similar to those in the right ventricle. The wall is smooth in the **vestibule,** or aortic outflow region. The two papillary muscles attached to the bicuspid valve by chordae tendineae usually are larger than those in the right ventricle. From the left ventricle, blood enters the aorta to supply the body through the systemic circulation. Between the left ventricle and the aorta is an **aortic semilunar valve.** This valve is located at the level of the third intercostal space, between the third and fourth ribs, on the left side of the sternum. Fig. 2-8 illustrates the surface projections of the heart valves.

The interventricular septum forms a partition between the right and left ventricles. The septum has an oblique orientation. Its position can be visualized on the surface of the heart by the anterior and posterior interventricular sulci, or grooves. Most of the septum is thick and muscular. A small, oval portion is thin and membranous. This is located just inferior to the right cusp of the aortic semilunar valve. The membranous portion of the interventricular septum is the part most frequently involved in ventricular septal defect. This defect, either singly or in combination with other defects, is present in about half of congenital cardiac abnormalities.

Valve location, as well as heart size and delineation, varies greatly depending on age, gender, body build, phase of respiration, and other factors. The locations and surface relationships stated here are for that "average" person who probably does not exist. The valve locations are anatomical projections and do not necessarily indicate the best position for listening to the heart sounds. Fig. 2-9 illustrates some of the features of the heart and the flow of blood through the heart.

QUICK CHECK

2.26   What is the name of the muscular ridges in the anterior wall of the right atrium?

2.27   Which valve associated with the heart usually is located most inferiorly?

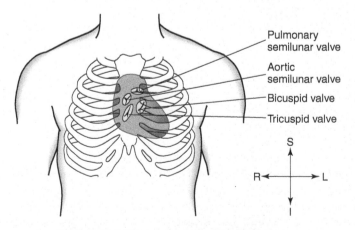

FIG. 2-8. Surface projections of the heart valves.

Blood Supply to the Heart.   The heart wall is muscle and requires a continuous supply of oxygenated blood to function effectively. Blood supply to the muscular wall of the heart is by way of the **coronary arteries** and their branches. The right and left coronary arteries originate from the aortic sinus at the root of the ascending aorta, immediately superior to the aortic semilunar valve. Fig. 2-10 illustrates the coronary arteries.

Right Coronary Artery.   The **right coronary artery** passes slightly forward and to the right to emerge between the root of the pulmonary trunk and the right auricle. It then descends in the atrioventricular sulcus (coronary sulcus) to the inferior border. During its course the right coronary artery gives off branches to the wall of the right atrium. Near the inferior border the right coronary artery gives off a **marginal branch** that proceeds toward the apex. The marginal branch supplies the right ventricle. After giving off the marginal branch, the right coronary artery continues in the coronary sulcus to the posterior surface, where it gives off a **posterior interventricular branch** that descends toward the apex in the posterior interventricular sulcus. This vessel gives off branches to supply the posterior wall of both ventricles and a portion of the interventricular septum.

Left Coronary Artery.   The **left coronary artery** is very short, usually only 2 to 3 cm long. It emerges between the left auricular appendage and the pulmonary trunk and then divides. The **anterior interventricular (descending) branch** descends toward the apex in the anterior interventricular sulcus and then turns toward the posterior surface to anastomose with the posterior interventricular branch of the right coronary artery. This branch supplies portions of both ventricles and the interventricular septum. The **circumflex branch** of the left coronary artery follows the left atrioventricular (coronary) sulcus around the left margin of the heart to the posterior surface, where it anastomoses with the right coronary artery. During its course, the circumflex branch gives off vessels to the left atrium and also supplies a portion of the left ventricle. The right coronary artery and its branches supply the right atrium, portions of both ventricles, and the posterior portion of the interventricular septum. The anterior interventricular branch of the left coronary artery supplies both ventricles and a portion of the interventricular septum, whereas the circumflex branch supplies the left atrium and a portion of the left ventricle. It should be understood that variations in the branching patterns of the coronary arteries are very common.

Venous Drainage.   The primary venous drainage of the heart wall is through veins that empty into the **coronary sinus,** which drains into the right atrium. The coronary sinus is a thin-walled venous dilation in the coronary sulcus on the posterior surface of the heart. The main tributary of the coronary sinus is the **great cardiac vein,** which begins at the apex and ascends in the anterior interventricular sulcus. When it reaches the atrioventricular sulcus (coronary sulcus), it passes to the left to enter the left end of the coronary sinus. Another vessel, the **middle cardiac vein,** is on the posterior surface and enters the coronary sinus on the right. It drains the

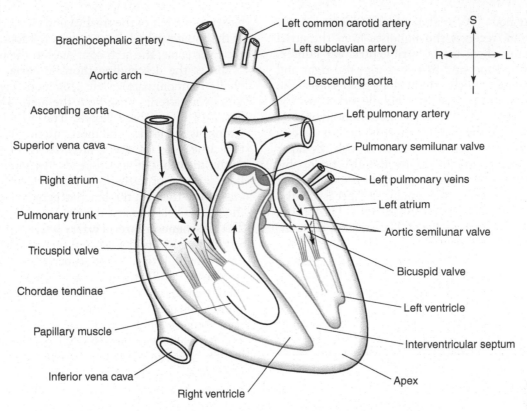

FIG. 2-9. Features of the heart.

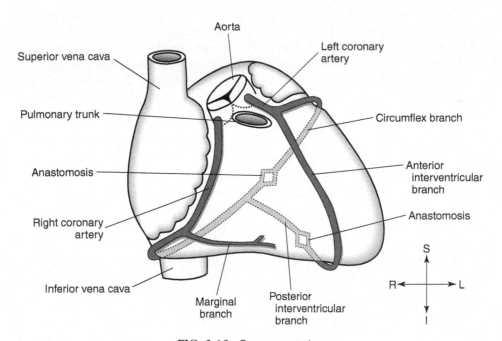

FIG. 2-10. Coronary arteries.

posterior wall of both ventricles. Other small vessels may empty directly into chambers of the heart.

Conduction System of the Heart. The conduction system of the heart consists of specialized cardiac muscle fibers that initiate and coordinate the contractions of the chambers. Impulses for contraction are initiated in the **sinoatrial node** (SA node), which is located in the wall of the right atrium near the superior vena cava. Because it initiates the impulses, the SA node is called the pacemaker. From the SA node the impulses spread through the cardiac muscle cells of the atria, causing them to contract. The

atrioventricular node (AV node), which is located in the interatrial septum, receives the impulses from the atrial cells and transmits them to the **atrioventricular bundle.** The AV bundle is short and branches into the **right** and **left bundle branches,** which extend along both sides of the interventricular septum. From the bundle branches, the impulses are transmitted by way of **conduction myofibers,** or **Purkinje fibers,** to the papillary muscles and to the cardiac muscle cells of the ventricles. Even though the heart has its own rhythm, established by the SA node, this rhythm can be altered by stimulation from the autonomic nervous system. Sympathetic stimulation speeds up the action of the SA node, and parasympathetic (vagal) stimulation reduces the heart rate. Fig. 2-11 illustrates the conduction system of the heart.

QUICK CHECK

2.28 What are the two main branches of the left coronary artery?

2.29 Which portion of the conduction system of the heart is located in the interatrial septum?

Great Vessels of the Heart

Aorta.   For descriptive purposes, the **aorta** is divided into the ascending aorta in the middle mediastinum, the aortic arch in the superior mediastinum, and the descending aorta in the posterior mediastinum. The ascending aorta originates at the outflow orifice from the left ventricle. An **aortic semilunar valve** at the aortic orifice prevents backflow of blood from the aorta into the left ventricle. The right and left coronary arteries originate from the ascending aorta immediately superior to the aortic orifice in the region of the semilunar valve. The ascending aorta passes superiorly to the level of the sternal angle, at the level of the disc between the fourth and fifth thoracic vertebrae, where it continues as the arch of the aorta. In the superior mediastinum the **aortic arch** ascends to the middle of the manubrium and then arches posteriorly and to the left so that it

passes to the left of the trachea and esophagus. At the level of the intervertebral disc between the fourth and fifth thoracic vertebrae, the arch continues in the posterior mediastinum as the **descending thoracic aorta.** The brachiocephalic (innominate), left common carotid, and left subclavian arteries arise from the arch. The angiogram in Fig. 2-12 shows these vessels. The brachiocephalic artery (trunk) is the largest and most anterior of the three vessels that arise from the aortic arch. At its origin it is anterior to the trachea, but as it ascends, the vessel becomes more lateral. Posterior to the right sternoclavicular joint and lateral to the trachea, the brachiocephalic artery divides into the right subclavian and the right common carotid arteries. The **left common carotid artery** is the middle branch of the aortic arch. It is to the left and slightly posterior to the brachiocephalic artery. In the superior mediastinum the left common carotid artery is at first anterior to the trachea and then becomes more lateral. As it passes posterior to the left sternoclavicular joint to ascend in the neck region, it follows a course similar to the right common carotid artery. The **left subclavian artery** is the third and most posterior branch from the aortic arch. As the vessel passes through the superior mediastinum, it lies very near the pleura and left lung. In fetal circulation, a vessel called the **ductus arteriosus** extends from the left pulmonary artery to enter the inferior aspect of the aortic arch. This allows fetal blood to pass directly from the pulmonary artery into the aorta and bypass the lungs, which are not yet functioning. The fetal ductus arteriosus usually closes by the end of the third month after birth to become the **ligamentum arteriosum.**

Numerous variations can occur in the arch of the aorta and the origins of its branches. Some of these are conditions are asymptomatic, but others are not compatible with life and must be corrected surgically.

Pulmonary Trunk.   Arising from the right ventricle, the **pulmonary trunk** ascends on the left side of the ascending aorta to the level of the aortic arch. At its origin from the right ventricle, the pulmonary trunk is anterior to the ascending aorta, but as it ascends, the trunk becomes more posterior. When it reaches the aortic arch, at the level of the sternal angle, the pulmonary trunk divides into the right and left pulmonary arteries. The **right pulmonary artery** is longer and larger in diameter than the left pulmonary artery. As it proceeds to the lungs, the right pulmonary artery passes posterior to the superior vena cava and the ascending aorta but anterior to the right bronchus. The **left pulmonary artery** courses horizontally to the left, anterior to the left bronchus and the descending aorta. At the hilus of the lung, the pulmonary arteries divide according to the divisions of the bronchial tree.

Venae Cavae.   The superior vena cava (SVC) is formed in the superior mediastinum by the union of the right and left brachiocephalic veins. The left brachiocephalic vein crosses horizontally anterior to the aorta and pulmonary trunk to join with the vein on the right. The superior vena cava descends on the right side of the superior mediastinum to enter the right atrium vertically from above. The lower half of the vessel is enclosed within the pericardium

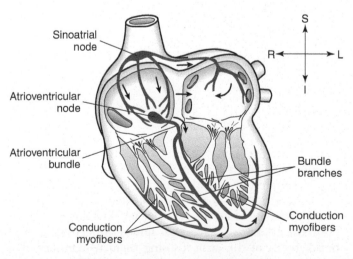

Sinoatrial node

Atrioventricular node

Atrioventricular bundle

Conduction myofibers

Bundle branches

Conduction myofibers

S
R — L
I

FIG. 2-11. Conduction system of the heart.

FIG. 2-12. Angiogram of the branches from the aortic arch.

in the middle mediastinum. It is located to the right of the aorta and anterior to the trachea and esophagus. The superior vena cava returns blood to the heart from structures above the diaphragm except the lungs.

The inferior vena cava ascends through the abdominal cavity to the right of the midline. It penetrates the diaphragm at vertebral level T8 and enters the middle mediastinum of the thoracic cavity. Here it enters the lowest part of the right atrium, almost in a vertical line with the superior vena cava. The inferior vena cava returns blood from the region below the diaphragm.

QUICK CHECK

2.30 What is the most anterior branch of the aortic arch?

2.31 Which vessel is located more to the right, the ascending aorta or the superior vena cava?

2.32 Where is the origin of the right and left coronary arteries?

Other Structures Associated with the Thoracic Region

Thymus.   The **thymus** gland is located immediately behind the manubrium of the sternum in the superior mediastinum. In infancy and early childhood, the gland is a prominent mass of lymphoid tissue that may extend downward into the anterior mediastinum. After puberty it gradually decreases in size and is replaced by fatty tissue, until it may be hardly recognizable in the adult. The thymus plays a major role in the development and maintenance of the immune system.

Trachea.   Beginning as a continuation of the larynx in the neck, the trachea descends in front of the **esophagus** to enter the superior mediastinum a little to the right of midline. At the level of the sternal angle, the trachea bifurcates into the **right** and **left primary bronchi.** Each bronchus is posterior to its corresponding pulmonary artery. The region of bifurcation is known as the **carina.**

A series of C-shaped cartilages keeps the trachea open for the passage of air. The posterior soft tissue of the trachea allows for expansion of the esophagus during swallowing.

Esophagus.   The esophagus extends from the pharynx at the level of the cricoid cartilage (C6) in the neck to the stomach in the upper left quadrant of the abdomen. As it descends through the neck and superior mediastinum, the esophagus is in a near midline position between the trachea anteriorly and the vertebral bodies posteriorly. The left bronchus passes anterior to the esophagus. In the posterior mediastinum the esophagus descends anterior and to the right of the descending aorta. In this region its anterior relationships are to the pericardium and the **left atrium.** In the lower regions of the posterior mediastinum, the esophagus curves to the left to penetrate the diaphragm at the T10 vertebral level. As it curves, the esophagus passes anterior to the aorta.

The esophagus has four clinically significant constrictions: (1) at its beginning, (2) at the level of the aortic arch, (3) at the level of the carina where the left bronchus crosses it, and (4) where it passes through the diaphragm. Objects tend to lodge in these constricted areas.

QUICK CHECK

2.33 Which is more anterior, the trachea or the esophagus?

2.34 Which is more anterior, a bronchus or its corresponding pulmonary artery?

2.35 In the posterior mediastinum, what is immediately anterior to the esophagus?

Thoracic Duct.   The **thoracic duct** is the primary duct of the lymphatic system. It collects lymph from the entire body except the upper right quadrant. The thoracic duct begins in the abdomen as the **cisterna chyli.** From there it ascends on the right side of the aorta, just anterior to the vertebral column. At level T12 it passes through the diaphragm in the same opening as the descending aorta and enters the posterior mediastinum of the thorax. The relative position of the thoracic duct in the posterior mediastinum of the lower thoracic region is illustrated in Fig. 2-13. At the level of the fifth thoracic vertebra, it deviates to the left, posterior to the esophagus, and enters the superior mediastinum, where it ascends into the neck on the left side. The thoracic duct empties into the venous system at the junction of the left internal jugular and left subclavian veins.

Azygos Vein.   The **azygos vein** begins in the abdomen and enters the posterior mediastinum of the thorax along with the thoracic duct. In the thorax the azygos vein ascends just anterior to the vertebral column. It is posterior to the esophagus and to the right of the aorta and thoracic duct. The relative position of the azygos vein is illustrated in Fig. 2-13. At the level of T4, it arches over the root of the right lung to enter the **superior vena cava** in the superior mediastinum. A smaller **hemiazygos vein** ascends on the left side to the level of T9 and then crosses the midline posterior to the aorta and esophagus to empty into the azygos vein. These veins drain the thoracic wall and posterior abdominal wall.

Brachial Plexus.   The brachial plexus is a network of nerves formed by the ventral rami, or branches, of spinal nerves C5 to C8 and T1. It extends from the posterior triangle of the neck into the axilla and supplies innervation to the arm. Portions of the brachial plexus are clearly evident in transverse sections, between the anterior scalene and middle scalene muscles (see Fig. 2-16). Five nerves supplying innervation to the arm emerge from the brachial plexus. These are the **musculocutaneous, median, ulnar, axillary,** and **radial nerves.**

Injuries to the brachial plexus may be caused by disease, trauma, or stretching. These injuries result in paralysis and/or anesthesia. The extent of the signs and symptoms depends on the part of the plexus injured.

Breast
General Breast Anatomy.   The breast is located in the superficial fascia of the pectoral region overlying the pectoralis major muscle. Mammary glands for the production of milk are located in the breast; normally, these become well developed and functional only in the female. The breast normally extends from the lateral margin of the sternum to the anterior border of the axilla between the second and sixth ribs. Breast tissue is separated from the deep fascia of the underlying muscle by a retromammary layer of loose connective tissue. Some breast carcinomas may invade the loose connective tissue and deep fascia and become fixed to the underlying muscle. This restricts the movement of the breast.

At birth and throughout early childhood, the male and female breasts are similar. Externally, near the center of the breast, a circular area of pigmented skin, known as the **areola,** surrounds an elevated nipple. Numerous sebaceous glands in the areola appear as small nodules under the skin and secrete an oily substance to keep the tissues soft. Internally, a few rudimentary ducts radiate from the nipple. At puberty the mammary gland in the female undergoes developmental changes, but the male gland usually remains rudimentary.

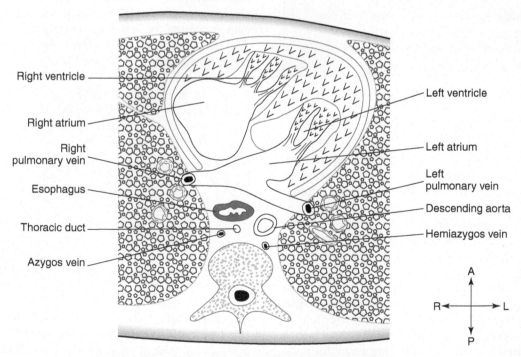

FIG. 2-13. Relationships of structures in the posterior mediastinum.

In the adult male, the breast consists of a few small ducts without any milk-secreting cells and some supporting adipose and fibrous tissue. The ducts in the male may become fibrous cords.

In the adult female, the breast includes glandular **parenchyma** and connective tissue **stroma.** The glandular parenchyma consists of 15 to 20 lobes of **alveoli,** or milk-producing cells, arranged radially around the centrally located nipple. An excretory **lactiferous duct** extends from each lobe to the nipple, where it terminates in a tiny opening at the surface. The glandular lobes are embedded in the connective tissue stroma, which contains varying amounts of fat. Condensations of connective tissue, known as **suspensory ligaments** or **Cooper's ligaments,** extend from the underlying deep fascia through the breast to the skin. These ligaments provide support for the breasts. The components of the female breast are illustrated by the line drawing in Fig. 2-14 and the mammogram in Fig. 2-15.

Lymphatic Drainage From the Breast. Although there are several routes of lymphatic drainage from the breast, about 75% of the drainage is by way of the **axillary lymph nodes,** In addition to the axillary nodes, other avenues of lymphatic drainage include the **parasternal, supraclavicular,** and **abdominal lymph nodes.** The drainage of one breast may also join the drainage of the opposite breast. The lymphatic drainage of the breast is of clinical significance in the diagnosis and treatment of breast cancer. As the cancer cells break loose, they travel through the lymphatic channels until they become trapped. Because 75% of the lymphatic drainage is through the axillary nodes, this is the most common site of metastases from breast carcinoma.

QUICK CHECK

2.36 From right to left, what is the sequence of the descending aorta, azygos vein, and thoracic duct?

2.37 In transverse sections, between which two muscles is the brachial plexus often visualized?

2.38 What is the primary lymphatic drainage from the breast?

Sectional Anatomy of the Thorax

Transverse Sections

Section Through the Thoracic Inlet Sections through the superior thoracic aperture, or thoracic inlet, illustrated in Figs. 2-16 and 2-17, show the structures passing through the root of the neck into the thorax. These sections also show the shoulder region with the pectoral girdle and upper extremity. Because the superior thoracic aperture slopes inferiorly from posterior to anterior, a transverse section through the first thoracic vertebra typically does not intersect the manubrium of the sternum.

Anteriorly in sections through the thoracic inlet, the **sternocleidomastoid** muscles are thin straps anterior to the lobes of the **thyroid gland.** The horseshoe-shaped **tracheal**

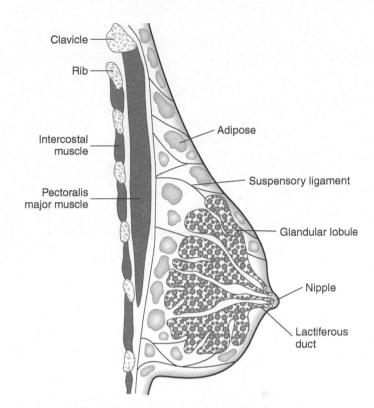

FIG. 2-14. Sagittal section of the female breast.

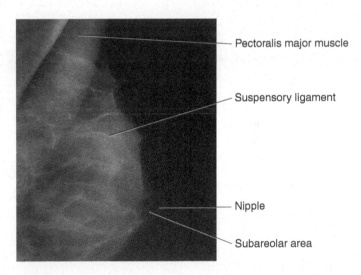

FIG. 2-15. Mammogram of the left breast of a premenopausal woman. (Modified from Weir J, Abrahams PH: *Imaging atlas of human anatomy,* ed 3, St Louis, 2003, Elsevier/Mosby.)

cartilage is between the lobes of the thyroid gland and the **esophagus.** The internal jugular veins are lateral to the common carotid arteries. Also of interest at this level are the **clavicle, scalene muscles, brachial plexus,** and **first rib.**

The components of the humeroscapular joint are discussed in more detail in a later chapter, but because of their relationship to the wall of the thorax, they are mentioned here.

At the level of the thoracic inlet, the most superficial muscle of the back is the **trapezius muscle** as it travels

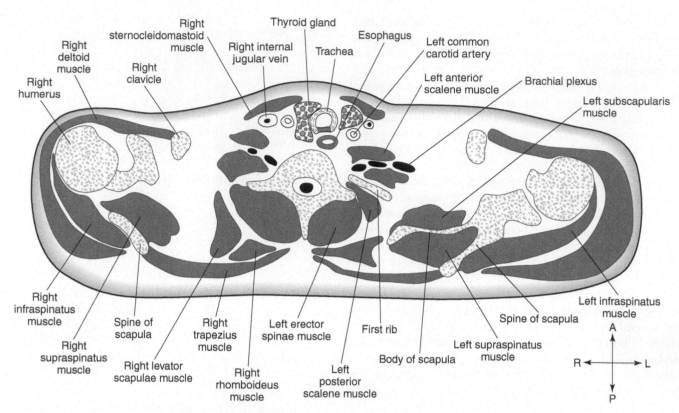

FIG. 2-16. Section through the thoracic inlet.

FIG. 2-17. Transverse CT image through the thoracic inlet. (Modified from Bo WJ et al: *Basic atlas of sectional anatomy: with correlated imaging,* ed 4, St Louis, 2007, Elsevier/Saunders.)

from the vertebral column to the scapula. Lying directly beneath the trapezius muscle are the **rhomboideus muscles.** Throughout the length of the vertebral column, the **erector spinae muscles** are seen in the groove between the spinous and transverse processes. The large **deltoid muscle** forms a semicircle around the humerus from the clavicle to

the spine of the scapula. Depending on the angle of the slice, either two or three muscles directly related to the scapula are seen. At some angles, when only the spine of the scapula is seen, there is a more superficial **infraspinatus muscle** and a deeper **supraspinatus muscle.** When the cut is below the scapular spine, through the blade or body of the scapula, the more superficial muscle is still the infraspinatus, but the muscle deep to the body is the **subscapularis.** Occasionally the angle of the slice is such that both the spine and the body of the scapula are seen. In this case, all three muscles are present. The infraspinatus appears superficial to the spine, the supraspinatus appears to be between the spine and the body, and the subscapularis is deep to the body of the scapula. These muscles are illustrated in Fig. 2-16.

QUICK CHECK

2.39 In transverse sections through the thoracic inlet, what tissue is immediately adjacent to the trachea?

2.40 In transverse sections through the thoracic inlet, which vessel is more lateral, the internal jugular vein or the common carotid artery?

Section Through the Apex of the Lung. Particular attention should be given to vascular relationships in this and the following few sections. As the aorta goes from the ascending to the descending portion, it arches in an anterior-posterior direction, as well as in a right-to-left direction. This means that the vessels closely associated with the aortic arch assume corresponding arch-shaped positions. At the level of the apex of the lung, illustrated in Fig. 2-18, the **right common carotid artery** and the **right subclavian artery** are seen as two separate vessels close together on the right side of the trachea. The proximity of the two vessels indicates that they are near the bifurcation of the brachiocephalic artery.

In sections inferior to this, illustrated in Fig. 2-19, the single **brachiocephalic (innominate) artery** is seen. The brachiocephalic artery is the first and most anterior branch from the arch of the aorta. On the left the anterior vessel is the **left common carotid** artery. The **left subclavian** artery is also on the left but is more posterior. This is the third and most posterior branch from the aortic arch. The **subclavian vein** is seen joining with the **internal jugular vein** to form the **left brachiocephalic (innominate) vein** on the left. On the right the brachiocephalic vein has already formed. The computed tomography (CT) image in Fig. 2-20 shows the relationships of the common carotid and subclavian arteries.

The anterior thoracic wall at the level of the lung apex is formed by the **pectoralis major** and **minor** muscles and the two clavicles joined by an **interclavicular ligament.** A **subclavius muscle** is associated with each clavicle.

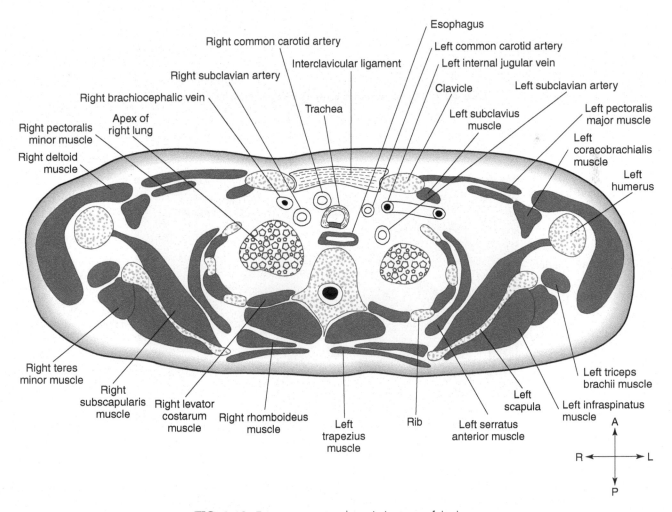

FIG. 2-18. Transverse section through the apex of the lung.

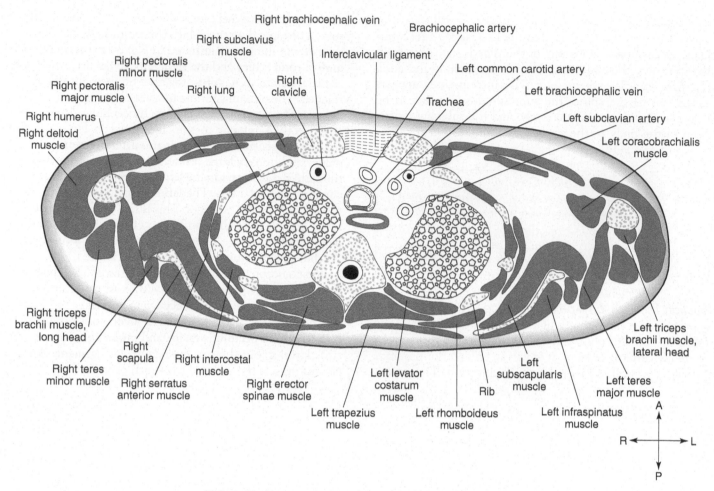

Right pectoralis minor muscle
Right subclavius muscle
Right brachiocephalic vein
Brachiocephalic artery
Interclavicular ligament
Left common carotid artery
Right pectoralis major muscle
Right lung
Right clavicle
Trachea
Left brachiocephalic vein
Right humerus
Left subclavian artery
Right deltoid muscle
Left coracobrachialis muscle
Right triceps brachii muscle, long head
Left triceps brachii muscle, lateral head
Right scapula
Right intercostal muscle
Left subscapularis muscle
Left teres major muscle
Right teres minor muscle
Right serratus anterior muscle
Right erector spinae muscle
Left levator costarum muscle
Rib
Left trapezius muscle
Left rhomboideus muscle
Left infraspinatus muscle

A
R ← → L
P

FIG. 2-19. Transverse section showing the brachiocephalic artery.

Right brachiocephalic vein
Sternum
Left brachiocephalic vein
Right common carotid artery
Left common carotid artery
Right subclavian artery
Left subclavian artery
Lung
Trachea
Scapula

A
R ← → L
P

FIG. 2-20. CT image showing the common carotid and subclavian arteries.

In addition to the intercostal muscles, two other muscles associated with the rib cage are illustrated in Figs. 2-18 and 2-19. The **serratus anterior** muscles that form the medial walls of the axillae appear much like parentheses enclosing the ribs and intercostal muscles. The **levator costarum** muscle connects a rib to its appropriate transverse vertebral process. Muscles associated with the scapula and upper extremity include the **teres major** and the **teres minor.** The teres minor is closely associated with the **infraspinatus** muscle, and it is sometimes difficult to distinguish between them except by location. The teres minor is at the lateral end of the infraspinatus muscle. The teres major is lateral to the teres minor. Both of these muscles are illustrated in Fig. 2-19.

QUICK CHECK

2.41 What two vessels result from the bifurcation of the brachiocephalic artery?

2.42 In transverse sections through the apex of the lung, what vessel appears closest to the left lung?

Section Through the Aortic Arch.   A section through the arch of the aorta probably will intersect the manubrium of the sternum. When looking at an inferior view through the arch of the aorta, as illustrated in Fig. 2-21, three holes should be seen in the arch, representing the three branches, the anterior **brachiocephalic artery,** the posterior **left subclavian artery** and, in the middle, the **left common carotid artery.** The **left brachiocephalic vein** crosses anterior to the aortic arch to join the **right brachiocephalic vein.** The right and left brachiocephalic veins join to form the **superior vena cava.** The CT image in Fig. 2-22 shows the right and left brachiocephalic veins and the three vessels from the aortic arch.

Section Through the Sternal Angle.   The **sternal angle** (angle of Louis), at the T4/T5 vertebral level, is an easily palpable landmark. Transverse sections at this level show an anteriorly located **ascending aorta** and a posteriorly situated **descending aorta** on the left side of the mediastinum. This is illustrated in Fig. 2-23. The right-sided **superior vena cava** is opposite the ascending aorta. Posterior to the ascending aorta and superior vena cava, the **trachea** begins to bifurcate into the **mainstem (primary) bronchi.** The **esophagus** is between the tracheal bifurcation and the descending aorta. The **azygos vein** is seen for the first time at this level as it makes a loop over the root of the right lung to enter the superior vena cava. The CT image in Fig. 2-24 shows the vessels and the bifurcation of the trachea.

Section Through the Pulmonary Trunk.   The **pulmonary trunk** appears on the left side within the pericardium at approximately level T5. In sequence from right to left, the great vessels are the **superior vena cava, ascending aorta,** and **pulmonary trunk,** as shown in Fig. 2-25. At this level the pulmonary trunk may be slightly posterior to the ascending aorta, but at more inferior levels it becomes anterior. Even though the pulmonary trunk is the outflow from the right ventricle, it is the most left sided of the three great vessels. The **right pulmonary artery,** as it branches from the pulmonary trunk, must pass horizontally, posterior to the ascending aorta and superior vena cava, to enter the right lung (see Fig. 2-25). Because the pulmonary trunk is on the left, the right pulmonary artery is longer and more horizontal than the left. The right and left pulmonary arteries are anterior to the right and left mainstem bronchi, respectively. In the posterior mediastinum the large vessel on the left is the **descending aorta.** The **esophagus** is anterior and slightly to the right of the descending aorta, and

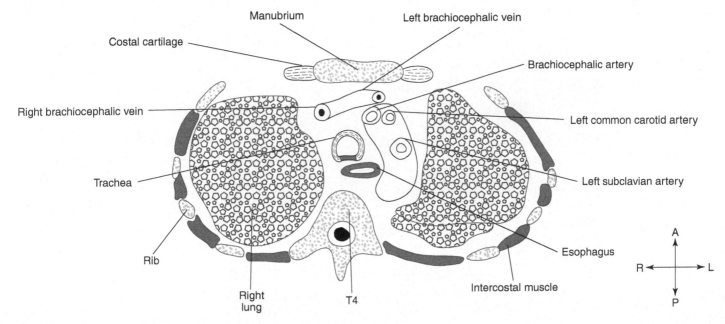

FIG. 2-21. Transverse section through the aortic arch.

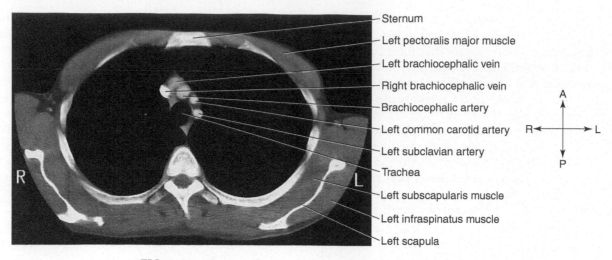

Sternum
Left pectoralis major muscle
Left brachiocephalic vein
Right brachiocephalic vein
Brachiocephalic artery
Left common carotid artery
Left subclavian artery
Trachea
Left subscapularis muscle
Left infraspinatus muscle
Left scapula

FIG. 2-22. CT image showing the three vessels from the aortic arch.

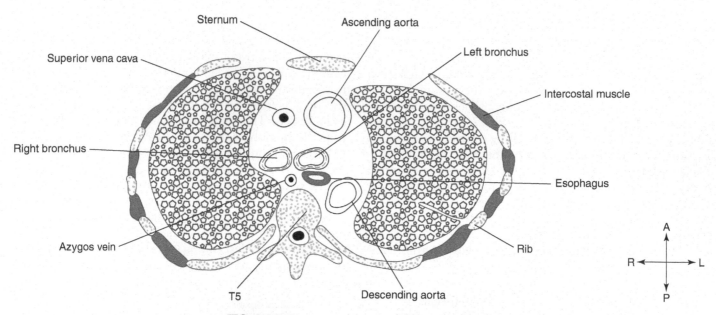

Sternum
Ascending aorta
Superior vena cava
Left bronchus
Intercostal muscle
Right bronchus
Esophagus
Azygos vein
Rib
T5
Descending aorta

FIG. 2-23. Transverse section through the sternal angle.

Superior vena cava
Sternum
Ascending aorta
Right bronchus
Left pulmonary artery
Esophagus
Azygos vein
Descending aorta

FIG. 2-24. CT image through the sternal angle.

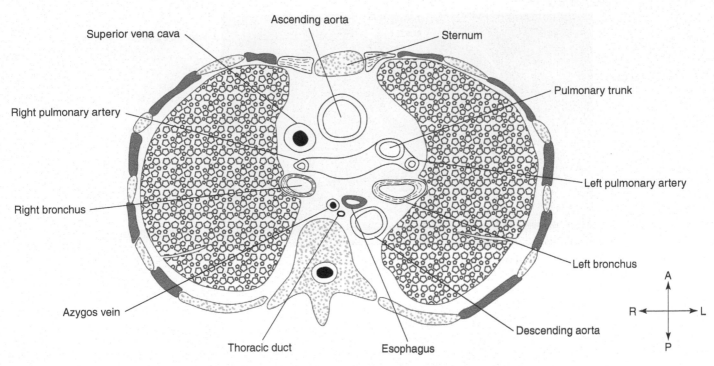

FIG. 2-25. Transverse section through the pulmonary trunk.

the **azygos vein** is to the right of the esophagus. The **thoracic duct** usually is between the azygos vein and the descending aorta but may be difficult to locate. The CT image in Fig. 2-26 shows the right pulmonary artery as it passes horizontally, posterior to the superior vena cava and the ascending aorta.

QUICK CHECK

2.43 In transverse sections through the aortic arch, what specific vessel is typically anterior to the brachiocephalic artery?

2.44 In transverse sections through the sternal angle, what major vessel is to the right of the ascending aorta?

2.45 What vessel is posterior to the ascending aorta and superior vena cava but anterior to the right bronchus?

Section Through the Base of the Heart. Sections through the base of the heart show the three great vessels at or near their attachment to the heart. As you follow the three great vessels from higher levels down to their origin from the chambers of the heart, you will notice that they keep the same right-to-left sequence (superior vena cava, ascending aorta, pulmonary trunk), but the anterior-posterior relationship of the ascending aorta and pulmonary trunk appears to change. At higher levels the ascending aorta is anterior to the pulmonary trunk (see Fig. 2-25). At lower levels the ascending aorta is posterior to the pulmonary trunk, as shown in Fig. 2-27. The pulmonary trunk courses in a posterior direction as it ascends

from the right ventricle. The outflow orifice is guarded by the **pulmonary semilunar valve.** The superior vena cava remains on the right side as it enters the right atrium, the most right-sided chamber of the heart. The **left atrium** is the most posterior chamber of the heart, and the vessels entering the left atrium are the **pulmonary veins** carrying freshly oxygenated blood from the lungs. The **esophagus, azygos vein,** and **descending aorta** are in the posterior mediastinum. The CT image in Fig. 2-28 shows the relationships of the superior vena cava, ascending aorta, pulmonary trunk, and left atrium.

Section Through the Chambers of the Heart. Transverse sections through the chambers of the heart show the **left atrium** to be the most posterior chamber. Posteriorly the left atrium is related to the **esophagus.** Anteriorly the left atrium is related to the centrally located aortic outflow region of the left ventricle. The **right atrium** is the most right-sided chamber. The cavity of the right atrium is anterior and perpendicular to that of the left atrium, therefore the **interatrial septum** is in a coronal plane. The most anterior chamber is the **right ventricle,** which is immediately to the left of the right atrium. Blood flow from the right atrium through the **tricuspid valve** into the **right ventricle** is primarily passive and is directed to the left and slightly anteriorly. The **bicuspid valve** between the left atrium and **left ventricle** is directed inferiorly, anteriorly, and to the left. The thick **interventricular septum** is predominately in a coronal plane. The **right coronary artery** is seen in the fat-filled sulcus between the right atrium and right ventricle. The **coronary sinus** is a venous dilation that receives blood from the coronary circulation and empties into the

FIG. 2-26. CT image showing the right pulmonary trunk.

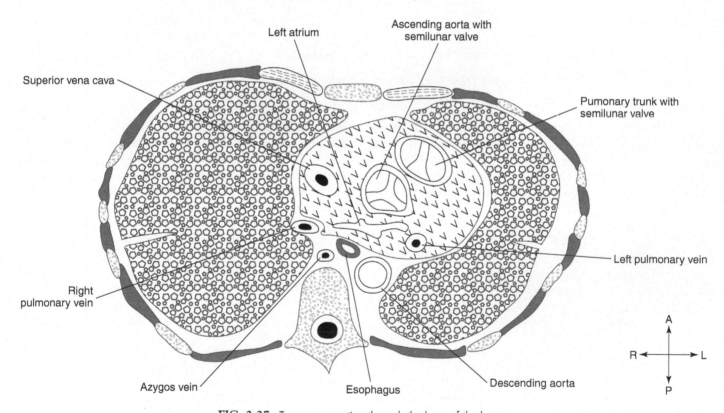

FIG. 2-27. Transverse section through the base of the heart.

right atrium. It is located in the left atrioventricular sulcus along the posterior surface of the heart. These features of the heart are illustrated in Fig. 2-29 and by the CT scan and sonogram in Fig. 2-30.

QUICK CHECK

2.46 At the base of the heart, which vessel is most anterior, the SVC, pulmonary trunk, or ascending aorta?

2.47 What is the most anterior chamber of the heart?

Sagittal Sections

Section Through the Right Lung. Sagittal sections to the right of the midline that intersect the **right lung** show the upper lobe separated from the middle lobe by a **horizontal (minor) fissure.** The middle lobe is separated from the lower lobe by an **oblique (major) fissure.** Sections in this region usually show the relationship of the scapula to the **infraspinatus, supraspinatus,** and **subscapularis muscles.** The infraspinatus muscle fills the fossa below the scapular spine, and the supraspinatus fills the space above the scapular spine. The subscapularis muscle is deep to the

FIG. 2-28. CT image through the base of the heart.

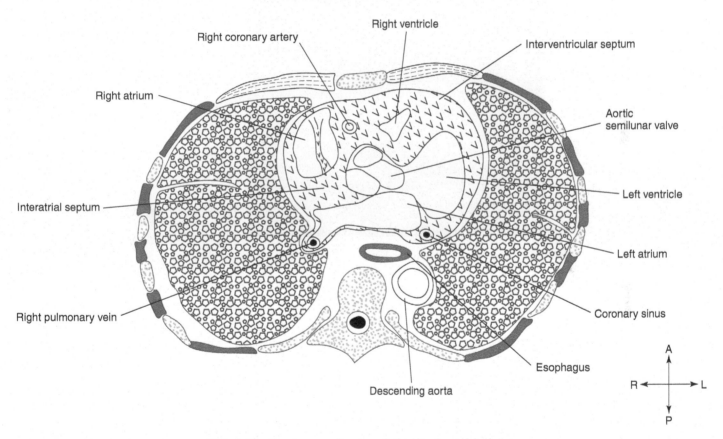

FIG. 2-29. Transverse section through the chambers of the heart.

plate or body of the scapula. Anteriorly the **pectoralis major** and **minor** muscles form the thoracic wall. **Axillary vessels,** which are a continuation of the subclavian vessels, are deep to the pectoralis muscles. These features are shown in Fig. 2-31.

Section Through the Right Atrium. Because the right atrium is the most right-sided chamber of the heart, it is the first chamber seen when serial sagittal sections are made from right to left. The sagittal section illustrated in

Fig. 2-32 is approximately 2 cm to the right of the midline. It shows the **inferior vena cava** and **superior vena cava** draining into the cavity of the **right atrium.** A continuation of the right atrium into the pectinate region of the **right auricle** is evident. The **left atrium** is seen as a posterior chamber with a **pulmonary vein** draining into it. Just superior to the left atrium, the **right pulmonary artery** and **right main bronchus** are sectioned as they course to the right, posterior to the superior vena cava. The artery is anterior to the bronchus. This section also shows the

FIG. 2-30. **A,** CT image through the chambers of the heart. **B,** Sonogram of the heart.

azygos vein as it enters the superior vena cava. The myocardium in the anterior region of the heart is the **right ventricle.** The **right coronary artery** is in the sulcus between the right atrium and right ventricle.

Midsagittal Section.   A midsagittal section through the thorax, illustrated in Fig. 2-33, usually cuts through the **aorta** as it ascends from the left ventricle. Remember that the aorta is to the right of the pulmonary trunk as they ascend from the heart. A portion of the **tricuspid valve,** between the right atrium and right ventricle, should be seen, because it is near the midline or slightly to the right. It is the most inferior of the four valves of the heart and generally is at the level of the intercostal space between the fourth and fifth ribs. The sound of the tricuspid valve is heard over the right half of the inferior portion of the body of the sternum. Near the bottom of the ascending aorta, at the level of the third intercostal space, the **aortic semilunar valve** guards the orifice between the left ventricle and aorta. The sound of the aortic valve is heard on the right edge of the sternum in the second intercostal space. More superiorly, where the aorta arches,

are the openings for the **left subclavian, left common carotid,** and **brachiocephalic arteries.** The **left brachiocephalic vein** is cut as it courses horizontally in front of the aorta to meet its counterpart on the right side. The **right pulmonary artery** is located posterior to the aorta. Recall that the right pulmonary artery passes posterior to the aorta and superior vena cava as it travels toward the right lung.

> **QUICK CHECK**
> 2.48   In sagittal sections through the right atrium, what vessel is posterior to the superior vena cava but anterior to the right bronchus?
> 2.49   In sagittal sections, what valve is seen in the right ventricle?

Section Through the Pulmonary Trunk.   Just to the left of the midline, the **pulmonary trunk** exits the **right ventricle** and curves posteriorly over the **left atrium.** This is illustrated in Fig. 2-34. Remember that the pulmonary trunk is to the left of the aorta as the vessels emerge from the heart.

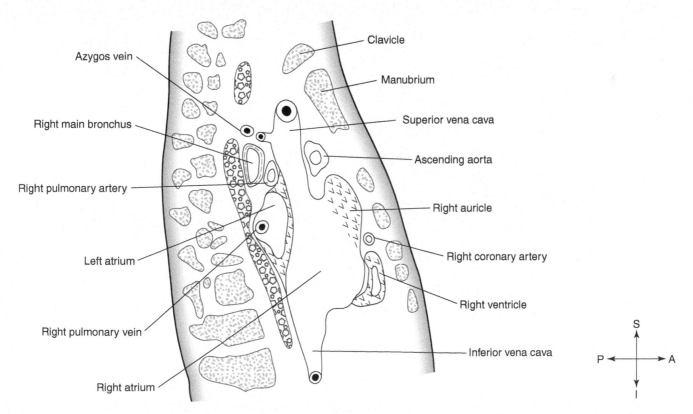

FIG. 2-31. Sagittal section through the right lung.

FIG. 2-32. Sagittal section through the right atrium.

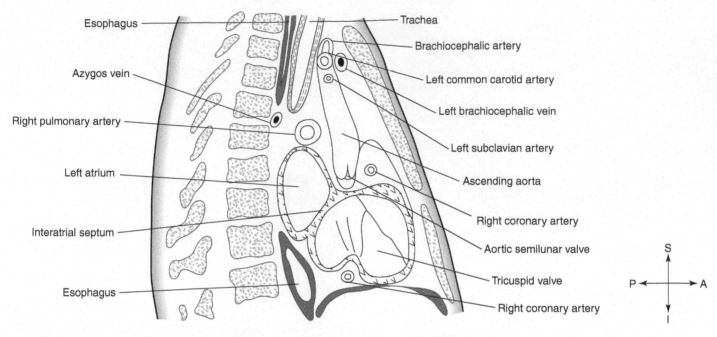

FIG. 2-33. Midsagittal section through the thorax.

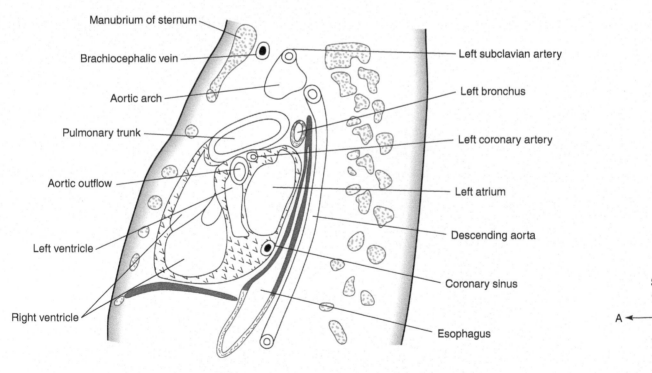

FIG. 2-34. Sagittal section through the pulmonary trunk.

Because the aortic arch curves to the left, you may see a portion of the arch continuous with the **descending aorta.** The **left brachiocephalic vein** passes horizontally anterior to the pulmonary trunk and aortic arch, therefore the vein is cut in cross section. The **left bronchus** is also cut in cross section as it courses on its path to the left lung. It is anterior to the descending aorta and posterior to the pulmonary trunk. After the short **left coronary artery** branches from the aorta, it follows a horizontal path posterior to the pulmonary trunk. The **coronary sinus** is in the fat-filled sulcus inferior to the posteriorly located left atrium. Both the left coronary artery and coronary sinus are seen in cross section in sagittal sections to the left of median (see Fig. 2-34).

Section Through the Bicuspid Valve. Sagittal sections showing the bicuspid valve are 4 to 5 cm left of midline. These sections, illustrated in Fig. 2-35, show the **right ventricle** in an anterior position and separated from the **left ventricle** by an **interventricular septum.** Two cusps (anterior and posterior) of the bicuspid (mitral) valve are between the left atrium and left ventricle. Sections in this region usually show the two branches of the left coronary artery, the **anterior interventricular (anterior descending) branch** in the fat of the interventricular sulcus and the **circumflex branch** in the anterior part of the atrioventricular sulcus. The **coronary sinus** is still evident on the posterior aspect of the heart. Because this section is to the left of the pulmonary trunk, the **left pulmonary artery** is seen anterior to the descending aorta and superior to the left bronchus. The elongated but narrow left lung is divided into two lobes by the oblique fissure.

QUICK CHECK

2.50   In sagittal sections through the pulmonary trunk, what structure is posterior to and closely related to the left atrium?

2.51   Are parasagittal sections through the bicuspid valve on the right side or the left side?

Coronal Sections

The anterior-posterior relationships of the mediastinal structures evidenced in the transverse and sagittal sections should be kept in mind when you study a coronal series. Structures that have a definite anterior-posterior curvature, such as the azygos vein as it curves over the root of the lung and the aortic arch, are cut perpendicular to their axis, as illustrated in Fig. 2-36. The posterior chamber of the heart, the left atrium, is seen in posterior coronal sections, but the right ventricle is not seen because it is an anterior chamber. The muscles that may be present are discussed in Chapter 7.

Section Through the Left Atrium. The **left atrium** is the most posterior chamber of the heart. It receives newly oxygenated blood from the lungs via the pulmonary veins. If the section is just right, these veins may be seen entering the left atrium (see Fig. 2-36). Superior to the left atrium, the **trachea** descends slightly to the right of midline. In some sections through the left atrium the bifurcation of the trachea into right and left mainstem bronchi may be evident. The CT and magnetic

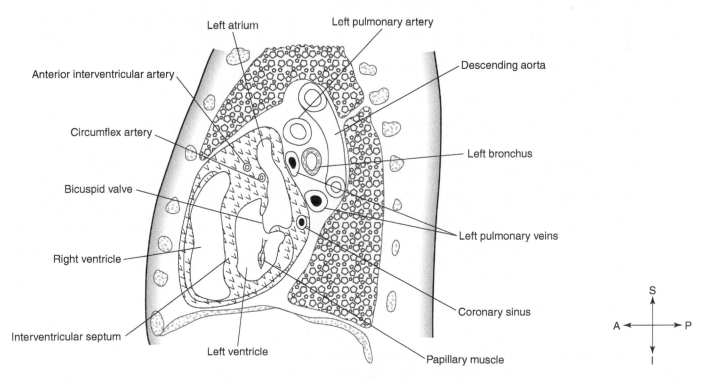

FIG. 2-35. Sagittal section through the bicuspid valve.

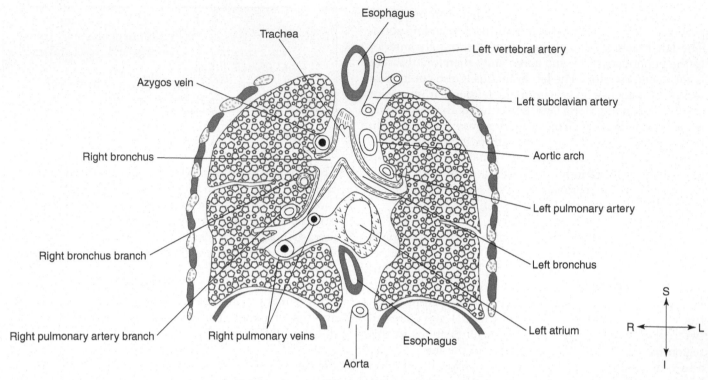

FIG. 2-36. Coronal section through the left atrium.

resonance (MR) images in Fig. 2-37 show the left atrium and the bifurcation of the trachea. In more posterior sections the esophagus is seen instead of the trachea. To the left of the trachea, the posterior part of the **aortic arch** is evident as it is cut across its axis. The most posterior of the three aortic arch tributaries, the **left subclavian artery,** may be seen as it branches from the arch. This vessel is in close relationship to the left lung. The **left vertebral artery** branches from the left subclavian artery and ascends in the neck. The **left pulmonary artery** is inferior to the aortic arch and to the left of the trachea. In some views the right pulmonary artery may also be seen. The descending aorta is evident as it enters the abdomen through the diaphragm. The azygos vein parallels the aorta in this region. Superiorly the azygos vein arches over the root of the right lung to empty into the superior vena cava.

Section Through the Right Atrium and the Left Ventricle. Figs. 2-38 and 2-39 illustrate a plane through the right atrium and left ventricle. They show the **superior vena cava** in a straight line with the **right atrium** on the right side of the heart. The superior vena cava is formed when the **right** and **left brachiocephalic veins** join. The azygos vein empties into the superior vena cava. Because the apex of the heart, formed by the **left ventricle,** displaces the left lung, the left lung is narrower than the right lung. The right-to-left arrangement of the superior vena cava, ascending aorta, and pulmonary trunk is evident in the two figures.

> **QUICK CHECK**
>
> **2.52** When visualizing serial coronal sections, starting at the posterior and progressing anteriorly, which chamber of the heart do you see first?

Working with Images of the Thorax

Fig. 2-40 is a reconstructed three-dimensional (3D) CT image of the heart with all surrounding bone and soft tissue removed. Three large vessels emerge from the base of the heart: the superior vena cava on the right, the ascending aorta in the middle, and the pulmonary trunk on the left. Three of the four chambers can be seen: the right atrium, the right ventricle, and the left ventricle. The left atrium is not visible because it is on the posterior surface. The right and left pulmonary veins, which are visible, enter the left atrium. The right coronary artery is visible in the right atrioventricular sulcus. The anterior descending (interventricular) coronary artery is one of the two branches of the left coronary artery and is visible in the interventricular sulcus. The other branch, the circumflex artery, curves posteriorly in the left atrioventricular sulcus.

Fig. 2-41 is a 3D CT image of the aortic arch and its branches. The brachiocephalic artery (trunk) divides into the right common carotid artery and the right subclavian artery. Normally, the left common carotid artery branches directly from the arch, but in this patient, the left common carotid artery has a common origin with the brachiocephalic artery. The third and most posterior branch is the

FIG. 2-37. Coronal MR and CT images through the left atrium. **A,** Coronal MR image. **B,** Coronal CT image with intravenous contrast. (Modified from Bo WJ et al: *Basic atlas of sectional anatomy: with correlated imaging,* ed 4, St Louis, 2007, Elsevier/Saunders.)

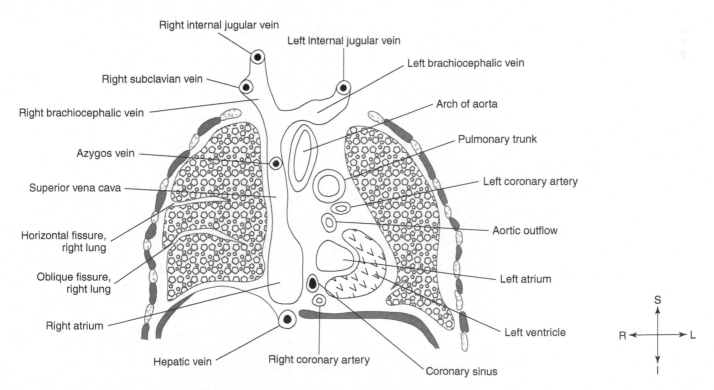

FIG. 2-38. Coronal section through the right atrium and left ventricle.

Pulmonary trunk

Left coronary artery

Aortic semilunar valve

Right atrium

Left ventricle

Papillary muscle

Diaphragm

Right brachiocephalic vein

Superior vena cava

Ascending aorta

Right atrium

Pulmonary trunk

Left ventricle

Diaphragm

FIG. 2-39. Coronal CT image through the right atrium and left ventricle with intravenous contrast. (Modified from Bo WJ et al: *Basic atlas of sectional anatomy: with correlated imaging,* ed 4, St Louis, 2007, Elsevier/Saunders.)

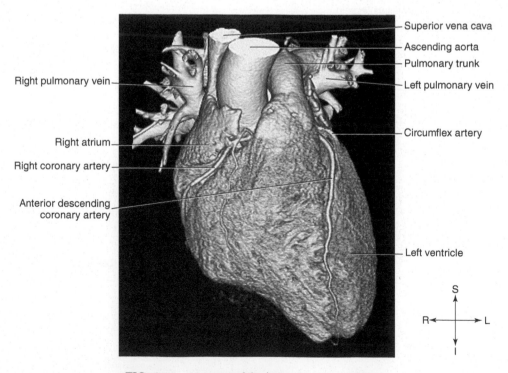

Right pulmonary vein

Right atrium

Right coronary artery

Anterior descending coronary artery

Superior vena cava

Ascending aorta

Pulmonary trunk

Left pulmonary vein

Circumflex artery

Left ventricle

FIG. 2-40. CT image of the heart, 3D reconstruction.

left subclavian artery. The vertebral arteries branch from the subclavian arteries. The common carotid arteries divide into external and internal carotid arteries.

The 3D CT image in Fig. 2-42 shows the ascending aorta with the aortic semilunar valve at its origin. The right and left coronary arteries branch from the aorta immediately superior to the valve. The short left coronary artery divides into the anterior descending (interventricular) and circumflex arteries.

The 3D CT image in Fig. 2-43 shows the trachea as it bifurcates into the right and left bronchi, which enter the lung and continue to divide into secondary and tertiary bronchi.

Fig. 2-44 is a 3D CT image of the aortic arch and the branches from the arch. Note the anterior brachiocephalic artery, which branches into the right common carotid artery and the right subclavian artery, the middle left

common carotid artery, and the posterior left subclavian artery. Each common carotid artery bifurcates into an external carotid artery and an internal carotid artery. Internal thoracic (mammary) arteries branch from the subclavian arteries.

Fig. 2-45 is a transverse CT image in the region of the aortic arch and is similar to the line drawing in Fig. 2-21 and the image in Fig. 2-22. The structures in the mediastinum are the left subclavian artery, the left common carotid artery, the brachiocephalic artery, the right brachiocephalic vein, the left brachiocephalic vein that passes anterior to the arch, the trachea, and the esophagus. Note the spinous process on the vertebra and the spine on the scapula. Numerous muscles are present. Note the anterior pectoralis major and minor. The intercostal muscles are between the ribs, and the serratus anterior muscle appears to enclose the ribs and intercostal muscles like parentheses.

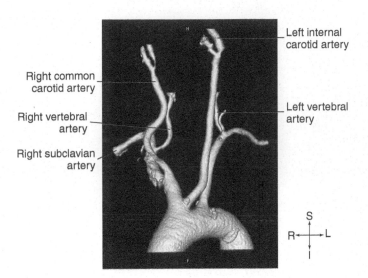

FIG. 2-41. CT image of the aortic arch and its branches, 3D reconstruction.

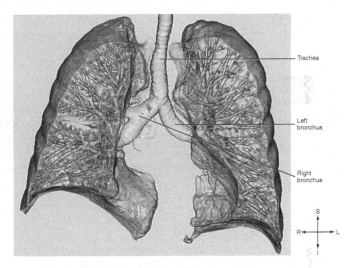

FIG. 2-43. CT image of the tracheal bifurcation.

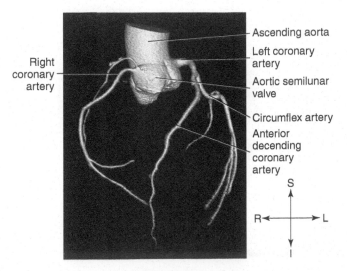

FIG. 2-42. CT image of the ascending aorta, 3D reconstruction.

FIG. 2-44. CT image of the aortic arch and its branches.

FIG. 2-45. Transverse CT image in the region of the aortic arch.

FIG. 2-46. Transverse CT image at the level of the sternal angle.

Scapular muscles are the subscapularis, infraspinatus, supraspinatus, and teres minor, which collectively form the rotator cuff. The trapezius muscle is superficial in the posterior region.

Transverse sections at the level of the sternal angle (angle of Louis), illustrated in Fig. 2-46, show an anteriorly positioned ascending aorta and a posteriorly positioned descending aorta. The superior vena cava is to the right of the ascending aorta. The trachea and esophagus are anterior to the vertebral body. Note the azygos vein posterior to the esophagus. Three of the four rotator cuff muscles are present. This section is inferior to the spine of the scapula, therefore the supraspinatus muscle is not present.

Sections at more superior levels showed the trachea in a central location among the great vessels. Fig. 2-47 illustrates the bifurcation of the trachea into right and left bronchi. The esophagus is posterior to the left bronchus in

FIG. 2-47. Transverse CT image at the level of the tracheal bifurcation.

FIG. 2-48. Transverse CT image through the bifurcation of the pulmonary trunk.

this view. The left pulmonary artery is seen entering the left lung at the hilus. The expected muscles are present. Note the sternopericardial ligament that attaches the pericardium to the sternum.

Fig. 2-48 illustrates the bifurcation of the pulmonary trunk into the right and left pulmonary arteries. Observe that the right pulmonary artery passes horizontally to the right, posterior to the ascending aorta and superior vena cava. It is anterior to the right bronchus. Note the articulation of the ribs with the facets on the vertebral body and on the transverse processes. The left pulmonary artery has two branches, one going to the superior lobe and one going to the inferior lobe.

Fig. 2-49 shows the anterior-to-posterior and the right-to-left relationships of the superior vena cava, ascending aorta, and pulmonary trunk. As it emerges from the right ventricle, the pulmonary trunk is anterior to the other vessels. The ascending aorta is in the middle, and the superior vena cava is more posterior. The right ventricle is the most

anterior chamber of the heart, therefore it follows that when the pulmonary trunk emerges from the ventricle, it will be anterior to the other vessels. As it ascends, the pulmonary trunk curves posteriorly such that at more superior levels, it is posterior to the aorta. The anterior-to-posterior positions of the vessels may change, but the right-to-left sequence of superior vena cava, ascending aorta, and pulmonary trunk remains fairly constant.

The image in Fig. 2-50 is similar to the line drawing in Fig. 2-27. It shows the left atrium as the most posterior chamber. Pulmonary veins enter the left atrium. On the right side, the superior vena cava enters the right atrium. Note that the right atrium is perpendicular to the left atrium. The ascending aorta and pulmonary trunk maintain their relative positions as seen in the previous figure. These positions are the result of the relative locations of the chambers from which they emerge. The esophagus, although difficult to see in the image, is posterior to the left atrium and to the right of the descending aorta.

Fig. 2-51 shows the four chambers of the heart. The left atrium, with the visible right pulmonary vein entering it, is the most posterior chamber. The right atrium is on the right side. The right ventricle is the most anterior chamber, and the left ventricle forms the apex and indents the left lung. The interventricular septum is between these two chambers. The esophagus is closely related to the left atrium.

Images at the level of Fig. 2-52 are inferior to the atria of the heart and illustrate the apex of the heart. The inferior vena cava appears in the section as it enters the right atrium. The right and left ventricles are separated by the interventricular septum.

The sagittal CT image in Fig. 2-53 shows the right ventricle with the left atrium posterior to it. The right pulmonary artery is superior to the left atrium and posterior to the ascending aorta. The left brachiocephalic vein is viewed in cross section as it passes anterior to the ascending aorta. The brachiocephalic artery branches from the aorta and is

FIG. 2-49. Transverse CT image near the base of the heart.

FIG. 2-50. Transverse CT image through the base of the heart.

Superior vena cava

Left pulmonary vein

Esophagus

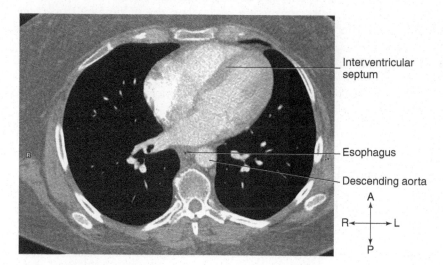

FIG. 2-51. Transverse CT image through the chambers of the heart.

Interventricular septum

Esophagus

Descending aorta

FIG. 2-52 Transverse CT image through the apex of the heart.

Esophagus

Descending aorta

Azygos vein

Trachea
Brachiocephalic artery
Manubrium of sternum
Sternal angle
Body of sternum
Esophagus
Xiphoid
Diaphragm

FIG. 2-53 Sagittal CT image through the sternum and mediastinum.

Left common
carotid artery
Left bronchiocephalic
vein
Left bronchus
Left ventricle

FIG. 2-54 Sagittal CT image through the arch of the aorta and the pulmonary trunk.

slightly superior to the vein. Note the diaphragm between the heart and the liver. The normal thoracic curvature of the vertebral column should be observed.

The sagittal CT image in Fig. 2-54 shows the pulmonary trunk ascending and curving posteriorly as it emerges from the right ventricle. The left common carotid artery branches from the aortic arch. The left bronchus is superior to the left atrium.

Fig. 2-55 shows a coronal CT image that is similar to the line drawing in Fig. 2-36. In this section, the trachea bifurcates into the right and left bronchi. Branches of the right bronchus are also evident. From superior to inferior on the left side, the left subclavian artery, aortic arch, and left pulmonary artery are visualized. Note the proximity of the left subclavian artery to the left lung. On the right, the azygos vein loops over the right bronchus and is cut in cross

section. The most posterior chamber of the heart, the left atrium, is present in this section.

The coronal CT image in Fig. 2-56 shows the right and left pulmonary arteries superior to the left atrium. On the left side, the aortic arch is superior to the pulmonary artery. The esophagus is superior to the arch, and the trachea is to the right of the arch.

Fig. 2-57 is a coronal CT image. The superior vena cava, with contrast medium, is clearly evident on the right side. To the left of the superior vena cava, the left subclavian artery branches from the arch of the aorta. Note the vertebral artery branching from the subclavian artery.

Fig. 2-58 shows the left ventricle, which forms the apex of the heart, indenting the left lung. The ascending aorta emerges from the left ventricle. The pulmonary trunk is to

FIG. 2-55 Coronal CT image showing the bifurcation of the trachea.

Left subclavian artery

Azygos vein

Right pulmonary vein

Descending aorta

FIG. 2-56 Coronal CT image through the left atrium.

Trachea

Left atrium

FIG. 2-57 Coronal CT image showing the superior vena cava.

Superior vena cava

Pulmonary trunk

Left ventricle

FIG. 2-58 Coronal CT image through the left ventricle and ascending aorta.

FIG. 2-59 Coronal CT image rotated to show the three branches from the aortic arch.

the left of the aorta, and the right atrium is adjacent to the right lung.

The coronal CT image in Fig. 2-59 is rotated slightly to show the arrangement of the three main branches from the arch of the aorta more clearly. The most anterior branch is the brachiocephalic artery, the middle branch is the left common carotid artery, and the posterior branch is the left subclavian artery. Note the close relationship of the left subclavian artery to the lung.

Important Anatomical Relationships in the Thorax

- The internal jugular vein is lateral to the common carotid artery (see Figs. 2-16 to 2-18).
- In the region of the thoracic inlet, the internal jugular vein is lateral to the common carotid artery and may also be anterior to it (see Figs. 2-16 and 2-17).
- The brachial plexus is posterior to the clavicle and is between the anterior scalene and middle scalene muscles (see Fig. 2-16).
- The left subclavian artery is near the apex of the left lung (see Figs. 2-19 and 2-20).
- The subclavian veins join with the internal jugular veins to form the brachiocephalic veins (see Fig. 2-38).
- The three vessels that branch from the aortic arch assume an arch-shaped arrangement near their origins (see Figs. 2-19 to 2-21).
- The brachiocephalic artery is the most anterior branch from the aortic arch (see Figs. 2-19 to 2-21).
- The left subclavian artery is the most posterior branch from the aortic arch (see Figs. 2-19 to 2-21).
- The left common carotid artery is the middle branch from the aortic arch (see Figs. 2-19 to 2-21).
- The left brachiocephalic vein passes anterior to the aortic arch to reach the vein on the right side to form the superior vena cava (see Figs. 2-21 and 2-22).
- The thoracic duct is in the posterior mediastinum, posterior to the esophagus and to the left of the azygos vein (see Figs. 2-13 and 2-25).
- The superior vena cava is to the right of the ascending aorta (see Figs. 2-23 to 2-26).
- The azygos vein curves over the right bronchus to empty into the superior vena cava (see Fig. 2-32).
- The right pulmonary artery passes horizontally to the left and is posterior to the superior vena cava and the ascending aorta (see Figs. 2-25 and 2-26).
- Pulmonary arteries are anterior to bronchi at the same level of division (see Figs. 2-25 and 2-32).
- Near the level of the sternal angle, the pulmonary trunk is posterior and to the left of the ascending aorta (see Fig. 2-25).
- The left atrium is the most posterior chamber of the heart (see Figs. 2-27 to 2-30 and 2-32).
- At lower levels, near the base of the heart, the pulmonary trunk becomes anterior to the ascending aorta (see Figs. 2-27 and 2-28).
- The pulmonary semilunar valve is the most superior of the heart valves (see Figs. 2-7 and 2-8).
- Pulmonary veins drain into the left atrium (see Figs. 2-27, 2-28, and 2-32).
- The right atrium is the most right-sided chamber of the heart (see Figs. 2-29, 2-30, and 2-32).
- The aortic semilunar valve is a centrally located structure within the heart (see Fig. 2-29).
- The left atrium is related posteriorly to the esophagus and anteriorly to the aortic outflow region of the left ventricle (see Figs. 2-27 to 2-29).
- The right ventricle is the most anterior chamber of the heart and is to the left of the right atrium (see Figs. 2-29 and 2-30).
- In sequence from right to left, the vessels at the base of the heart are the superior vena cava, ascending aorta, and pulmonary trunk (see Figs. 2-25 to 2-27).

Pathology

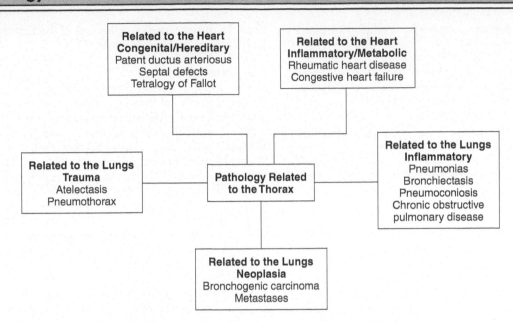

**Related to the Heart
Congenital/Hereditary**
Patent ductus arteriosus
Septal defects
Tetralogy of Fallot

**Related to the Heart
Inflammatory/Metabolic**
Rheumatic heart disease
Congestive heart failure

**Related to the Lungs
Trauma**
Atelectasis
Pneumothorax

**Pathology Related
to the Thorax**

**Related to the Lungs
Inflammatory**
Pneumonias
Bronchiectasis
Pneumoconiosis
Chronic obstructive
pulmonary disease

**Related to the Lungs
Neoplasia**
Bronchogenic carcinoma
Metastases

Patent Ductus Arteriosus

A patent ductus arteriosus results if the lumen of the ductus arteriosus persists after birth. The ductus arteriosus, a channel between the aorta and pulmonary trunk, is open during the prenatal period to allow most of the blood to bypass the lungs. Normally this channel closes shortly after birth. When it remains open, much of the cardiac output is diverted from the aorta to the pulmonary circulation, causing the left ventricle to work harder to maintain systemic circulation. This may result in cardiomegaly and increased vascular congestion. Symptoms may be slight and unnoticed in the infant, but as the child grows older and becomes more active, there may be evidence of dyspnea.

Septal Defects

A defect in either the interatrial or interventricular septum allows blood to pass between the chambers, usually from left to right because of the higher pressures on the left side. The more common type of septal defect is an opening in the interventricular septum, often described as a hole in the heart. The opening may be small and of little significance. Larger openings permit blood to flow from the left ventricle into the right ventricle, placing an increased load on the right ventricle with subsequent enlargement. Bacterial endocarditis also may develop around the edges of the opening. In these cases, surgical repair may be indicated.

Tetralogy of Fallot

Tetralogy of Fallot is a congenital defect of the heart that combines four structural anomalies: (1) pulmonary stenosis resulting in an obstruction to pulmonary flow; (2) ventricular septal defects, or abnormal opening between the right and left ventricles; (3) dextroposition of the aorta in which the aortic opening overrides the ventricular septum and receives blood from both the right and left ventricles; and (4) hypertrophy of the right ventricle. Infants with this condition are sometimes referred to as blue babies because of the presence of cyanosis. The cyanosis occurs because poorly oxygenated blood from the right ventricle enters the overriding aorta and mixes with the oxygenated

blood from the left ventricle. Treatment involves surgical correction whenever possible.

Rheumatic Heart Disease

Rheumatic heart disease is the most important and constant cardiac complication of rheumatic fever. It begins as endocarditis, an inflammation of the inner lining of the heart, including the membrane covering the valves. As the inflammation heals, scar tissue forms on the valves, usually the mitral (bicuspid) and aortic valves, causing damage in the form of stenosis, insufficiency, and/or incompetency. Stenosis results when the scarred valve cusps adhere to one another. If blood leaks through the valve, it is classified as insufficiency. If the valve does not close properly, allowing blood to reflux during contraction, it is classified as incompetency. These conditions usually are manifest only in the adult because it takes several years for the scarring to develop enough to alter valve function. If the condition becomes severe, the compromised valve may have to be surgically replaced with an artificial valve.

Congestive Heart Failure

Congestive heart failure is an inclusive term for conditions in which the heart is unable to pump blood at a sufficient rate and volume to maintain good blood supply to the tissues. It may be caused by any disease process that overburdens the heart, may involve either side of the heart, and may develop gradually or quickly. Left ventricular failure occurs when the left ventricle fails to pump an amount of blood equal to venous return on the right side. As a result, blood backs up in the pulmonary circulation with subsequent increased pulmonary venous pressure, and fluid leaks from the capillaries into the interstitial tissue of the lungs (pulmonary edema). In addition, there is decreased output to the systemic circulation, which decreases kidney perfusion, resulting in increased sodium and water retention and increased blood volume. Left side failure is often due to coronary artery disease, valvular disease, or hypertension. Right ventricular failure occurs when the right ventricle is unable to pump an amount of blood equal to the venous return in the right atrium. As a result, there

Pathology—cont'd

is increased venous pressure in systemic circulation as blood backs up in the superior vena cava, inferior vena cava, and systemic veins. The liver may enlarge and become tender because blood accumulates in its substance. Ascites and edema in the extremities may be evident. Common causes of right side failure include pulmonary valve stenosis and emphysema.

Atelectasis

Atelectasis is a collapsed or airless state of the lung. It is not a disease process, but is the result of an abnormal process and occurs when the lungs fail to expand properly or when there is excessive resorption of air from the alveoli. Fetal atelectasis is common in premature births when the lungs do not fully expand. In the adult, atelectasis is commonly the result of an obstruction by foreign objects or mucus, or compression of the airways by tumors, pleural effusion, or air. It may also occur as a complication following chest or abdominal surgery caused by a lack of deep breathing.

Pneumothorax

Pneumothorax is the accumulation of air in the pleural cavity. The air may come from inside the lungs, usually when a weakened area of the lung, such as an emphysematous bulla, ruptures. Air may also enter the pleural cavity from the outside as the result of a perforating wound or fractured rib. In any case, the presence of air compresses the lung and may lead to collapse (see atelectasis).

Pneumonias

Pneumonia refers to an inflammation of the lung tissue and may be caused by any irritant that results in inflammation. The most common causative agents are bacteria and viruses. Three main categories of pneumonia are recognized: lobar or bacterial pneumonia, lobular or bronchopneumonia, and interstitial or viral pneumonia. Lobar or bacterial pneumonia affects the alveoli or a segment of or an entire lobe of a lung and is usually caused by *Streptococcus pneumoniae* (pneumococcus) bacteria. The onset is rapid with cough, chest pain, blood-streaked sputum, rapid pulse and respiration, and high fever. Lobular pneumonia or bronchopneumonia, usually caused by *Streptococcus pneumoniae, Streptococcus hemolyticus*, or *Staphylococcus aureus*, begins in the bronchi and may progress into the bronchioles and alveoli. It appears in patchy areas rather than involving an entire segment or lobe. Bronchopneumonia is more common than lobar pneumonia, and the onset of symptoms is more gradual and less dramatic. Interstitial or viral pneumonia differs from the other two types because it is caused by a virus and no exudate is formed in the alveoli. It is the most common type and may occur in epidemic proportions; however, it is usually less severe than the others. Viral pneumonia also occurs as a complication of other viral diseases such as measles, influenza, and chickenpox.

Bronchiectasis

Bronchiectasis is a dilation of a weakened area in the wall of the smaller bronchi, similar to an aneurysm of an artery. The weakened area in the wall is caused by chronic inflammation. As the bronchus dilates, it forms a sac in which infection can occur. In chronic conditions the wall of the bronchus may be destroyed and an abscess results.

Pneumoconiosis

Pneumoconiosis refers to a group of lung diseases caused by long-continued irritation by certain substances, usually industrial dusts, that results in chronic interstitial inflammation. Examples of pneumoconiosis include silicosis, caused by silica dust, anthracosis (black lung), caused by coal dust, and asbestosis, caused by asbestos dust.

Chronic Obstructive Pulmonary Disease (COPD)

Chronic obstructive pulmonary disease (COPD) is a general term for a group of conditions that result in a chronic obstruction of airflow in the bronchi. It is associated with long-term respiratory disorders such as asthma, chronic bronchitis, and emphysema. Bronchial asthma is marked by dyspnea, wheezing, and difficulty with expiration caused by spasmodic constriction of the bronchi. The attacks often are in response to allergens but may also occur as a result of emotional disturbances and bronchial infections. Chronic bronchitis produces inflammation in the bronchi with increased secretion of mucus, which interferes with airflow and causes persistent coughing and shortness of breath. It appears to be common in individuals who smoke cigarettes over a period of years. Pulmonary emphysema also is associated with long-term cigarette smoking and often exists concurrently with chronic bronchitis, although it is anatomically different. Emphysema is characterized by a destruction of the alveolar walls to create large saccules, some of which may resemble large balloons called bullae (see pneumothorax). As the alveolar walls deteriorate and coalesce, the lungs become less efficient and gaseous exchange between alveoli and pulmonary capillaries is compromised. The individual may develop an enlarged or barrel chest, and cardiac complications eventually occur.

Bronchogenic Carcinoma

Bronchogenic carcinoma is the most common fatal primary malignancy in the United States. Statistical evidence indicates that the degree of risk for developing bronchogenic carcinoma is directly proportional to the number of cigarettes smoked. The tumors arise in the major bronchi and metastasize by way of the lymph nodes and bloodstream. One of the devastating features of lung cancer is the formation of metastases to the lymph nodes, liver, brain, bone marrow, and adrenal gland. Often the first indication of lung cancer is a dysfunction caused by a secondary tumor outside the lungs. The symptoms of bronchogenic carcinoma are due to obstruction of the airways and metastases.

Metastases

It is important to remember that not all tumors in the lungs are primary tumors (bronchogenic carcinoma). Many primary malignancies in other organs develop metastases in the lungs. These secondary lung tumors often arise from the breast, kidneys, and colon. By the time these tumors are identified, it is often too late for therapeutic measures to be of benefit.

Summary

- The skeleton of the thorax is formed by the sternum, the 12 thoracic vertebrae, and the ribs with their costal cartilages.
- The jugular notch is at the level of the disc between T2 and T3; the sternal angle is at the level of the disc between T4 and T5; the xiphisternal junction is at the level of T9.
- The superior thoracic aperture is formed by T1, the first pair of ribs and costal cartilages, and the manubrium of the sternum.
- The margin of the inferior thoracic aperture is formed by T12, the twelfth rib and costal margin, and the xiphisternal junction.
- The diaphragm, intercostal muscles, and levator costarum muscles form the thoracic boundaries.
- Muscles of the pectoral region include the pectoralis major and minor muscles, subclavius muscle, and serratus anterior muscle.
- The trapezius muscle and latissimus dorsi muscle are superficial muscles of the back.
- Deep back muscles include the levator scapulae muscle, rhomboideus major muscle, rhomboideus minor muscle, and serratus anterior muscle.
- The muscles of the scapular region act on the shoulder joint. These muscles are the supraspinatus muscle, infraspinatus muscle, subscapularis muscle, teres minor muscle, teres major muscle, and deltoid muscle.
- The pleura is a serous membrane. The parietal pleura lines the thoracic wall, and the visceral pleura adheres intimately to the surface of the lung. The minute space between the two layers of pleura is the pleural cavity.
- The right lung is divided into three lobes by an oblique fissure and a horizontal fissure. It is shorter and wider and has a greater volume than the left lung.
- The left lung is divided into two lobes by an oblique fissure and has an indentation, called the *cardiac notch*, for the apex of the lung.
- The central portion of the thoracic cavity, between the lungs, is the mediastinum. It is divided into superior and inferior regions. The inferior region is further subdivided into anterior, middle, and posterior regions.
- The superior mediastinum contains all the structures passing from the neck into the thorax; the middle mediastinum contains the heart and great vessels; the anterior mediastinum contains connective tissue, lymph nodes, and a portion of the thymus gland; the posterior mediastinum contains the descending thoracic aorta, azygos and hemiazygos veins, thoracic duct, and esophagus.
- The pericardial sac is a fibroserous sac that encloses the heart in the middle mediastinum. The outer layer is tough, fibrous connective tissue called the *fibrous pericardium*, and the inner layer is the parietal layer of the serous pericardium.
- The serous pericardium has a parietal and a visceral layer. The parietal layer lines the pericardial sac. The visceral layer is closely adherent to the surface of the heart. A small space, the pericardial cavity, is present between the two layers.
- The outer layer of the heart wall, the epicardium, is the visceral serous pericardium; the middle layer, the myocardium, is a thick layer of cardiac muscle; the inner layer, or endocardium, is a thin, smooth layer of simple squamous epithelium.
- The apex of the heart points downward and to the left and is the most inferior portion of the heart. It is formed by the left ventricle. The broad superior base formed by the two atria is opposite the apex and projects superiorly, anteriorly, and to the right.
- The sternocostal surface is anterior and is formed by the right atrium and right ventricle. The two ventricles form the diaphragmatic surface.
- The right atrium, superior vena cava, and inferior vena cava form the right border of the heart. The left border is outlined by the left ventricle. The inferior border is formed by the right ventricle and a small portion of the left ventricle. The superior border at the base of the heart is formed by the two atria.
- The four chambers of the heart are the right atrium, right ventricle, left atrium, and left ventricle. Blood flows through the heart in this sequence.
- The tricuspid valve is between the right atrium and right ventricle. The pulmonary semilunar valve is between the right ventricle and the pulmonary trunk. The bicuspid, or mitral, valve is between the left atrium and left ventricle. The aortic semilunar valve is between the left ventricle and the ascending aorta.
- The right and left coronary arteries branch from the ascending aorta just superior to the semilunar valve. The right coronary artery descends in the right atrioventricular sulcus to the border and supplies the right atrium.
- The left coronary artery is very short and divides into a circumflex artery and an anterior interventricular artery. These vessels supply the left atrium, left ventricle, and a portion of the interventricular septum.
- Venous drainage of the heart is through veins that empty into the coronary sinus.
- The sinoatrial node is the pacemaker of the heart. From there impulses travel through the atria to the atrioventricular node, then to the atrioventricular bundle and the right and left bundle branches. From the bundle branches the impulses travel to the conduction myofibers and into the cardiac muscle cells of the ventricles.
- The great vessels of the heart are the superior vena cava, inferior vena cava, ascending aorta, and pulmonary trunk.
- From the right atrium, blood flows through the tricuspid valve into the right ventricle and then is pumped out through the pulmonary semilunar valve into the pulmonary trunk and pulmonary arteries to the lungs. From the lungs blood flows through pulmonary veins to the left atrium, then through the bicuspid valve into the left

ventricle. The left ventricle pumps the blood through the aortic semilunar valve into the ascending aorta. From there it is distributed throughout the body.

- The thymus is immediately posterior to the manubrium of the sternum in the superior mediastinum.
- The trachea descends anterior to the esophagus in the superior mediastinum. It divides into right and left bronchi at the level of the sternal angle.
- The esophagus extends from the pharynx at the level of C6 to the stomach in the abdomen. In the superior mediastinum it is near the midline, posterior to the trachea. In the posterior mediastinum it is posterior to the left atrium and anterior to the descending aorta.
- The azygos vein is posterior to the esophagus and to the right of the descending aorta in the posterior mediastinum. The hemiazygos vein ascends on the left

side to the level of T9, then crosses over the midline posterior to the esophagus and descending aorta, to enter the azygos vein.

- The brachial plexus is a network of nerves formed by the ventral branches of spinal nerves C5 to C8 and T1. The musculocutaneous, median, ulnar, axillary, and radial nerves emerge from the brachial plexus to provide innervation to the upper extremity.
- The female breast is composed of glandular parenchyma and connective tissue stroma. Fifteen to 20 lobes of alveoli are capable of producing milk in the parenchyma. The supporting stroma contains varying amounts of fat.
- About 75% of the lymphatic drainage from the breast is through the axillary lymph nodes. Other avenues of drainage are through the parasternal, supraclavicular, and abdominal lymph nodes.

• REVIEW QUESTIONS •

1. What bones form the thoracic cage?
2. Where is the sternal angle relative to the jugular notch?
3. What marks the anterior boundary of the inferior thoracic aperture?
4. What are the three muscles that form thoracic boundaries?
5. Numerous muscles are evident in transverse sections through the thorax; (a) name four muscles in the pectoral region; (b) name two superficial back muscles; (c) name four deep back muscles; and (d) name six muscles in the scapular region.
6. Name five nerves that emerge from the brachial plexus.
7. Where is the pleural cavity (pleural space) located?
8. Indicate whether each of the following is a feature of the right lung or the left lung:
   a. Cardiac notch
   b. Three lobes
   c. Horizontal fissure
   d. Larger volume
   e. Narrow and longer
9. Identify the specific portion of the mediastinum that contains each of the following:
   a. Brachiocephalic veins
   b. Superior vena cava
   c. Descending thoracic aorta
   d. Heart
   e. Esophagus

10. Identify the chamber of the heart described by each of the following:
    a. Posterior chamber
    b. Pectinate muscle
    c. Chamber on the right side
    d. Receives oxygenated blood through pulmonary veins
    e. Most anterior chamber
    f. Forms the apex of the heart
    g. Has the thickest wall
    h. Blood passes through the aortic semilunar valve when it leaves this chamber
    i. Blood passes through the tricuspid valve to enter this chamber
    j. Receives blood from the superior vena cava
11. Where do the right and left coronary arteries originate?
12. List in sequence, from fastest to slowest, the components of the conduction system of the heart.
13. What are the three branches of the aortic arch?
14. List in sequence, from right to left, the three large vessels at the base of the heart.
15. What is the function of the azygous vein?

• CHAPTER QUIZ •

Name the Following:

1. The junction between the manubrium and body of the sternum
2. The anterior boundary of the inferior thoracic aperture
3. The layer of the heart wall that contains cardiac muscle
4. The two major branches of the left coronary artery
5. The most posterior chamber of the heart
6. The pacemaker of the heart
7. The nerve plexus that supplies innervation to the arm
8. The muscles between the ribs
9. The blood vessels that return oxygenated blood from the lungs to the left atrium
10. The most posterior branch of the aortic arch

True/False:

1. The left lung is longer and narrower than the right lung and is divided into three lobes.
2. The middle mediastinum is a subdivision of the inferior mediastinum and contains the heart.
3. The parietal layer of serous pericardium lines the fibrous pericardium of the pericardial sac.
4. The right ventricle makes up most of the right border of the heart.
5. The pulmonary semilunar valve is on the left side of the sternum at the level of the third costal cartilage.
6. The most posterior chamber of the heart is the left atrium, which receives oxygenated blood from the pulmonary arteries.
7. The vessel that passes horizontally posterior to the aorta and the superior vena cava is the right pulmonary artery.
8. The ascending aorta is to the right of the pulmonary trunk.
9. The left bronchus is posterior to the esophagus.
10. The azygos vein drains into the superior vena cava.

Answers to the Review Questions and Chapter Quiz questions can be found at http://evolve.elsevier.com/Applegate/SAlearning/

CHAPTER THREE

The Abdomen | 3

**Anatomical Review
of the Abdomen**
Surface Markings
Osseous Components
Muscular Components
Vascular Components
Peritoneum
Viscera of the Abdomen

Sectional Anatomy of the Abdomen
Transverse Sections
Sagittal Sections
Coronal Sections
Working with Images of the Abdomen
**Important Anatomical Relationships
in the Abdomen**

OBJECTIVES

Upon completion of this chapter, the student should be able to do the following:
- State the boundaries of the abdomen.
- Define the transpyloric, subcostal, transumbilical, interiliac, median, and midclavicular planes and then use these planes to divide the abdomen into four quadrants and nine regions.
- Describe the features of lumbar vertebrae.
- Describe the structure of the diaphragm, name and give the vertebral levels of the three major openings in the diaphragm, and identify the structures that pass through each opening.
- Name the four muscles that form the anterolateral abdominal wall and the three muscles associated with the posterior abdominal wall.
- Discuss the topography of the posterior abdominal wall and the effect this has on organ position and fluid accumulation.
- State the level of origin of the visceral branches of the abdominal aorta and identify the regions each one supplies.
- Identify and trace the pathway of the tributaries of the inferior vena cava.
- Trace the pathway of blood through the hepatic portal system of veins.
- Discuss the peritoneum and its extensions, including mesentery, omenta, ligaments, and cul-de-sacs.
- Discuss the structure and relationships of the liver, including its lobar subdivisions and blood supply.
- Discuss the visceral relationships of the gallbladder.
- Describe the external features of the stomach, its peritoneal extensions, its relationships, and its blood supply.
- Name the regions of the small intestine and discuss the relationships of each region.
- Identify the regions of the large intestine and discuss the relationships of each region.
- Describe the location of the spleen and its relationship to other organs.
- Discuss the location and relationships of the head, neck, body, and tail of the pancreas.
- Describe the location and relationships of the kidneys, ureters, and suprarenal glands.
- Identify the abdominal viscera, muscles, and blood vessels on transverse, sagittal, and coronal sections.

Key Terms, Structures, and Features to Be Identified and/or Described

Abdominal aorta
Aortic hiatus
Aponeurosis
Ascending colon
Caudate lobe
Caval hiatus
Celiac trunk
Common hepatic artery
Descending colon

Diaphragm
Duodenum
Epigastric region
Esophageal hiatus
Esophagus
External iliac artery
External iliac vein
External oblique muscle
Falciform ligament

Gallbladder
Gastroduodenal artery
Gonadal vessels
Greater omentum
Hepatic artery
Hepatic ducts
Hepatic flexure of the colon
Hepatic portal vein
Hypochondriac region

Hypogastric region	Middle sacral artery	Right gastric artery
Ileum	Omentum	Sigmoid colon
Iliac crest	Pancreas, head, neck, body, tail	Small intestine
Iliac region	Pancreatic duct	Spleen
Iliacus muscle	Peritoneum	Splenic artery
Inferior mesenteric artery	Portal triad	Splenic flexure of the colon
Inferior mesenteric vein	Psoas major muscle	Splenic vein
Inferior vena cava	Quadrate lobe	Stomach
Interiliac plane	Quadratus lumborum muscle	Subcostal plane
Internal iliac artery	R & L common iliac arteries	Superior mesenteric artery
Internal iliac vein	R & L common iliac veins	Superior mesenteric vein
Internal oblique muscle	R & L hepatic veins	Superior pelvic aperture
Jejunum	R & L kidneys	Transpyloric plane
Left branch of the portal vein	R & L lobes of the liver	Transtubercular plane
Left gastric artery	R & L renal arteries	Transumbilical plane
Lesser omentum	R & L renal veins	Transverse colon
Ligamentum teres	R & L suprarenal arteries	Transversus abdominis muscle
Ligamentum venosum	R & L suprarenal glands	Umbilical region
Linea alba	R & L suprarenal veins	Umbilicus
Lumbar region	Rectum	Ureter
Mesentery	Rectus abdominis muscles	
Midclavicular plane	Retroperitoneal	

Anatomical Review of the Abdomen

Surface Markings

The ventral body cavity is divided into two distinct subdivisions that are separated by the dome-shaped diaphragm (Fig. 3-1). The upper portion, superior to the diaphragm, is the thoracic cavity. The lower portion, inferior to the diaphragm, is the abdominopelvic cavity. For the sake of convenience, the large abdominopelvic cavity may be divided into an upper abdominal cavity and a lower pelvic cavity. This is an artificial division, because no partition separates the two cavities, and some structures may move from one region to the other.

Boundaries. The **abdominal cavity,** the upper portion of the abdominopelvic cavity, extends from the **diaphragm** superiorly to the **superior pelvic aperture** inferiorly. Because the dome of the diaphragm extends superiorly under the ribs to the level of the fifth intercostal space, the contents of the superior portion of the abdominal cavity are protected by the thoracic cage. Portions of the liver, stomach, and spleen are in this region. Inferiorly, the large wings, or **alae,** of the iliac bones offer some protection for the soft tissue. The superior peripheral boundaries are the **xiphoid process** of the sternum and the sloping **costal cartilages** of the false ribs. The inferior peripheral margins of the cavity are the **iliac crest, inguinal ligament,** and **symphysis pubis.** The iliac crest is the highest portion, or margin, of the ilium bone, and it terminates anteriorly in the anterior-superior iliac spine. The inguinal ligament is the folded inferior margin of the broad, flat tendon, or **aponeurosis,** of the **external oblique muscle.** This ligament extends from the anterior-superior iliac spine to the pubic tubercle, a small elevation about 2 cm lateral to the

pubic symphysis. Just superior to the pubic tubercle, an opening in the aponeurosis forms the inguinal canal.

Umbilicus. The most obvious surface marking on the anterior abdominal wall is the **umbilicus,** or navel. The umbilicus is the scar that results from the closure of the umbilical cord shortly after birth. It represents the site of attachment of the umbilical cord in the fetus. The position of the umbilicus varies, depending on such factors as muscle tone, obesity, body build, and age. In general, however, it is located at the level of the intervertebral disc between the third and fourth lumbar vertebrae.

Linea Alba. When the skin of the abdomen is removed, a light-colored line that extends from the xiphoid process to the symphysis pubis is evident. This is the **linea alba,** and its position is indicated on the surface by a shallow groove in the midline. The linea alba is formed by the fusion of the sheets of tendon that extend from the anterolateral muscles of the abdominal wall.

QUICK CHECK

3.1 What muscle forms the superior boundary of the abdominal cavity?

3.2 What is the name of the vertical white line that extends from the xiphoid to the symphysis pubis?

Abdominal Planes. Superficial landmarks are used to identify the various abdominal planes, which are used as indicators of vertebral levels and to describe the location of deeper structures. Vertical and horizontal planes divide the abdomen into regions, which are used to describe the

FIG. 3-1. Divisions of the ventral body cavity.

FIG. 3-2. Vertical planes of the abdominal cavity.

location of organs or, in the clinical setting, the location of pain, tenderness, swelling, or abnormal growths. Five horizontal and three vertical planes are described. These planes are summarized in Table 3-1.

Vertical Planes.   The **right midclavicular plane** extends vertically from the midpoint of the right clavicle to the midpoint of a line joining the right anterior-superior iliac spine and symphysis pubis, or midinguinal point. The **left midclavicular plane** is in the same position as the right midclavicular plane except that it is on the left side. It extends from the midpoint of the left clavicle to the left midinguinal point. The **midsagittal plane,** or **median plane,** is a vertical plane through the umbilicus. It divides the body into right and left halves. These planes are illustrated in Fig. 3-2.

Horizontal Planes.   The **transpyloric plane** is the most superior of the horizontal planes. It is located about halfway between the jugular notch and the symphysis pubis or, more simply, midway between the xiphoid and umbilicus. This plane typically intersects the **pyloric region of the stomach,** which accounts for the name. Passing laterally to the right on this plane gives the location of the **first part of the duodenum** and the top of the **head of the pancreas.** Proceeding farther to the right, this plane intersects the **ninth costal cartilage,** which gives the location of the **fundus of the gallbladder** and then the upper portion of the hilus of the **right kidney.** Going to the left of the midline, the transpyloric plane gives the location of the **neck of the pancreas** and middle portion of the **hilar region of the left kidney.** Usually this plane marks the level of the **first lumbar vertebra.**

A line through the most inferior point of the rib cage gives the position of the subcostal plane, which marks the level of the **third lumbar vertebra.** The subcostal plane intersects the **third part of the duodenum** and **lower border of the pancreatic head.** There is no good method of locating the L2 vertebral level except that it is halfway between the transpyloric and subcostal planes.

TABLE 3-1   **Horizontal and Vertical Abdominal Planes**

Plane	Description	Vertebral Level
Transpyloric	Horizontal plane halfway between the xiphoid and the umbilicus	Indicates vertebral level L1
Subcostal	Horizontal plane through the most inferior point of the rib cage	Indicates vertebral level L3
Transumbilical	Horizontal plane through the umbilicus	Indicates the disc between L3 and L4
Interiliac	Horizontal plane between the highest points of the iliac crests	Indicates vertebral level L4
Transtubercular	Horizontal plane between the tubercles of the iliac crests	Indicates vertebral level L5
Midclavicular	Vertical plane from the midpoint of the clavicle to the midpoint of the inguinal ligament; right and left	
Median	Vertical plane through the umbilicus; divides body into right and left halves	

The transumbilical plane passes horizontally through the umbilicus. In individuals with relatively normal abdominal contour, this marks the level of the intervertebral disc between the third and fourth lumbar vertebrae. The interiliac plane passes through the most superior point of the iliac crests. This plane marks the level of the **fourth lumbar vertebra.** The transtubercular plane passes through the tubercles of the iliac crests. The tubercles are small projections on the crests about 5 cm posterior to the anterior-superior iliac spine. This plane marks the level of the **fifth lumbar vertebra.** The horizontal planes are illustrated in Fig. 3-3.

Abdominal Quadrants and Regions

Abdominal Quadrants. The horizontal transumbilical plane and the vertical median plane divide the abdomen into four quadrants for descriptive purposes. For example, the pain of acute appendicitis usually localizes in the lower right quadrant (see Fig. 1-6 for an illustration of the four abdominopelvic quadrants.

Abdominal Regions. Nine abdominal regions are described using the horizontal subcostal and transtubercular planes and the vertical right and left midclavicular planes. On the right and left sides the regions are, from superior to inferior, the hypochondriac region, the lumbar (or lateral) region, and the iliac (or inguinal) region. The three regions in the midline are, from superior to inferior, the epigastric region, the umbilical region, and the hypogastric region (see Fig. 1-7 for an illustration of the nine abdominopelvic regions).

QUICK CHECK

3.3 What horizontal plane marks the vertebral level L1?
3.4 What are the two planes that divide the abdomen into quadrants?

Osseous Components

The only osseous components of the abdomen are the lumbar vertebrae in the posterior wall. Some abdominal organs extend upward under the thoracic cage, but the components of the thoracic cage are not considered part of the abdomen.

Five large lumbar vertebrae with their intervertebral discs form the skeletal support for the posterior abdominal wall. A lumbar vertebra (Fig. 3-4) has a large body with short, thick, blunt spinous processes. The transverse processes are also thicker than in other vertebrae. The shape of the lumbar vertebrae and discs gives a normal lumbar curvature that is convex anteriorly. This curvature develops during the second year as a child begins to walk and puts increased weight on the lumbar region. An exaggeration of or increase in the convex curvature is called **lordosis.**

The spinal cord within the vertebral foramen ends at the level of the third lumbar vertebra at birth. Because of the different growth rates of the cord and the vertebral column, the spinal cord ends at the level of the **second lumbar vertebra** in the adult. Even though the spinal cord ends at L2, the meninges, subarachnoid space, and cerebrospinal fluid continue to the second sacral vertebra. This is clinically important when a spinal tap is performed to remove cerebrospinal fluid for laboratory examination. The needle is inserted between the third and fourth lumbar vertebrae, or sometimes between the fourth and fifth lumbar vertebrae, to remove the fluid from the subarachnoid space. This minimizes the possibility of damage to the spinal cord. Remember that the location of L4 is determined by the interiliac plane, through the superior points of the iliac crests.

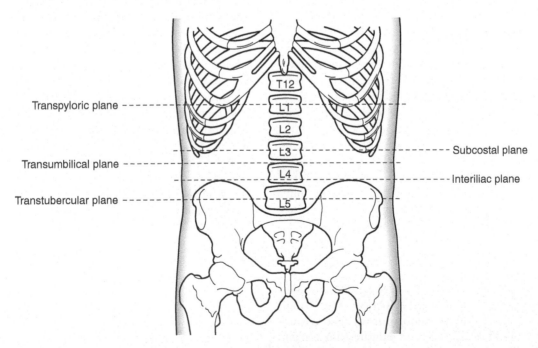

FIG. 3-3. Horizontal planes of the abdominal cavity.

QUICK CHECK

3.5   What bones form the skeleton of the abdomen?
3.6   At what vertebral level does the spinal cord end in
the adult?

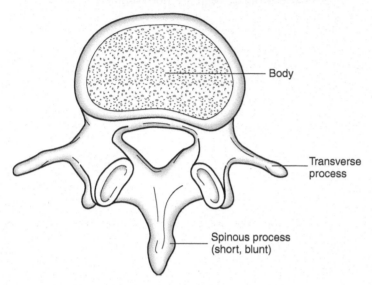

Body

Transverse
process

Spinous process
(short, blunt)

FIG. 3-4. Lumbar vertebra.

Muscular Components

The muscular components of the abdomen include the diaphragm, the muscles of the anterolateral wall, and the muscles of the posterior wall. The musculotendinous diaphragm forms a movable partition between the thoracic and abdominal cavities. The anterolateral abdominal wall is formed by four muscles and their aponeuroses. The posterior abdominal wall is formed primarily by two pairs of muscles and their attachments to the vertebrae, ribs, and ilium.

Diaphragm. The musculotendinous diaphragm extends superiorly under the rib cage to the level of the fifth intercostal space when the individual is supine. Because of the large right lobe of the liver, the diaphragm usually rises to a slightly higher level on the right side than on the left. The central portion of the diaphragm consists of tendinous fibers that form a strong **central tendon.** All the muscular fibers of the diaphragm converge and insert on the central tendon. The muscular portion of the diaphragm is divided into three regions according to the origin of its fibers. A short and narrow **sternal portion** arises from the back of the xiphoid process. The extensive **costal portion** originates from the inner surface of the lower six costal cartilages. These costal muscular fibers form the two domes, or **hemidiaphragms.** The **vertebral** (or **lumbar**) **portion** arises from the upper lumbar vertebrae as a pair of **muscular crura.** Each crus is a thick, fleshy, muscular bundle that tapers inferiorly and becomes tendinous. Fibers from each crus

spread out and ascend to attach to the central tendon. The right crus encircles the esophagus.

Because structures passing from the thoracic cavity into the abdominal cavity must penetrate the diaphragm, its continuity is interrupted by three large and several small apertures. Each opening is called a *hiatus.* At the level of the eighth thoracic vertebra, the wide caval hiatus for the inferior vena cava is located within the central tendon about 3 cm to the right of the median plane. Not only is the caval hiatus the most superior of the three openings, it is also the most anterior. In addition to the inferior vena cava, this opening transmits the right phrenic nerve and lymph vessels. Occasionally, the right hepatic vein passes through this opening before it enters the inferior vena cava.

The oval esophageal hiatus, at the level of the tenth thoracic vertebra, is an opening in the muscular diaphragm posterior to the central tendon. It is 2 or 3 cm to the left of the midline and is surrounded by the right crus of the diaphragm. In addition to the esophagus, the esophageal hiatus transmits the vagus nerve and esophageal branches of the left gastric blood vessels.

The long, oblique aortic hiatus is located between the right and left crura of the diaphragm and begins at the level of the twelfth thoracic vertebra. The aortic hiatus is the most posterior of the three large openings in the diaphragm. Technically, the aorta does not penetrate the diaphragm; rather, it passes between the crura slightly to the left of the midline. In addition to the aorta, this opening transmits the azygos vein and thoracic duct.

Muscles of the Anterolateral Abdominal Wall. The anterior and lateral abdominal wall consists of four muscles and their aponeuroses with a covering of fascia and skin. The muscles, illustrated in Fig. 3-5 and by the computed tomography (CT) image in Fig. 3-6, are the rectus abdominis, the external oblique, the internal oblique, and the transverse abdominis. The skin and muscles of the anterior and lateral abdominal wall are innervated by intercostal nerves.

Anteriorly, on each side of the linea alba, the long, vertical rectus abdominis muscles extend the length of the abdominal wall from the symphysis pubis to the xiphoid process. The rectus abdominis is enclosed in a rectus sheath formed by the aponeuroses of the three lateral muscles.

The outermost layer of the lateral muscles is formed by the external oblique. Fibers of this muscle originate from the ribs and extend downward and medially. Most of the fibers terminate in a broad aponeurosis that inserts on the linea alba, iliac crest, and pubic tubercle. The inferior margin of this aponeurosis forms the inguinal ligament.

In contrast to the external oblique muscle, the fibers of the internal oblique muscle extend upward and medially, perpendicular to the external oblique, from the iliac crest to the inferior borders of the ribs. Medially the aponeurosis of the internal oblique muscle splits into two layers to enclose the rectus abdominis muscle.

FIG. 3-5. Muscles of the abdominal wall.

FIG. 3-6. CT image of the abdominal wall muscles.

The transverse abdominis muscle is the innermost of the three flat muscles. These fibers pass in a transverse or horizontal direction. This arrangement of the three flat muscles provides maximum support for the abdominal viscera and diminishes the risk of tearing of the muscles.

Muscles of the Posterior Abdominal Wall. The paired psoas major and quadratus lumborum muscles, with their attachments to the vertebrae, ribs, and ilium form the musculature of the posterior abdominal wall. The long, thick psoas major muscles are lateral to the lumbar region of the vertebral column. Their fibers originate on the transverse processes, borders, and intervertebral discs of the lumbar vertebrae, pass

along the brim of the pelvis, and enter the thigh to insert on the lesser trochanter of the femur. In transverse sections the psoas major muscles appear as large muscular masses adjacent to the lumbar vertebral bodies. The psoas major muscles are innervated by branches of the lumbar nerves.

The second pair of muscles associated with the posterior abdominal wall is the pair of quadratus lumborum muscles. This thick muscular sheet originates on the iliac crest and transverse processes of the lower lumbar vertebrae and ascends to insert on the transverse processes of the upper lumbar vertebrae and twelfth rib. They are innervated by branches of the lumbar nerves. In transverse sections these muscles appear lateral and posterior to the psoas major muscles. The arrangement of the posterior wall muscles is illustrated in Figs. 3-5 and 3-6 with the anterolateral muscles.

The iliacus muscle is a large, triangular sheet of muscle in the iliac fossa on the medial side of the alae, or wings, of the ilium. It originates in the iliac fossa and inserts with the psoas major on the lesser trochanter. This muscle is a part of the posterior abdominopelvic wall but does not appear in sections of the abdomen. It is located in the false pelvis and is evident in pelvic sections. The iliacus and psoas major muscles are closely associated, and together they often are referred to as the *iliopsoas*. The **iliopsoas** is the most powerful flexor of the thigh.

Examination of the posterior abdominal wall reveals a single longitudinal ridge and two oblique ridges. The **longitudinal ridge line,** sometimes called the *longitudinal divide*, is especially evident in transverse sections (see Figs. 3-5 and 3-6). It is formed by the **lumbar vertebrae,** the **normal lumbar lordosis,** the **psoas major muscles,** the **inferior vena cava,** and the **aorta.** On either side of the elevated longitudinal ridge is a paravertebral groove, or gutter. In superior regions of the abdomen, this groove is occupied by the liver on the right side and the spleen on the left side. The kidneys, ureters, and portions of the colon also are located in the paravertebral grooves. Whenever an organ crosses the midline, it is moved anteriorly because of the elevation of this longitudinal ridge. For example, the right lobe of the liver is rather posterior in position, whereas the left lobe is more anterior because it is moved forward by the longitudinal ridge. The pancreas offers another example of this anterior displacement. The tail of the pancreas is in a relatively posterior position, near the spleen. As the gland courses to the right, it is pushed forward by the longitudinal ridge so that the head and neck are more anteriorly situated.

Inferiorly, the longitudinal ridge divides to form two **oblique ridges** that mark the location of the pelvic inlet. These oblique ridges are formed by the **bony pelvic inlet,** the **psoas major muscles,** and the **iliac blood vessels.**

In addition to influencing organ position, the longitudinal and oblique ridges to some extent determine regions of fluid accumulation. Fluids tend to flow off the sides of the longitudinal ridges to accumulate in the paravertebral "valleys," or grooves. The paravertebral grooves slope posteriorly from the oblique ridges so that fluids tend to flow down the abdominal portions of the oblique ridges and accumulate in the superior regions of the paravertebral grooves when the patient is supine.

QUICK CHECK

3.7   Which hiatus is in the central tendon of the diaphragm?

3.8   What muscle of the anterolateral abdominal wall has fibers that extend vertically from the symphysis pubis to the xiphoid?

3.9   What is the most medial muscle of the posterior abdominal wall?

Vascular Components

Vasculature of the Abdominal Wall. The principal arterial supply of the anterolateral abdominal wall comes from branches of the internal thoracic arteries and the parietal branches of the abdominal aorta. In addition to these, branches of the intercostal and subcostal arteries contribute to the arterial supply at higher levels. All of these vessels branch and anastomose freely. Venous drainage is accomplished primarily through branches of the superficial epigastric and lateral thoracic veins. The posterior abdominal wall is supplied and drained by lumbar arteries and veins. These are direct tributaries of the aorta and inferior vena cava, respectively. Azygos veins also contribute to the venous drainage of the abdominal wall.

Abdominal Aorta and Its Branches. The abdominal aorta begins about 2.5 cm above the transpyloric line at the aortic hiatus in the diaphragm. At this level it is usually slightly left of the midline, but as the aorta descends, it assumes a more midline position. At the L4 vertebral level, marked by the interiliac line, the aorta bifurcates into the right and left common iliac arteries. The branches of the abdominal aorta may be divided into four groups: unpaired visceral, paired visceral, unpaired parietal, and paired parietal. The visceral branches supply the viscera or organs of the abdominal cavity, whereas the parietal branches supply the abdominal wall. The branches of the abdominal aorta are illustrated in Fig. 3-7.

Unpaired Visceral Branches. The unpaired visceral branches of the abdominal aorta are the celiac trunk, the superior mesenteric artery (SMA), and the inferior mesenteric artery. The celiac trunk (artery) is the first major branch of the abdominal aorta. It arises from the ventral surface of the aorta just above the transpyloric line, near the upper margin of the first lumbar vertebra. The celiac trunk is only 1 to 2 cm long before it divides into the **left gastric, hepatic,** and **splenic arteries.** The **left gastric artery,** the smallest branch of the celiac trunk, passes to the left to supply the cardiac region of the stomach and then descends along the lesser curvature. Its branches anastomose with those of the right gastric artery, a branch of the hepatic artery. Intermediate in size, the common hepatic artery is directed to the right and enters the porta of the liver, where it divides into right and left branches. During its course, the common hepatic artery gives off the **right gastric, gastroduodenal,** and **cystic arteries.** The third and largest branch of the celiac trunk is the splenic artery. This long, tortuous vessel passes horizontally to the left, behind the stomach and along the upper border of the pancreas, to enter the hilus of the spleen. As it passes along the upper border of the pancreas, the splenic artery gives off numerous **pancreatic branches.**

The second unpaired visceral branch of the aorta is the superior mesenteric artery. This vessel arises just below

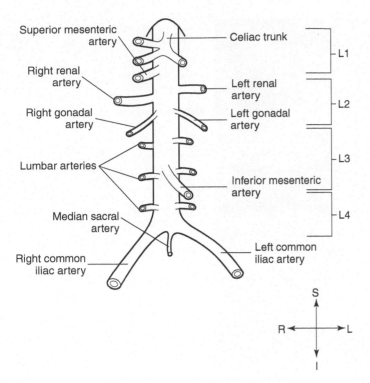

FIG. 3-7. Abdominal aorta and its branches.

the transpyloric line at the level of the lower border of the first lumbar vertebra. It branches and anastomoses freely to supply all of the small intestine except the duodenum. In addition, it supplies the cecum, ascending colon, and most of the transverse colon. At its origin the superior mesenteric artery is separated from the aorta by the left renal vein. The splenic vein and body of the pancreas are anterior to the superior mesenteric artery. The sonogram in Fig. 3-8 and the CT image in Fig. 3-9 show the celiac trunk and superior mesenteric artery as they branch from the aorta.

The third unpaired visceral vessel arising from the aorta is the inferior mesenteric artery. This vessel originates from the ventral surface of the abdominal aorta at the L3 vertebral level marked by the subcostal plane. Near its origin the inferior mesenteric artery descends anterior to the aorta and then curves to the left to supply the distal portion of the transverse colon and all of the descending colon, sigmoid colon, and rectum.

Paired Visceral Branches.   The paired visceral branches of the aorta are the suprarenal, renal, and gonadal arteries. The small **suprarenal arteries** arise from the aorta, one vessel on each side, at the level of the superior mesenteric artery. The suprarenal arteries course laterally and slightly superiorly to supply the suprarenal (adrenal) gland.

A large **renal artery** arises from each side of the aorta at the upper L2 vertebral level, just inferior to the superior mesenteric artery. Each vessel passes laterally at right angles to the aorta and enters the hilus of the kidney on that side. Because the aorta is slightly left of the midline, the right renal artery is longer than the left. As it proceeds to the right kidney, the right renal artery passes posterior to the inferior vena cava, the right renal vein, the head of the pancreas, and the second, or descending, part of the duodenum. The right renal artery is usually at a slightly lower level than the left renal artery, because the right kidney generally is displaced downward by the liver and is at a lower level than the left kidney. As it passes to the kidney, the left renal artery lies posterior to the body of the pancreas, the left renal vein, and the splenic vein. One or two accessory renal arteries may be present. These usually arise directly from the aorta.

The paired visceral **gonadal vessels**, testicular arteries in the male and ovarian arteries in the female, branch from the aorta just inferior to the renal vessels. This places their origin in the lower margin of the second lumbar vertebra. Each testicular artery descends along the psoas muscle and passes over the ureters and the lower part of the external iliac artery to reach the deep inguinal ring, where it enters the spermatic cord. Along with the other contents of the spermatic cord, the testicular artery enters the scrotum to supply the testes. In the female the ovarian arteries descend along the psoas muscle to the pelvic brim. Here they cross over the external iliac vessels to enter the pelvic cavity, where they continue in the suspensory ligament to supply the ovary.

Unpaired Parietal Branch.   The unpaired parietal branch of the abdominal aorta is the **middle sacral artery**. This vessel arises from the posterior surface of the aorta, just proximal to the aortic bifurcation. As it descends along the anterior surface of the L4 and L5 vertebrae, the middle sacral artery gives off a pair of lumbar arteries, which supply a portion of the posterior abdominal wall.

Paired Parietal Branches.   Four pairs of **lumbar arteries** constitute the paired branches of the aorta. These vessels arise from the posterolateral surface of the aorta along the

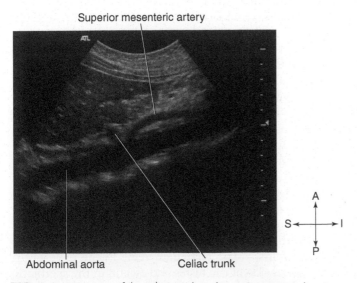

FIG. 3-8. Sonogram of the celiac trunk and superior mesenteric artery.

FIG. 3-9. CT image showing the celiac trunk and superior mesenteric artery.

upper four lumbar vertebrae. Lumbar arteries supply the posterolateral abdominal wall.

Bifurcation of the Aorta.   At the L4 vertebral level the aorta divides into the right and left **common iliac arteries**, which diverge along the bodies of the fourth and fifth lumbar vertebrae. At the level of the disc between the fifth lumbar vertebra and the sacrum, each common iliac artery divides into internal and external branches. The **internal iliac artery** supplies the wall and viscera of the pelvis, perineum, and gluteal region. The **external iliac artery** supplies the lower limb.

QUICK CHECK

3.10   Name the three unpaired visceral branches of the abdominal aorta.

3.11   Name the three paired visceral branches of the abdominal aorta.

3.12   At L4 the abdominal aorta divides into what two vessels?

Inferior Vena Cava and Veins of the Abdomen.   Anterior to the fifth lumbar vertebra, the right and left common iliac veins join to form the inferior vena cava (IVC), which is the largest vein in the body. The inferior vena cava receives tributaries as it ascends through the abdomen along the vertebral column. After passing along the posterior surface of the liver, the IVC passes through the caval hiatus of the diaphragm at the T8 vertebral level. In the mediastinum it penetrates the pericardium to drain into the lower

part of the right atrium. There are no valves in the inferior vena cava, but a rudimentary semilunar valve is located at its atrial orifice.

In general the inferior vena cava is slightly to the right of the aorta. Near its origin at the L5 vertebral level, the inferior vena cava is posterior to the aorta, but as it ascends, it becomes more anterior so that in superior regions of the abdomen, it is anterior to the aorta. As the IVC ascends the abdomen, it is anterior to the right psoas muscle, the right renal artery, the right suprarenal gland, and the right crus of the diaphragm. The inferior vena cava is retroperitoneal and is posterior to the superior mesenteric vessels, the head of the pancreas, and the horizontal third part of the duodenum. Tributaries of the IVC include the common iliac, lumbar, right gonadal, renal, right suprarenal, inferior phrenic, and hepatic veins.

Common Iliac Veins.   Anterior to the sacroiliac joint, the **external** and **internal iliac veins** join to form a **common iliac vein**. The right and left common iliac veins drain the regions supplied by the arteries of the same name. The common iliac veins pass obliquely upward from the sacroiliac joint to the fifth lumbar vertebra, where they join to form the inferior vena cava.

Lumbar Veins.   The **lumbar veins** consist of four or five pairs of vessels that collect blood from the muscles and skin of the abdominal wall. The arrangement of these veins varies. Some drain directly into the inferior vena cava, whereas others may enter the azygos system.

Gonadal Veins.   The **testicular veins** in the male begin on the dorsal side of the testes and ascend in the spermatic cord to enter the abdomen. In the abdominal cavity the veins ascend retroperitoneally along the psoas muscle and anterior to the ureter. On the right side the testicular vein opens directly into the inferior vena cava. On the left side it opens into the left renal vein. The **ovarian veins** in the female follow the same pattern as the testicular veins in the male, except they begin at the ovaries.

Renal Veins.   The **renal veins** drain the kidneys and empty into the inferior vena cava at the L2 vertebral level. They are usually anterior to the renal arteries, because the inferior vena cava is anterior to the aorta at this level. Because the inferior vena cava is to the right side of the midline, the left renal vein is considerably longer than the right. The left renal vein passes posterior to the splenic vein and the body of the pancreas. It crosses anterior to the aorta, just inferior to the origin of the superior mesenteric artery, so that the left renal vein is posterior to the superior mesenteric artery but anterior to the aorta. The sonogram in Fig. 3-10 shows the relationship of the left renal vein to the superior mesenteric artery and the aorta. The left renal vein receives the left gonadal (testicular or ovarian) vein and the left suprarenal vein before it enters the inferior vena cava. The right renal vein is slightly more inferior than the left because the right kidney is lower than the left kidney in position. The right renal vein passes posterior to the second or descending part of the duodenum.

Suprarenal Veins.   The right suprarenal vein is a short vessel emerging from the right suprarenal gland and emptying directly into the posterior aspect of the inferior vena cava. The left suprarenal vein is usually longer and drains into the left renal vein. The arrangement of the suprarenal veins can vary considerably.

Inferior Phrenic Veins.   The inferior phrenic veins drain blood from the inferior, or abdominal, surface of the diaphragm. The left inferior phrenic vein usually joins the left suprarenal vein, but the right inferior phrenic vein generally drains directly into the inferior vena cava.

Hepatic Veins.   The **hepatic veins** drain blood from the liver and return it to the inferior vena cava. The **central veins** of the liver lobules collect blood from the **intralobular venous sinusoids.** The central veins merge to form the hepatic veins, which exit from the posterior surface of the liver and empty immediately into the inferior vena cava. Sometimes the right hepatic vein passes through the caval hiatus before entering the inferior vena cava. The sonogram in Fig. 3-11 shows the right, left and middle hepatic veins as they drain into the inferior vena cava.

Hepatic Portal System.   Blood from the digestive system is carried to the liver by a hepatic portal system of veins before it enters the inferior vena cava. Blood from the inferior mesenteric vein, superior mesenteric vein, and splenic vein enters the hepatic portal vein (Fig. 3-12). In the liver the hepatic portal vein branches until it ends in small, capillary-like spaces, called *sinusoids*, within the liver lobule. From the sinusoids the blood enters the central veins, which merge to form the hepatic veins as described previously.

The inferior mesenteric vein drains blood from the descending colon, sigmoid colon, and rectum. The vessel begins at the rectum and ascends to the left of the inferior mesenteric artery. As it courses upward, it is retroperitoneal and anterior to the left psoas muscle. The inferior mesenteric vein usually empties into the splenic vein posterior to the body of the pancreas.

The superior mesenteric vein collects blood from the small intestine, cecum, ascending colon, and transverse colon. It begins in the right iliac fossa and ascends on the right side of the superior mesenteric artery. Both the superior mesenteric artery and superior mesenteric vein, along with their numerous branches, are enclosed within the layers of the mesentery. The superior mesenteric vein

Superior mesenteric vein   Superior mesenteric artery

Inferior vena cava   Left renal vein   Abdominal aorta

FIG. 3-10. Sonogram showing the relationship of the left renal vein to the superior mesenteric artery and the aorta.

Middle hepatic vein   Left hepatic vein

Right hepatic vein   Inferior vena cava

FIG. 3-11. Sonogram showing the right, left, and middle hepatic veins near their entry into the inferior vena cava.

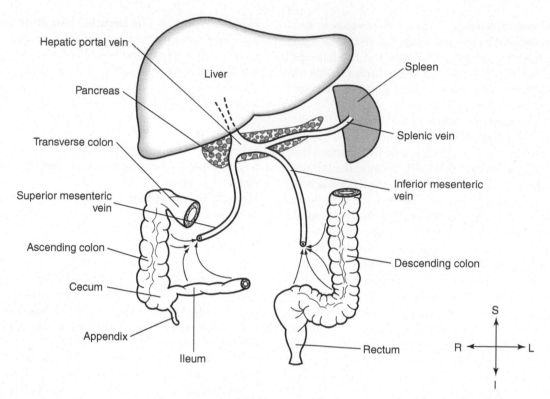

Hepatic portal vein

Liver

Pancreas

Transverse colon

Superior mesenteric vein

Ascending colon

Cecum

Appendix

Ileum

Spleen

Splenic vein

Inferior mesenteric vein

Descending colon

Rectum

FIG. 3-12. Hepatic portal system.

terminates behind the neck of the pancreas, where it joins the splenic vein to form the hepatic portal vein.

Four or five small vessels emerge from the hilus of the spleen and join to form a single splenic vein. As it courses to the right, inferior to the splenic artery and posterior to the body of the pancreas, the splenic vein receives numerous tributaries from the pancreas. The splenic vein

terminates behind the neck of the pancreas, where it joins the superior mesenteric vein to form the portal vein. The CT image in Fig. 3-13 shows the formation of the portal vein.

Some important vascular relationships must be noted in this region. As the splenic vein courses to the right from the spleen to the hepatic portal vein, it passes anterior to

Inferior vena cava

Portal vein

Abdominal aorta

Splenic vein

Inferior mesenteric vein

FIG. 3-13. CT image showing the formation of the portal vein.

the superior mesenteric artery near that vessel's origin from the aorta. As mentioned earlier, at this level the superior mesenteric artery is separated from the aorta by the left renal vein. Sections at this level show, in order from anterior to posterior, the **splenic vein, superior mesenteric artery, left renal vein,** and **aorta.**

The hepatic portal vein is formed behind the neck of the pancreas at the L2 vertebral level by the union of the **superior mesenteric vein** and the **splenic vein.** From this point the hepatic portal vein ascends obliquely to the right, posterior to the duodenum and anterior to the inferior vena cava. It is usually 7 to 8 cm long and is enclosed in the free border of the lesser omentum, along with the hepatic artery and **bile duct.** At the porta of the liver, the hepatic portal vein divides into right and left branches and enters the substance of the liver. Because the left lobe of the liver is more anterior than the right, the left branch of the portal vein is more anterior in position than the right. In the lesser omentum the portal vein is posterior to the hepatic artery and bile duct, and the bile duct is to the right of the artery. The portal vein typically is surrounded by connective tissue, which makes it quite echogenic and easy to identify.

QUICK CHECK

3.13 Through what opening and at what vertebral level does the inferior vena cava pass from the abdomen into the mediastinum?

3.14 What two vessels join to form the inferior vena cava?

3.15 Superior to its formation, what veins drain directly into the inferior vena cava?

3.16 At the level of the origin of the superior mesenteric artery, what is the artery's relationship to the splenic vein and left renal vein?

Peritoneum

The wall of the abdominal cavity is lined with a thin, translucent, serous membrane called the **parietal peritoneum.** This forms a peritoneal sac and a peritoneal cavity, both enclosed within the abdominal cavity, which is delineated by the muscular abdominal walls.

Peritoneal Sac.   During development, some organs of the abdominal cavity protrude from the abdominal wall into the peritoneal cavity and carry a covering of peritoneum with them. The layer around the organs is called the **visceral peritoneum** and is continuous with the parietal peritoneum lining the walls. The space between the two layers of peritoneum is the peritoneal cavity. As the organs continue to develop, the peritoneal cavity is obliterated, leaving only a potential space between the visceral and parietal layers of peritoneum. The two layers of peritoneum are separated only by a capillary film of serous fluid for lubrication. This permits the organs to move against each other without friction. Normally the peritoneal cavity has

a very small volume and contains only a few drops of serous fluid. Abnormal accumulations of serous fluid, called ascites, may exaggerate the volume to form a real space of several liters in volume. In males the peritoneal cavity is a closed cavity, but in females it communicates with the exterior through the uterine tubes, uterus, and vagina.

Terminology Relating to the Peritoneum.   The extent and character of the **peritoneum** are complex, and specific terms are used to describe different parts. **Mesentery** is the double layer of peritoneum that encloses the intestine and attaches it to the posterior abdominal wall in a vertical attachment. Blood and lymphatic vessels, nerves, lymph nodes, and fat cells are found between the two layers of a mesentery. An omentum is a mesentery, or double layer of peritoneum, that is attached to the stomach. The lesser omentum joins the lesser curvature of the stomach and the proximal duodenum to the liver. The space behind the lesser omentum and stomach is the **omental bursa,** or **lesser sac.** The remainder of the peritoneal cavity is the **greater sac.** The omental bursa is closed at the end near the spleen but open at the right edge. The opening into the omental bursa is the **epiploic foramen,** which allows communication between the lesser and greater sacs of the peritoneal cavity. The **hepatic artery,** the **portal vein,** and the **bile duct** are enclosed within the layers of peritoneum at the free margin of the lesser omentum. The greater omentum hangs from the greater curvature of the stomach like an apron over the intestines.

Anything that is not a mesentery or an omentum usually is referred to as a **peritoneal ligament.** These are double layers of peritoneum that connect one organ to another or to the anterior abdominal wall. An example of this is the falciform ligament, which extends from the liver to the anterior abdominal wall. Fig. 3-14 illustrates the continuity of the peritoneum and its extensions, the mesenteries and omenta.

As might be expected, numerous exceptions exist to these generalizations. This is particularly true with the peritoneal attachments associated with the stomach. Although called *ligaments*, many of these actually are a part of the omenta.

Cul-de-sacs.   In certain places peritoneal folds form blind pouches, or cul-de-sacs. The largest of these is the omental bursa, or lesser sac, described previously. In the pelvic region of the female peritoneal cavity, a cul-de-sac is found between the rectum and the uterus; this is the **rectouterine pouch,** or pouch of Douglas. A **vesicouterine pouch** is formed by the reflection of peritoneum from the uterus to the superior surface of the bladder. In males a **rectovesical pouch** lies between the rectum and the posterior surface of the bladder.

Retroperitoneal Structures.   Some organs of the abdominal cavity are not included within the peritoneal sac but are found behind the peritoneum, as illustrated in Fig. 3-14. Their location is described as retroperitoneal. Only the anterior surfaces of these organs are covered with peritoneum. The kidneys, pancreas, duodenum, ascending and descending colon, abdominal aorta, and inferior vena cava are retroperitoneal.

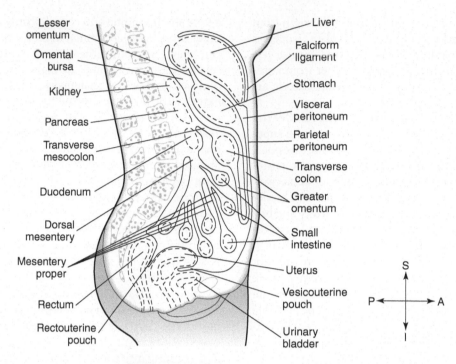

FIG. 3-14. Peritoneum and its extensions.

Viscera of the Abdomen

Liver.   The liver is the largest organ in the abdominal cavity. The large right lobe occupies the right hypochondriac region and fills the right paravertebral groove. From the right hypochondriac region, the liver extends across the epigastric region into the left hypochondriac region. As the liver mass extends across the midline, it is moved forward by the longitudinal ridge line, therefore the smaller left lobe is positioned more anteriorly.

Surfaces and Aspects.   The anterior, superior, and posterior aspects of the liver are related to the diaphragm and follow its configuration. The convex superior aspect usually bulges upward more on the right side than on the left. The inferior (or visceral) surface is flatter than the superior aspect but has depressions where it is in contact with the abdominal viscera. The inferior surface is not in a horizontal plane; rather, it is situated at a 45-degree angle to both the longitudinal and horizontal planes, so that the more inferior portions are more anteriorly positioned and the superior portions are more posteriorly located. The visceral surface of the right lobe is related to the right kidney, right colic flexure, gallbladder, and duodenum. The left lobe has a large depression for the stomach and a smaller one for the colon.

Peritoneal Relationships.   Most of the liver is enclosed in visceral peritoneum. An exception to this is a triangular space on the posterior surface, called the **bare area,** that is devoid of peritoneum and is in direct contact with the diaphragm. A deep groove exists in the bare area for the inferior vena cava. As the peritoneum around the bare area is reflected onto the diaphragm, it forms the **cardinal ligaments,** which represent the margins of the bare area.

A small space exists between the visceral peritoneum of the liver and the parietal peritoneum on the diaphragm, both anteriorly and posteriorly. Anteriorly, this space is part of the **greater sac** and is called the **subphrenic recess.** Posteriorly, to the left of the midline, the space is part of the **omental bursa,** or lesser sac (see Fig. 3-14).

On the right side the peritoneum is reflected from the liver over the surface of the right kidney, forming a **hepatorenal recess.** This recess is clinically significant because it represents the most posterior portion of the peritoneal cavity. Fluids and pus tend to accumulate in the hepatorenal recess when the patient is supine.

The lesser omentum from the lesser curvature of the stomach and the first part of the duodenum is continuous with the visceral peritoneum of the liver. The left portion, between the stomach and the liver, is called the **gastrohepatic (hepatogastric) ligament.** The right portion, between the duodenum and the liver, is called the **duodenohepatic (hepatoduodenal) ligament.** To state this another way, the gastrohepatic and hepatoduodenal ligaments make up the lesser omentum. The portal vein, hepatic artery, and bile duct are enclosed within the right margin of the lesser omentum.

The **falciform ligament** is a thin, anteroposterior fold of peritoneum attached to the convex surface of the liver, to the diaphragm, and to the anterior abdominal wall down to the level of the umbilicus. The falciform ligament marks the division between the right and left lobes on the anterior surface.

Configuration of the Visceral Surface. With a little imagination, examination of the inferior (visceral) surface of the liver reveals an H-shaped configuration separating the organ into four distinct regions. In addition to the right and left lobes, a caudate lobe and a quadrate lobe are present. The left arm of the H is formed by the **ligamentum teres** inferiorly and the **ligamentum venosum** superiorly. The ligamentum teres represents the obliterated umbilical vein, which carried blood from the placenta to the liver in fetal circulation. The ligamentum venosum is the remnant of the ductus venosus, which carried blood directly from the umbilical vein to the inferior vena cava to bypass the liver in fetal circulation. The left lobe is to the left of the line marked by the ligamentum teres and ligamentum venosum. The right arm of the H is formed inferiorly by the gallbladder and superiorly by the inferior vena cava. The right lobe is to the right of the line marked by these two structures. The caudate lobe and the quadrate lobe are between the two vertical lines. The crossbar of the H is formed by the porta hepatis, which includes the portal vein, hepatic artery, and hepatic duct. The caudate lobe is superior and posterior to the crossbar (porta hepatis) and the quadrate lobe is inferior and anterior to it (Fig. 3-15). The ligamentum venosum separates the left lobe from the caudate lobe, which is separated from the right lobe by the inferior vena cava. Inferiorly, the ligamentum teres separates the left lobe from the quadrate lobe, and the

gallbladder separates the quadrate lobe from the right lobe. In the central region, the caudate lobe is separated from the quadrate lobe by the porta hepatis.

A superficial anatomical examination indicates that the caudate and quadrate lobes are part of the right lobe. The falciform ligament anteriorly and the ligamenta teres and venosum posteriorly mark the surface division between the right and left lobes. An investigation of the internal morphology and vasculature reveals that functionally the caudate and quadrate lobes are more closely related to the left lobe than to the right.

Blood Supply. Blood is brought to the liver by the **hepatic artery** and the **hepatic portal vein.** Approximately 70% of the blood supply to the liver is nutrient-rich venous blood from the digestive system brought to the liver by the hepatic portal vein. The remaining 30% is oxygenated blood supplied by the hepatic artery. The blood passes through the **sinusoids of the liver** to enter the **central vein** of a liver lobule. The central veins converge to form **hepatic veins,** which transport the blood to the inferior vena cava.

QUICK CHECK

3.19　What anatomical structure marks the division between the right and left lobes of the liver on the anterior surface?

3.20　On the visceral surface of the liver, what separates the posterior caudate lobe from the more anterior quadrate lobe?

3.21　What two vessels bring blood into the liver? Which has a higher oxygen content?

Gallbladder. The gallbladder is a saclike reservoir for bile. It lies along the right edge of the quadrate lobe of the liver, as illustrated in Fig. 3-15. For descriptive purposes, it may be divided into the fundus, the body, and the neck. The fundus is the inferior extremity of the sac that usually protrudes from the inferior margin of the liver. It is in contact with the anterior abdominal wall, duodenum, and transverse colon. The body extends upward from the fundus and is in direct contact with the visceral surface of the liver. It is also related to the duodenum and transverse colon. The neck is a narrow, constricted portion directed toward the porta of the liver. It is continuous with the cystic duct, which joins the hepatic duct to form the common bile duct. A hormonal feedback system controls the flow of bile from the common bile duct into the duodenum.

Esophagus. Most of the esophagus lies is the thoracic cavity, with only the terminal portion located in the abdomen. The portion of the esophagus in the thoracic cavity lies anterior to the vertebral column and to the right of the descending aorta. At the T7 vertebral level, it deviates to the left, passing anterior to the aorta, on its way to the stomach. After penetrating the diaphragm at the T10 vertebral level, the abdominal portion of the esophagus forms

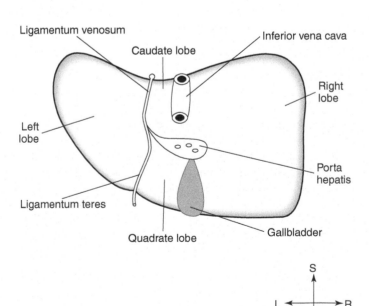

FIG. 3-15. Configuration of the visceral surface of the liver.

a groove in the left portion of the liver and enters the stomach at the **cardiac orifice.** The right margin of the esophagus is continuous with the lesser curvature of the stomach. A **cardiac notch** separates the left margin of the esophagus from the fundus of the stomach. The **lower esophageal sphincter** at the cardiac orifice slows the passage of food from the esophagus into the stomach and also prevents reflux of gastric contents into the esophagus.

Stomach.   The stomach pulverizes food and mixes it with gastric juice. It is located in the upper left quadrant of the abdomen. Under normal conditions the stomach cannot be palpated because the walls are rather flat and flabby. However, because the walls are distensible, the size and shape of the stomach varies with circumstances. Figure 3-16 illustrates features of the stomach.

Curvatures.   The stomach has two curvatures. The concave **lesser curvature** is directed to the right and superiorly. It is continuous with the right margin of the esophagus. The **greater curvature** is convex and forms the left and inferior margins of the stomach.

Regions.   For descriptive purposes, the stomach is divided into four regions. The limited **cardiac portion** lies adjacent to the cardiac orifice, where the esophagus enters. The **fundus** is the rounded portion above the gastroesophageal junction. The major portion is the **body** of the stomach, which is between the fundus and the pyloric region. The distal portion, which empties into the small intestine, is the **pyloric region.** The junction of the body and the pyloric region is marked by the **angular notch,** or **incisura angularis,** a notch on the lesser curvature. The pyloric region is divided into a wider portion, the **pyloric antrum,** and a narrow **pyloric canal.** The sphincter region at the orifice between the stomach and the duodenum is the **pylorus.** The radiograph in Fig. 3-17 illustrates the regions of the stomach.

Peritoneal Relationships.   The stomach is completely covered by peritoneum and is attached to other organs by peritoneal folds and ligaments. The **gastrohepatic portion**

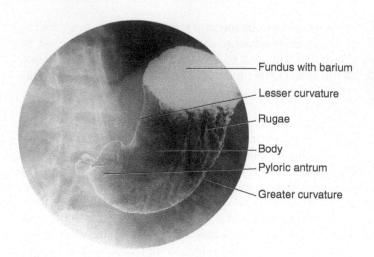

FIG. 3-17. Contrast-enhanced radiograph of the stomach. (Modified from Weir J, Abrahams PH: *Imaging atlas of human anatomy,* ed 3, St Louis, 2003, Elsevier/Mosby.)

of the lesser omentum radiates from the lesser curvature to attach to the liver. From the inferior and left greater curvature, the **greater omentum** falls like an apron over the intestines. A portion of the greater omentum is attached to the transverse colon and is called the **gastrocolic ligament.** The anterior surface of the stomach is related to the diaphragm, left lobe of the liver, and anterior abdominal wall. The posterior surface is related to many abdominal viscera, including the spleen, left kidney and suprarenal gland, pancreas, and transverse colon.

Blood Supply.   All three branches of the celiac trunk contribute to the vasculature of the stomach. The **left gastric artery** is the smallest branch of the celiac trunk. It courses to the left along the lesser curvature, giving off branches along the way, to supply that region. The **right gastric** and **right gastroepiploic arteries** are branches of the common hepatic artery. The splenic artery contributes the **left gastroepiploic artery** and numerous short **gastric arteries.** The veins of the stomach follow the same pattern as the arteries, both in name and distribution. The venous blood from the stomach, like blood from other parts of the digestive tract, is taken to the liver by way of the hepatic portal vein, but the way gastric veins enter the portal system varies considerably. From the liver, the blood enters the hepatic veins, which carry it to the inferior vena cava.

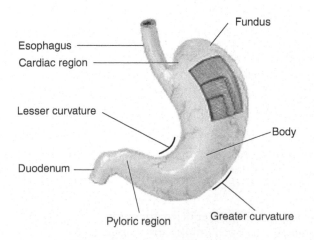

Esophagus
Cardiac region
Fundus
Lesser curvature
Body
Duodenum
Pyloric region
Greater curvature

FIG. 3-16. Features of the stomach.

QUICK CHECK
3.22   What lobe of the liver is marked on the right margin by the gallbladder?
3.23   At what vertebral level does the esophagus penetrate the diaphragm?
3.24   What region of the stomach typically is most superior?
3.25   What peritoneal structure is attached to the left and inferior margins of the stomach?

Small Intestine.   Most of the digestion of food and the absorption of nutrients takes place in the **small intestine.** This long, convoluted tube is usually 6 or 7 m long and is divided into the **duodenum, the jejunum,** and the **ileum.** The jejunum and ileum are enclosed in peritoneum and are suspended from the posterior abdominal wall by a vertical fanshaped **dorsal mesentery.** The duodenum is retroperitoneal except for a small portion near the pylorus of the stomach.

Duodenum.   The first part of the small intestine, beginning at the pyloric valve, is the **duodenum.** About 25 cm long, this portion presents a C-shaped pattern as it curves around the head of the pancreas to become continuous with the jejunum. The duodenum is the most fixed part of the small intestine. For descriptive purposes, the duodenum may be divided into four parts, as illustrated in Fig. 3-18.

The **first** (or **superior**) **part** of the duodenum is horizontal, beginning at the pylorus and extending to the gallbladder. Anteriorly, the first part is related to the quadrate lobe of the liver and the gallbladder. The inferior vena cava, portal vein, bile duct, and gastroduodenal artery course along the posterior surface. The inferior border of the first (horizontal) part of the duodenum courses along the upper margin of the pancreatic head.

Posterior to the gallbladder, the duodenum turns sharply downward to become the **second** (or **descending**) **part.** It is against the posterior abdominal wall in the paravertebral groove, along the right side of the first three lumbar vertebrae. As it descends, it is to the right and parallel to the inferior vena cava. As the second part descends, it passes anterior to the hilus of the right kidney and posterior to the transverse colon. The second part, then, is related anteriorly to the right lobe of the liver and the transverse colon; posteriorly to the right kidney, renal vessels, ureter, and psoas muscle; and medially to the bile duct and pancreas. The pancreatic and bile ducts enter the second part.

After descending to the inferior margin of L3 or the superior margin of L4, the duodenum again makes a sharp turn, this time to the left, to become the **third** (or **inferior**) **horizontal part.** As this part extends across the midline, from right to left, it is moved anteriorly by the longitudinal ridge. As it courses horizontally, the third part passes anterior to the inferior vena cava, aorta, right ureter, right gonadal vessels, and psoas muscles but posterior to the superior mesenteric vessels. Superiorly, this part is related to the pancreas and inferiorly to coils of the jejunum.

The **fourth** (or **ascending**) **part** ascends anterior and slightly to the left of the aorta. In addition to the aorta, the fourth part is related on its posterior aspect to the left psoas muscle and left renal and left gonadal vessels. To its left are the left kidney and ureter, and to its right is the pancreas. Superiorly, the fourth part is related to the body of the pancreas. The fourth part ascends only to the second lumbar vertebra and ends abruptly in the duodenojejunal flexure. This flexure is directed anteriorly and is attached to the posterior abdominal wall by a fibromuscular band called the *suspensory muscle* of the duodenum, or the *ligament of Treitz.* The radiograph in Fig. 3-19 illustrates the regions of the duodenum.

Jejunum.   The second division of the small intestine is the jejunum. This is a tightly coiled tube that begins at the duodenojejunal flexure and continues until it imperceptibly changes into the ileum. Most of the jejunum is located in the umbilical region of the abdomen.

Ileum.   No obvious structural changes occur at the junction between the jejunum and the ileum; however, the tissues that form the wall do change. The mucosa of the ileum lacks circular folds. Accumulations of lymphoid tissue, called *Peyer's patches,* also are evident in the wall of the ileum. Most of the ileum lies in the hypogastric region, with distal parts usually in the pelvis. The ileum terminates in the right iliac region by opening into the cecum through the ileocecal valve.

Both the ileum and the jejunum are enclosed in peritoneum and are suspended from the posterior abdominal wall by vertical fan-shaped folds of mesentery. The duodenojejunal flexure and the ileocecal valve are fixed points, but between these two points the jejunum and ileum are highly mobile and fill any available space in the abdominopelvic cavity. Because of their mobility, the jejunum and the ileum are the regions frequently involved in hernias.

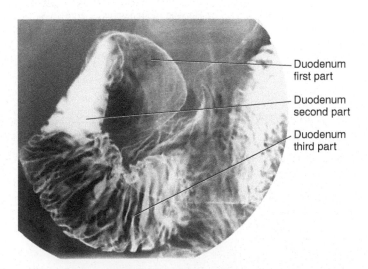

FIG. 3-19. Contrast-enhanced radiograph of the duodenum. (Modified from Weir J, Abrahams PH: *Imaging atlas of human anatomy,* ed 3, St Louis, 2003, Elsevier/Mosby.)

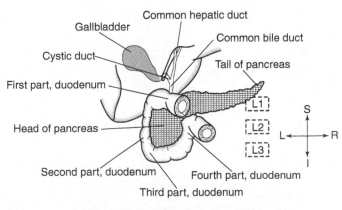

FIG. 3-18. Divisions of the duodenum.

QUICK CHECK

3.26 What portion of the small intestine encloses the head of the pancreas?

3.27 What regions of the small intestine are enclosed in peritoneum and are highly mobile?

Large Intestine. The large intestine extends from the ileocecal valve to the anus, a length of approximately 1.5 m. It consists of the cecum, colon, rectum, and anal canal (Fig. 3-20). The large intestine forms an arch for the loops of small intestine. Fig. 3-21 is a radiograph of the large intestine after barium application; it also illustrates the regions of the large intestine.

Cecum. Located in the right iliac region of the abdominopelvic cavity, the **cecum** is a blind saclike pouch that extends 5 to 7 cm below the ileocecal valve. The vermiform appendix is a blind tubular projection from the cecum. Although the position of the appendix varies considerably, it is commonly inferior and posterior to the cecum. The cecum is retroperitoneal and has no mesentery.

Ascending Colon. From the cecum, the large intestine passes superiorly on the right side of the abdominal cavity to the liver. When it reaches the visceral surface of the liver, the ascending colon bends sharply to the left in the right colic flexure, or hepatic flexure. The ascending colon lies on the posterior abdominal wall, where it is separated from the muscles by the right kidney. It is retroperitoneal and has no mesentery.

Transverse Colon. The transverse colon extends across the abdomen from the right colic (hepatic) flexure to the **left colic (splenic) flexure.** It is the longest part of the large intestine. Suspended by a mesentery, the **transverse**

mesocolon, the transverse colon is the most movable part of the large intestine. Between the two flexures the position of the transverse colon is variable, but it typically forms a loop that is directed inferiorly. This loop may be on the transpyloric plane or may extend down to the pelvic brim. As the transverse colon extends across the abdominal cavity, it becomes more superior and more posterior, therefore the **splenic flexure** is the most superior part of the large intestine and is also relatively posterior in position. At the left colic (splenic) flexure, the large intestine turns sharply downward and becomes the descending colon.

Descending Colon. The descending **colon** extends form the left colic flexure to the iliac crest. As it descends, it passes along the lateral border of the left kidney. The descending colon is smaller in diameter than either the ascending or transverse colon. It is retroperitoneal and has no mesentery. At the iliac crest, the descending colon becomes continuous with the sigmoid colon.

Sigmoid Colon. The sigmoid colon begins at the pelvic brim, crosses the sacrum, and then curves to the midline at the third sacral segment. It is enclosed in peritoneum and has a long mesentery, the **sigmoid mesocolon.** Because of its mesentery, the sigmoid colon is movable. It usually is located in the pelvis but may extend upward into the abdomen.

Rectum. The **rectum** extends from the third sacral segment to the pelvic diaphragm just below the tip of the coccyx, a length of about 12 cm. Here the rectum turns dorsally to become the anal canal. The rectum is partially covered with peritoneum but has no mesentery, therefore it is considered to be retroperitoneal.

Anal Canal. The **anal canal** is 2.5 to 4 cm long and represents the final portion of the intestinal tract. As the canal penetrates the pelvic diaphragm to terminate at the anus in the perineum, it is supported by the **levator ani muscles.**

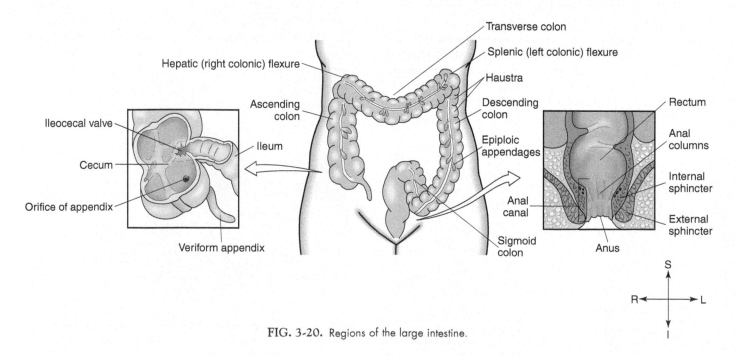

FIG. 3-20. Regions of the large intestine.

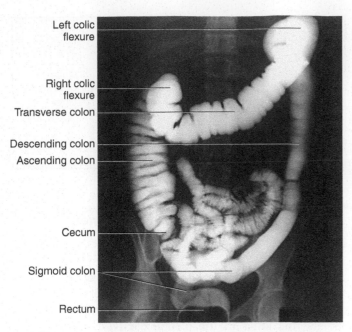

Left colic flexure

Right colic flexure

Transverse colon

Descending colon

Ascending colon

Cecum

Sigmoid colon

Rectum

FIG. 3-21. Contrast-enhanced radiograph of the large intestine. (From Frank ED, Long BW, Smith BJ: *Merrill's atlas of radiographic positioning and procedures,* ed 11, St Louis, 2007, Elsevier/Mosby.)

QUICK CHECK

3.28   Which portions of the large intestine are retroperitoneal?

3.29   The appendix is attached to what region of the large intestine?

Spleen.   The spleen is a highly vascular organ composed of lymphoid tissue that is located in the left hypochondriac region of the abdomen. It is posterior to the stomach and is protected by the ninth, tenth, and eleventh ribs. In addition to the stomach, the visceral surface of the spleen is related to the left kidney and the transverse colon. The hilus of the spleen is closely related to the tail of the pancreas. The spleen is enclosed in peritoneum except at the hilus and is held in place by two peritoneal ligaments. The gastrosplenic ligament attaches the hilus of the spleen to the greater curvature of the stomach, and the lienorenal ligament attaches the hilus to the left kidney. The spleen varies considerably in size and shape, depending on the distention of the stomach and colon. The vascular needs of the spleen are supplied by the splenic artery and vein, which penetrate the organ at the hilus.

Pancreas.   The pancreas is an elongated, soft, pliable gland that has both exocrine and endocrine functions. Because it is covered with peritoneum only on its anterior surface, it is considered to be retroperitoneal. The pancreas extends across the posterior surface of the abdomen from the duodenum to the spleen. For descriptive purposes, it is divided into the head, neck, body, and tail.

The head is the broad, flattened, right extremity of the pancreas, which lies within the curve of the duodenum

(see Fig. 3-18). A small **uncinate process** projects inferiorly and medially posterior to the duodenum, such that it rests on the inferior vena cava and left renal vein. The superior mesenteric vessels are anterior to the uncinate process. The neck is a constricted portion to the left of the head. The splenic and superior mesenteric veins join to form the hepatic portal vein posterior to the neck of the pancreas. The neck merges imperceptibly with the body. As the body of the pancreas extends to the left and superiorly across the aorta, its posterior surface is related to the superior mesenteric artery, splenic artery and vein, left suprarenal (adrenal) gland, and left kidney with its vessels. It is separated from the stomach by the omental bursa. The tail of the pancreas is the left extremity, which is close to the hilus of the spleen. The tail is the most superior and posterior portion of the pancreas.

The main pancreatic duct, or **duct of Wirsung,** begins in the tail of the pancreas, runs through the substance of the gland, and then empties into the descending second part of the duodenum. Blood supply is by way of the splenic artery, which is a branch of the celiac trunk. The splenic vein carries blood from the spleen to the hepatic portal circulation before it returns to the inferior vena cava.

Kidneys

Location and Position.   The **kidneys** are paired, reddish brown, bean-shaped organs just below the diaphragm in the superior part of the paravertebral grooves. They are behind the peritoneum (retroperitoneal) along the posterior body wall, against the psoas muscle, and adjacent to the vertebral column. The superior part of each kidney is protected by the ribs. Each adult kidney is approximately 12 cm long and 6 cm wide and extends from the level of the twelfth thoracic vertebra to the third lumbar vertebra. This level changes during respiratory movements and with changes in posture. Because it is pushed down by the liver, the right kidney is generally slightly lower than the left. A cushion of **perirenal fat** surrounds each kidney, and the ribs, muscles, and intestines serve as protective barriers. Occasionally a kidney slips from its normal position and is no longer held securely in place by adjacent organs or its covering of fat. This condition is known as *floating kidney,* or ptosis, and may cause a kinking or twisting of the ureter, with subsequent obstruction of urine flow. In addition, the kidneys become more susceptible to physical trauma when they drop below the rib cage.

Hilus.   The region where the blood vessels enter and leave and where the ureter begins its descent to the urinary bladder is called the **hilus of the kidney.** The hilus is generally at the level of the transpyloric plane, with the plane intersecting the midhilar region of the left kidney and the upper hilar region of the right kidney.

Relationships.   On its posterior (or dorsal) surface, the kidney is related to the diaphragm superiorly and to the quadratus lumborum and psoas muscles inferiorly. The CT image in Fig. 3-22 shows some of the relationships of the

FIG. 3-22. CT image showing some of the relationships of the kidney to surrounding structures.

kidneys to surrounding structures. The anterior and medial surface of the superior pole of each kidney is covered by a **suprarenal (adrenal) gland.**

The anterior (or ventral) relationships are different for the right and left kidneys. On the right, the kidney forms a renal impression on the visceral surface of the liver. The second (or descending) part of the duodenum descends across the hilar region, and the right colic (hepatic) flexure of the colon covers the inferior pole of the kidney. The anterior (or ventral) surface of the left kidney is related to the left suprarenal gland, stomach, pancreas, spleen, left colic (splenic) flexure, and coils of the small intestine.

Ureters.   The **ureters** are muscular ducts that transport urine from the kidneys to the urinary bladder. Originating at the renal pelvis, the ureters descend retroperitoneally along the psoas muscle. The right ureter is in close relationship with the inferior vena cava as it descends. The abdominal portion of the ureter crosses the pelvic brim and the external artery just distal to the bifurcation of the common iliac artery, then continues as the pelvic ureter to enter the posterior surface of the urinary bladder. The ureter is vulnerable during pelvic and abdominal surgery, because it sometimes resembles a blood vessel and because it is close to the pelvic organs.

Suprarenal Gland.   A **suprarenal (adrenal) gland** lies on each side of the vertebral column in close relation to the superior pole of the corresponding kidney. The suprarenal gland is separated from the kidney by fatty connective tissue. The right gland is somewhat pyramidal in shape, whereas the left is more semilunar. On the right, the suprarenal gland is limited by the liver laterally, the inferior vena cava anteriorly, and the diaphragm medially. The left suprarenal gland is related to the left crus of the diaphragm medially and the left kidney posteriorly and laterally. Anteriorly it is related to the stomach and pancreas. Each gland has an abundant blood supply from the suprarenal arteries, which branch directly from the aorta. Branches of the renal and inferior phrenic arteries also supply the suprarenal glands.

Sectional Anatomy of the Abdomen

Transverse Sections

Sections Through the Upper Abdomen, Level T9.   Transverse sections through the superior regions of the abdomen also intersect portions of the heart in the pericardial sac and the lungs in the pleural cavity, as illustrated in Fig. 3-23. The hiatus in the diaphragm for the inferior vena cava is at vertebral level T8, therefore in this region of the abdominal cavity, the inferior vena cava may be embedded in the substance of the liver. The right and left hepatic veins are short vessels that drain into the inferior vena cava near the caval hiatus in the diaphragm. Fig. 3-23 illustrates the right hepatic vein as it drains into the inferior vena cava. The left hepatic vein is slightly anterior to the right hepatic vein and inferior vena cava, because the left lobe of the liver is positioned more anteriorly. The sonogram in Fig. 3-24 shows the right and left hepatic veins entering the inferior vena cava. The middle hepatic vein drains blood from the caudate lobe.

Sections Through Level T10..   The three most noticeable structures in transverse sections at level T10 are the liver, stomach, and spleen. The relationships of these organs are illustrated in Fig. 3-25 and in the CT image in Fig. 3-26.

The right lobe of the liver fills the right paravertebral groove. The left lobe is moved anteriorly as it crosses the longitudinal ridge to the left side. The falciform ligament attaches the anterior surface of the liver to the anterior abdominal wall and separates the right and left lobes superficially. Posteriorly the bare area of the liver is closely related to the diaphragm. The inferior vena cava is on the posterior surface just to the right of the midline, near the vertebral body. The fissure for the ligamentum venosum separates the caudate lobe from the left lobe. Within the parenchyma of the liver, branches of the portal vein are surrounded by connective tissue.

Fig. 3-25 also shows the esophagus as it enters the cardiac region of the stomach. The stomach is related to the left lobe of the liver anteriorly and to the spleen posteriorly. The lateral surface is next to the diaphragm. The spleen is against the posterior abdominal wall in the left paravertebral groove, posterior to the stomach.

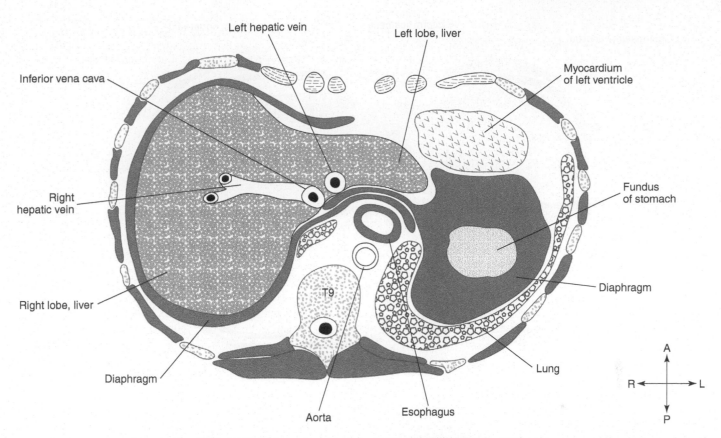

FIG. 3-23. Transverse section through the upper abdomen, level T9.

FIG. 3-24. Sonogram of the hepatic veins.

Sections Through the Porta Hepatis. The relationship of structures in transverse sections through the porta of the liver is significant. The most obvious structure at the porta hepatis is the hepatic portal vein. The portal vein is formed behind the neck of the pancreas and then courses obliquely toward the liver. It is enclosed in the free margin of the lesser omentum. At the porta hepatis, the portal vein is posterior to the hepatic arteries and hepatic ducts. The common hepatic artery, a branch of the celiac trunk, also ascends toward the

liver in the right free margin of the lesser omentum. Near the porta, the common hepatic artery branches to form the right and left hepatic arteries, which are anterior to the portal vein and to the left of the hepatic ducts. In the liver parenchyma, bile canaliculi merge to form progressively larger hepatic ducts until a right hepatic duct and a left hepatic duct emerge from the porta. The hepatic ducts are anterior to the portal vein and to the right of the hepatic arteries. A hepatic duct, portal vein, and hepatic artery make up a portal triad. These

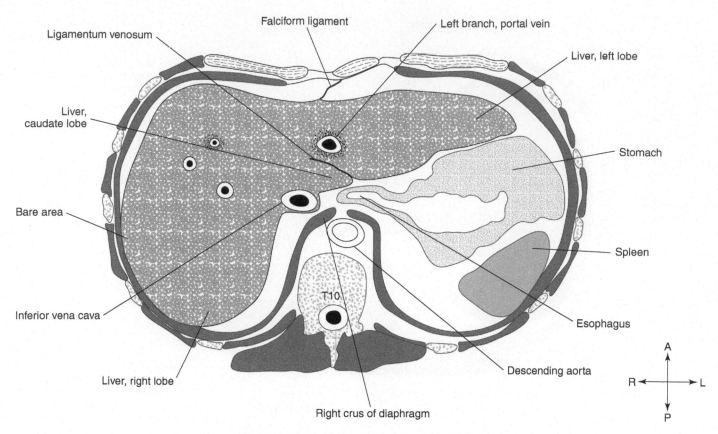

FIG. 3-25. Transverse section through level T10.

FIG. 3-26. CT image through level T10.

triads are visible throughout the parenchyma of the liver and are marked by the connective tissue that surrounds the portal vein. Posterior to the portal vein, a narrow piece of liver, the caudate process, connects the caudate lobe with the right lobe. These relationships are illustrated in Fig. 3-27.

Transverse sections at the level of the porta hepatis may also show suprarenal (adrenal) glands. The right suprarenal gland is somewhat pyramidal in shape. It is limited anteriorly by the inferior vena cava, posteriorly by the kidney, laterally by the liver, and medially by the right crus of the diaphragm. The left suprarenal (adrenal) gland is thinner and more semilunar in shape as it drapes along the margin of the kidney. Anteriorly and laterally it is related to the stomach and the pancreas, and medially it is related to the left crus of the diaphragm. These relationships are illustrated by the CT image in Fig. 3-28.

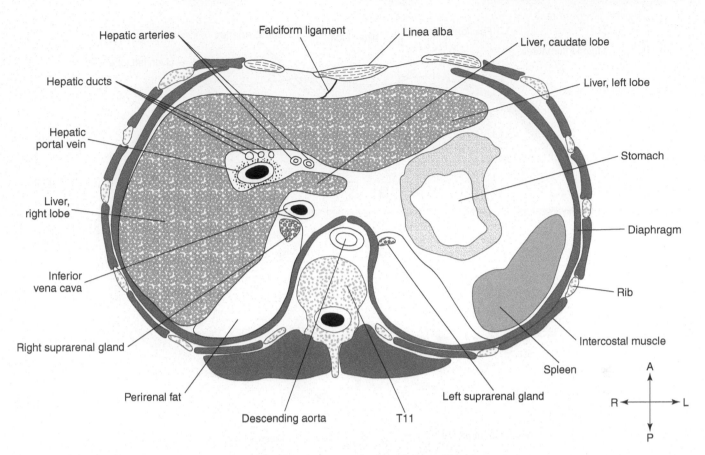

Hepatic arteries — Falciform ligament — Linea alba — Liver, caudate lobe

Hepatic ducts —

Hepatic portal vein —

— Liver, left lobe

— Stomach

Liver, right lobe —

— Diaphragm

Inferior vena cava —

— Rib

Right suprarenal gland —

— Intercostal muscle

Perirenal fat — Spleen

Descending aorta — T11 — Left suprarenal gland

A
R ← → L
P

FIG. 3-27. Transverse section through the porta hepatis.

Ligamentum teres —
Diaphragm right crus —
Hepatic duct —

— Hepatic atery

— Pancreas

Hepatic portal vein —
Inferior vena cava —
Right suprarenal gland —

— Spleen
— Aorta
— T11

FIG. 3-28. Transverse CT image through the porta hepatis and suprarenal glands.

QUICK CHECK

3.34 In transverse sections through the upper abdomen, what vessel is anterior to the inferior vena cava?

3.35 In transverse sections near the T10 vertebral level, what lobe of the liver is between the inferior vena cava and ligamentum venosum?

3.36 What are the relative positions of the vessels and ducts in the porta hepatis?

Sections Through the Gallbladder. Transverse sections inferior to the porta, through the gallbladder, show the anteriorly located quadrate lobe delineated by the gallbladder and the ligamentum teres. Relationships at this level are illustrated in Fig. 3-29. Because the celiac trunk branches from the aorta just above the transpyloric line, which intersects the gallbladder, the trunk or some of its three branches probably will be evident at this level. The tail of the pancreas frequently reaches this level, because it is the most

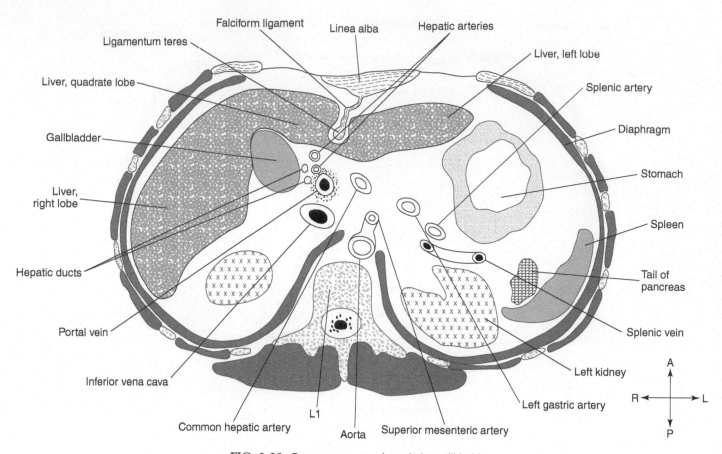

FIG. 3-29. Transverse section through the gallbladder.

FIG. 3-30. Transverse CT image through the gallbladder. (Modified from Bo WJ et al: *Basic atlas of sectional anatomy: with correlated imaging,* ed 4, St Louis, 2007, Elsevier/Saunders.)

superior portion of the pancreas. Fig. 3-30 is a transverse CT image that shows the gallbladder and the relationship of abdominal vessels.

Sections Through L1/L2. Numerous interesting relationships exist at the level of the lower part of the first lumbar vertebra and the upper part of the second lumbar vertebra.

The duodenum becomes evident next to the gallbladder. The head of the pancreas butts against the duodenum. The common bile duct forms a groove along the posterior surface of the pancreatic head, whereas the **gastroduodenal artery,** a branch of the common hepatic artery, courses along the anterior surface. The portal vein is formed posterior to the neck of the pancreas where the splenic and superior mesenteric veins join. These relationships are illustrated in Fig. 3-31.

A classic vascular arrangement evident at the L1/L2 level is also shown in Fig. 3-31. The long left renal vein passes between the aorta and superior mesenteric artery as the vein goes from the left kidney to the inferior vena cava. The left renal vein is anterior to the aorta and posterior to the superior mesenteric artery. The CT image in Fig. 3-32 is at a similar level and shows some of these relationships.

Sections Through the Head of the Pancreas. Fig. 3-33 shows the head of the pancreas between the second and fourth parts of the duodenum. The third part appears in

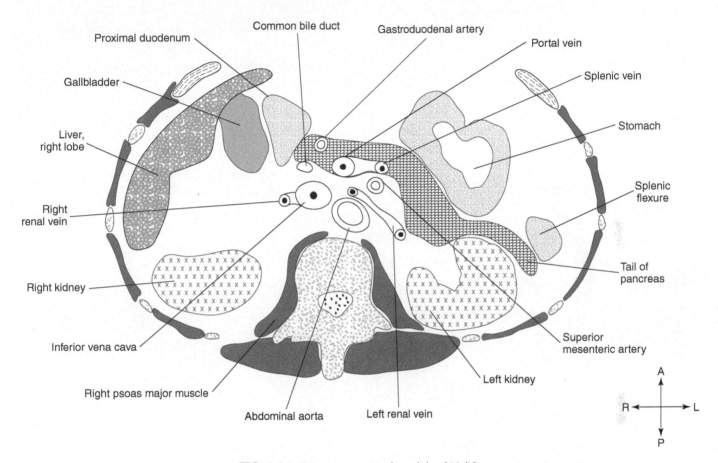

FIG. 3-31. Transverse section through level L1/L2.

FIG. 3-32. CT image through level L1/L2.

sections inferior to this level. The uncinate process of the pancreas projects from the pancreatic head and extends posterior to the superior mesenteric vessels. The descending colon appears in the left paravertebral groove. The larger ascending colon, in the right paravertebral groove, is more anterior than the descending colon. The kidneys are against the posterior abdominal wall and are related to the psoas and quadratus lumborum muscles. Notice also that the aorta and inferior vena cava add height to the longitudinal ridge line. The CT image in Fig. 3-34 also shows some of these relationships.

QUICK CHECK

3.37 In transverse sections through the gallbladder, what is between it and the ligamentum teres?

3.38 In transverse sections at the L1-L2 vertebral level, what vessel is along the anterior surface of the pancreas?

3.39 In transverse sections through the head of the pancreas, what structure is adjacent to the pancreas on the right?

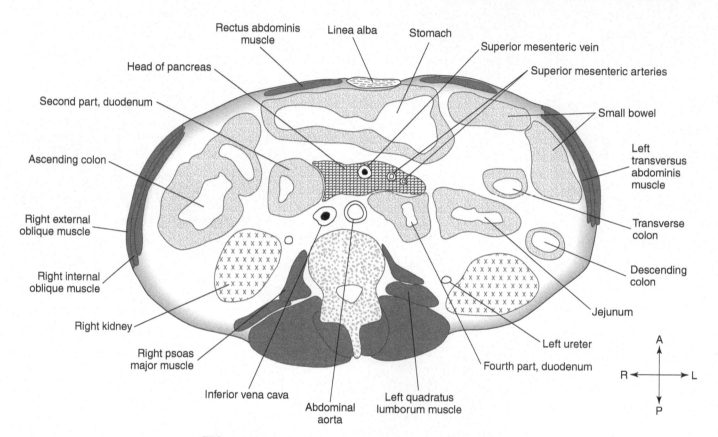

FIG. 3-33. Transverse section through the head of the pancreas.

FIG. 3-34. CT image through the head of the pancreas.

Sagittal Sections

Sections Through the Ascending Colon.   The most lateral sections on the right side of the abdomen show the right lobe of the liver conforming to the shape of the diaphragm and protected by the rib cage. Sections taken 2 cm or so more medially intersect the kidney and ascending colon. Fig. 3-35 illustrates the organ relationships in this region. The predominant structure is the right lobe of the liver. The right kidney forms an indentation on the posterior visceral surface of the liver. The ascending colon extends from the cecum to the hepatic flexure. The quadratus lumborum and iliacus muscles form the posterior wall of the abdomen. Anteriorly the external oblique, internal oblique, and transverse abdominis muscles form the abdominal wall.

Sections Through the Gallbladder. Saggital sections approximately 6 or 7 cm to the right of the midline typically intersect the gallbladder. A large portion of the right lobe of the liver with the right branch of the portal vein is visible. Fig. 3-36 illustrates the relationship of the duodenum to the gallbladder and the kidney. The descending second part of the duodenum is related to the gallbladder anteriorly and rests on the kidney posteriorly. This illustrates the posterior position of the second part of the duodenum. The large psoas muscle, adjacent to the vertebral bodies, is evident in this region.

Sections Through the Head of the Pancreas. Because the head of the pancreas is surrounded by the four parts of the duodenum, it is logical that saggital sections through this region will be medial to the descending second portion of the duodenum but will intersect the horizontal first and third parts. This is illustrated in Fig. 3-37, which shows the first part of the duodenum superior to the pancreatic head and the third part inferior to it. Also in this region, the right suprarenal (adrenal) gland is delineated by the right kidney and liver. The right renal artery and vein course to the right, posterior to the pancreatic head. Sections in this region show the anterior position of the transverse colon and the segmented nature of the rectus abdominis muscle. The porta of the liver separates the caudate lobe posteriorly from the quadrate lobe anteriorly.

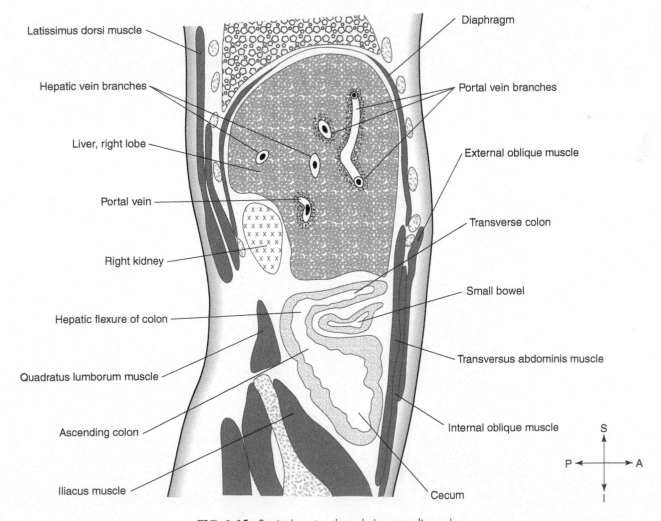

FIG. 3-35. Sagittal section through the ascending colon.

Diaphragm

Latissimus dorsi muscle

Right kidney

Quadratus lumborum muscle

Duodenum, second part

Erector spinae back muscles

Sacrum

Right lobe, liver

Hepatic vein

Portal vein

Gallbladder

Transverse colon

Small bowel

Psoas major muscle

S
P ← → A
I

FIG. 3-36. Sagittal section through the gallbladder.

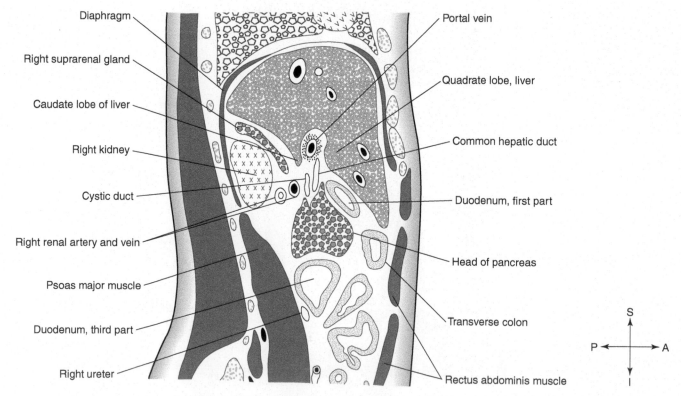

Diaphragm

Right suprarenal gland

Caudate lobe of liver

Right kidney

Cystic duct

Right renal artery and vein

Psoas major muscle

Duodenum, third part

Right ureter

Portal vein

Quadrate lobe, liver

Common hepatic duct

Duodenum, first part

Head of pancreas

Transverse colon

Rectus abdominis muscle

S
P ← → A
I

FIG. 3-37. Sagittal section through the head of the pancreas.

QUICK CHECK

3.40 What is the most predominant organ seen in sagittal sections through the ascending colon?

3.41 In sagittal sections through the gallbladder, what structure is posterior to the gallbladder?

3.42 In sagittal sections through the head of the pancreas, what specific portion of the duodenum is superior to the pancreas and what part is inferior?

Sections Through the Inferior Vena Cava. The inferior vena cava ascends to penetrate the diaphragm and empty into the right atrium of the heart 1 or 2 cm to the right of the midline. Fig. 3-38 illustrates the relationships of the inferior vena cava. It is related anteriorly to the caudate lobe of the liver, the pancreas, and the horizontal third part of the duodenum.

Midsagittal Section. A little to the left of the inferior vena cava, in more of a midline position, the aorta descends along the vertebral column. The classic relationship of the aorta, superior mesenteric artery, and left renal vein is usually evident in this region. Watch for the superior mesenteric artery as it branches from the aorta at approximately a 60-degree angle. The left renal vein is neatly tucked in the angle between the two vessels, as illustrated in Fig. 3-39. The horizontal third part of the duodenum, or possibly the ascending fourth part, is just inferior to the left renal vein. Anteriorly the pylorus of the stomach is related to the inferior portion of the left lobe of the liver.

Left Parasagittal Sections. Proceeding to the left from the midline, the relationships of the liver, stomach, spleen, pancreas, and kidney become evident. Fig. 3-40 illustrates some of these relationships. Centrally located in the superior portion of the abdomen, the stomach is related anteriorly to the left lobe of the liver and posteriorly to the spleen. Just inferior to the spleen, the left kidney rests along the posterior abdominal wall. The body of the pancreas courses to the left posterior to the stomach and anterior to the kidney. The splenic artery and vein are located along the posterior superior margin of the pancreas.

QUICK CHECK

3.43 Is a sagittal section through the inferior vena cava on the right side or the left side of the midline?

3.44 Is the abdominal aorta typically to the right or the left of the inferior vena cava?

3.45 In sagittal sections through the abdominal aorta, what are the relationships of the left renal vein to the aorta and superior mesenteric artery?

3.46 In left parasagittal sections, what is the relationship of the spleen to the stomach and the left kidney?

Coronal Sections

Sections Through the Vertebral Canal. When considering coronal sections of the abdomen, remember the anterior-posterior relationships of the abdominal viscera. Because the spleen, kidneys, and right lobe of the liver are

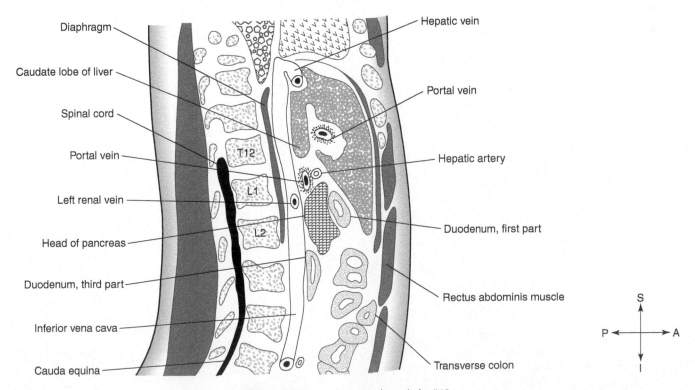

FIG. 3-38. Sagittal section through the IVC.

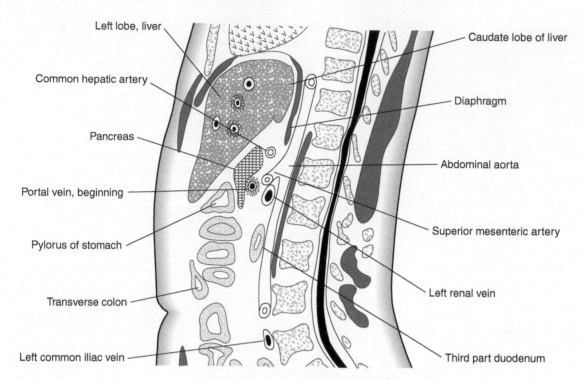

Left lobe, liver

Common hepatic artery

Pancreas

Portal vein, beginning

Pylorus of stomach

Transverse colon

Left common iliac vein

Caudate lobe of liver

Diaphragm

Abdominal aorta

Superior mesenteric artery

Left renal vein

Third part duodenum

FIG. 3-39. Midsagittal section through the abdomen.

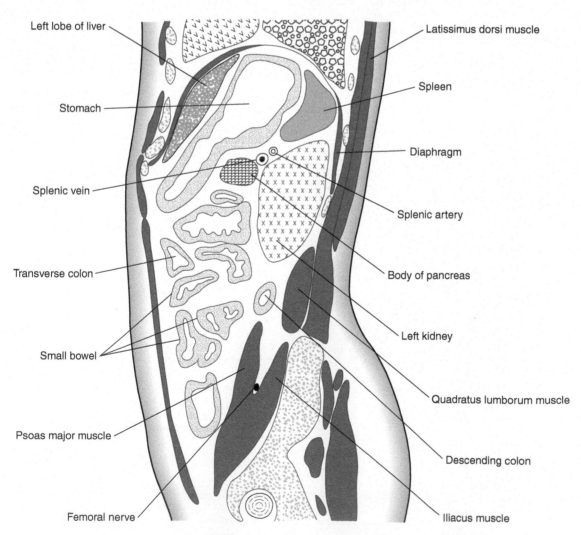

Left lobe of liver

Stomach

Splenic vein

Transverse colon

Small bowel

Psoas major muscle

Femoral nerve

Latissimus dorsi muscle

Spleen

Diaphragm

Splenic artery

Body of pancreas

Left kidney

Quadratus lumborum muscle

Descending colon

Iliacus muscle

FIG. 3-40. Left parasagittal section through the abdomen.

in the paravertebral grooves, against the posterior abdominal wall, they are seen in the most posterior sections. This is illustrated in Fig. 3-41, which depicts a coronal section through the vertebral canal. Fig. 3-42 is a coronal magnetic resonance (MR) image similar to the line drawing in Fig. 3-41.

Sections Through Vertebral Bodies.   Moving anteriorly from the vertebral canal to the vertebral bodies, structures related to the spleen become evident. These include the tail of the pancreas, the stomach, and the left colic (splenic) flexure. The splenic vessels typically are related to the superior margin of the pancreas, therefore whenever any part of the pancreas is present, look for splenic vessels. Posterior sections such as the one depicted in Fig. 3-43 also illustrate the relationship of the kidneys to the psoas muscle. Because lordosis of the vertebral column is normal, coronal sections through lumbar vertebral bodies are more anterior than those through the thoracic vertebrae. The CT image in Fig. 3-44 is similar to the line drawing in Fig. 3-43.

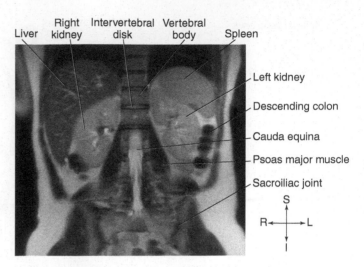

FIG. 3-42. Coronal MR image through the posterior abdomen. (Modified from Bo WJ et al: *Basic atlas of sectional anatomy: with correlated imaging,* ed 4, St Louis, 2007, Elsevier/Saunders.)

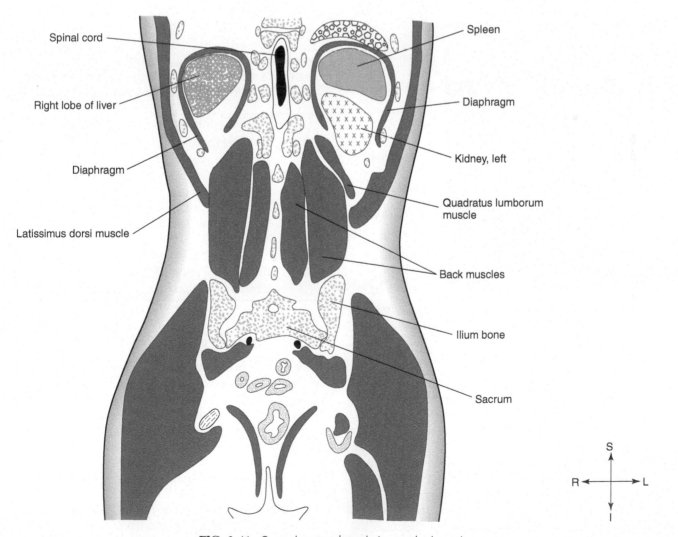

FIG. 3-41. Coronal section through the vertebral canal.

FIG. 3-43. Coronal section through the vertebral bodies.

FIG. 3-44. Coronal CT image through the vertebral bodies. (Modified from Bo WJ et al: *Basic atlas of sectional anatomy: with correlated imaging,* ed 4, St Louis, 2007, Elsevier/Saunders.)

Sections Through the Anterior Abdomen. Anterior sections of the abdomen (e.g., through the gallbladder) are likely to show both the right and left lobes of the liver and the structures related to them. The fundus of the gallbladder is the most anterior part. The body is slightly more posterior and is in contact with the visceral surface of the liver, as shown in Fig. 3-45. The gallbladder is related to the right colic (hepatic) flexure and the right side of the transverse colon. Medially the body of the gallbladder is related to the pylorus of the stomach and duodenum. Because the

pancreatic head is closely associated with the duodenum, it usually is seen in sections with the gallbladder. Coronal sections anterior to the gallbladder show only the liver.

Working with Images of the Abdomen

The transverse CT image in Fig. 3-46 is through the upper abdomen at approximately level T9. The inferior vena cava passes through the caval hiatus at T8 and is now adjacent to the right lobe of the liver. The right and left ventricles of the heart are enclosed by pericardium in the mediastinum. The diaphragm is visible on the left side, and the spleen occupies the left paravertebral groove. The esophagus is posterior to the left atrium and slightly anterior to the aorta.

The transverse CT image in Fig. 3-47 shows the inferior vena cava within the parenchyma of the liver. The caudate

Right lobe of liver

Left lobe of liver

Gallbladder

Stomach

Pylorus, stomach

Pancreas

Hepatic flexure of colon

Transverse colon

Duodenum

Left external
oblique muscle

Ascending colon

Left internal
oblique muscle

Loops of small bowel

Left transverse
abdominis muscle

Cecum

Descending colon

S
R ← → L
I

FIG. 3-45. Coronal section through the anterior abdomen.

Pericardium

Diaphragm

Left atrium

Descending aorta

A
R ← → L
P

FIG. 3-46. Transverse CT image through the upper abdomen.

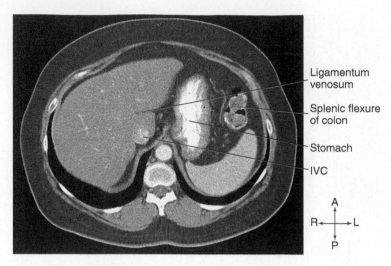

FIG. 3-47. Transverse CT image through vertebral level T10.

lobe of the liver is between the inferior vena cava and the ligamentum venosum. The crura of the diaphragm overlap anterior to the aorta. The spleen occupies the left paravertebral groove. A portion of the stomach is present in the space anterior to the spleen, and the splenic flexure of the colon is anterior to the left margin of the spleen.

The transverse CT image in Fig. 3-48 shows the pancreas with the tortuous splenic artery along its posterior border. Perirenal fat is adjacent to the diaphragm on either side, and a small portion of the suprarenal (adrenal) gland is present.

The CT image in Fig. 3-49 is approximately at the T12 vertebral level. The crura of the diaphragm are separated to form the aortic hiatus. The celiac trunk branches from the aorta and divides into the common hepatic artery, the left gastric artery, and the splenic artery.

The transverse CT image in Fig. 3-50 shows the splenic vein crossing the abdomen along the posterior margin of the pancreas to meet the portal vein. The splenic vein

and the superior mesenteric vein merge to form the portal vein. The superior mesenteric vein is present in images at levels inferior to this. The superior mesenteric artery branches from the aorta in the image.

The transverse CT image in Fig. 3-51 shows the gallbladder separating the right lobe of the liver from the quadrate lobe. Other structures to observe include the portal vein, superior mesenteric artery, superior mesenteric vein, inferior vena cava, aorta, and kidneys. The renal pyramids are clearly evident in the medulla of the kidney. The psoas major muscles are adjacent to the vertebral column, and the quadratus lumborum muscles are posterior and lateral to the psoas. The muscles of the lateral abdominal wall are clearly defined.

The transverse CT image in Fig. 3-52 shows the typical relationships of the left renal vein as it continues from the left kidney to the inferior vena cava. Because the inferior vena cava is on the right side, the left renal vein is longer than the right renal vein. From the left kidney, the

FIG. 3-48. Transverse CT image through the pancreas.

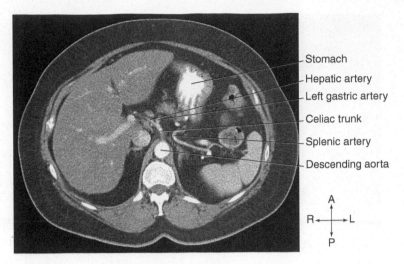

FIG. 3-49. Transverse CT image showing the branches of the celiac trunk.

Stomach
Hepatic artery
Left gastric artery
Celiac trunk
Splenic artery
Descending aorta

FIG. 3-50. Transverse CT image through the splenic vein and the portal vein.

Portal vein
Pancreas
Splenic vein
Superior mesenteric artery
Descending colon
Spleen
Pole of left kidney

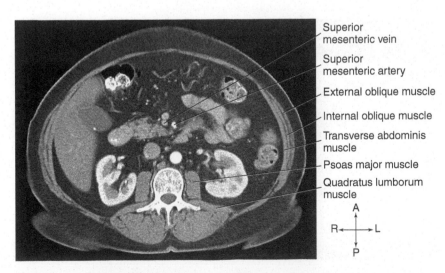

FIG. 3-51. Transverse CT image through the gallbladder.

Superior mesenteric vein
Superior mesenteric artery
External oblique muscle
Internal oblique muscle
Transverse abdominis muscle
Psoas major muscle
Quadratus lumborum muscle

Duodenum,
2nd part

Renal pelvis

Superior
mesenteric vein

Superior
mesenteric artery

Left renal vein

FIG. 3-52. Transverse CT image showing the left renal vein.

vein crosses the midline, where it is anterior to the aorta and posterior to the superior mesenteric artery. The renal pelvis is present in each kidney, and the second part of the duodenum is at the right margin of the head of the pancreas.

Fig. 3-53 shows many of the same features as Fig. 3-52, including the left renal vein, superior mesenteric artery, superior mesenteric vein, duodenum, and head of the pancreas. In addition, this figure shows the right and left renal arteries as they branch from the aorta. The renal arteries typically arise from the aorta at the upper L2 vertebral level.

The transverse CT image in Fig. 3-54 uses contrast to show the renal pelvis. The aorta, inferior vena cava, and numerous branches of the superior mesenteric vessels are present. The three muscle layers of the lateral abdominal wall are clearly defined. Posteriorly the psoas major muscle is adjacent to the vertebral body, and the quadratus lumborum muscle is posterolateral to the psoas.

In the preceding image, contrast medium highlighted the renal pelvis. Fig. 3-55 shows a section inferior to the renal pelvis. The contrast medium highlights the ureters in their typical position along the anterolateral margin of the psoas muscle. The rectus abdominis muscle forms the anterior wall of the abdominal cavity. Numerous loops of bowel fill the cavity. This section also illustrates the longitudinal ridge and paravertebral grooves of the abdominal cavity.

The interiliac line passes through the iliac crests and marks the L4 vertebral level. At this level the aorta typically bifurcates into the right and left common iliac arteries, evident in the CT image in Fig. 3-56. The iliacus muscle lines the ilium, and the gluteus medius muscle is on the posterior surface. The gluteus medius muscle has the most superior origin of the three gluteal muscles.

The coronal image in Fig. 3-57 is derived from a digital reconstruction of sequential axial CT sections. It shows the inferior vena cava as it ascends through the abdomen and

Superior mesenteric
artery

Pancreas, head

Descending colon

Left renal vein

FIG. 3-53. Transverse CT image showing the origin of the renal arteries.

FIG. 3-54. Transverse CT image with contrast to highlight the renal pelvis.

IVC

Right renal pelvis

Descending colon

Quadratus lumborum muscle

FIG. 3-55. Transverse CT image with contrast to highlight the ureters.

Transverse colon

Ascending colon

Rectus abdominis muscle

Left ureter

FIG. 3-56. Transverse CT image at the level of the iliac crests.

Left common iliac artery

Ilium

Iliacus muscle

L4 vertebra

Gluteus medius muscle

FIG. 3-57. Coronal CT image through the inferior vena cava.

— Stomach

— Inferior vena cava

— Descending aorta

Left common
iliac artery

Left common
iliac vein

FIG. 3-58. Coronal CT image through the lumbar vertebral bodies.

Left crus
of diaphragm

Splenic vein

Splenic artery

enters the liver before penetrating the diaphragm to drain into the right atrium. The large renal veins branch from the inferior vena cava. The aorta, to the left of the inferior vena cava, bifurcates into the right and left common iliac arteries. Common iliac veins are also present.

The coronal image in Fig. 3-58 shows the right and left crura of the diaphragm along the margins of the vertebral column. This illustrates the origin of the vertebral portion of the diaphragm. In addition to its vertebral origin, the diaphragm has a narrow sternal portion that arises from the xiphoid and an extensive costal portion that originates from the lower six costal cartilages. This figure also shows the psoas major muscles adjacent to the vertebral column. The liver, spleen, and kidneys are present, and splenic vessels are evident near the spleen.

The coronal CT digital reconstruction in Fig. 3-59 illustrates some significant vasculature of the abdomen. The

splenic vein carries blood from the spleen and pancreas and merges with the superior mesenteric vein that carries blood from the small intestine and part of the colon. This forms the hepatic portal vein, which enters the liver. The inferior mesenteric vein usually drains into the splenic vein.

The aorta and vessels in Fig. 3-60 are digitally reconstructed from sequential axial CT images of the thorax and abdomen. The aortic arch continues into the thoracic aorta, which passes through the aortic hiatus and continues as the abdominal aorta. In the abdomen, the celiac trunk and the superior mesenteric artery are the first two unpaired visceral branches.

The sonogram in Fig. 3-61 shows the common hepatic artery and the splenic artery branching from the short celiac trunk. The common hepatic artery goes to the right to enter the liver, and the larger splenic artery goes to the left to supply the pancreas and spleen. The celiac trunk,

Pancreas

Portal vein

Splenic vein

Inferior mesenteric
vein

Superior mesenteric
vein

Superior mesenteric
artery

FIG. 3-59. Coronal CT image showing the formation of the portal vein.

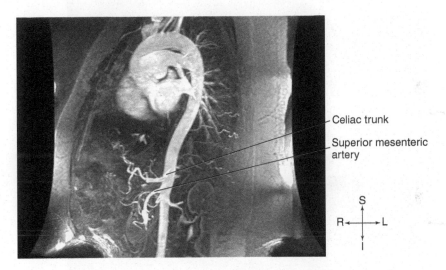

Celiac trunk

Superior mesenteric
artery

FIG. 3-60. "3D reconstruction of sequential axial CT slices showing the aorta with celiac trunk and superior mesenteric artery."

Celiac trunk

Descending aorta

FIG. 3-61. Sonogram of the celiac trunk.

the first unpaired visceral branch of the abdominal aorta, usually arises from the aorta at the upper L1 vertebral level.

The sonogram in Fig. 3-62 shows a sagittal view of the gallbladder with surrounding liver parenchyma. A small gallstone is present in the lumen of the gallbladder.

The sonogram in Fig. 3-63 is from a patient who entered the emergency department with midepigastric and right shoulder pain. The individual also had symptoms of nausea and indigestion. An ultrasound examination revealed multiple small stones in the lumen of the gallbladder. The gallstones cause the classic "shadows" seen in this sonogram. This shadow artifact is also present with the single gallstone in Fig. 3-62.

FIG. 3-62. Sonogram showing a sagittal view of the gallbladder.

FIG. 3-63. Sonogram of a gallbladder with multiple gallstones.

Important Anatomical Relationships in the Abdomen

- The left hepatic vein is anterior to the inferior vena cava because the left lobe of the liver is an anteriorly positioned lobe (see Figs. 3-23 and 3-24).
- The falciform ligament attaches the anterior surface of the liver to the anterior abdominal wall (see Figs. 3-25 and 3-27).
- The caudate lobe of the liver is between the inferior vena cava on the right and the ligamentum venosum on the left (see Figs. 3-15, 3-25, and 3-26).
- The spleen is posterior to the stomach in the left paravertebral groove (see Figs. 3-25 and 3-26).
- The bare area of the liver is in contact with the diaphragm (see Figs. 3-25 and 3-26).
- The right suprarenal gland is limited anteriorly by the inferior vena cava, laterally by the right lobe of the liver, and medially by the right crus of the diaphragm (see Figs. 3-27 and 3-28).
- The hepatic portal vein is anterior to the inferior vena cava (see Figs. 3-27 and 3-28).
- In superior regions of the abdomen, the inferior vena cava is anterior and to the right of the abdominal aorta (see Figs. 3-23, 3-25, and 3-26).
- In the porta of the liver and the free margin of the lesser omentum, the hepatic ducts are to the right of the hepatic arteries (see Figs. 3-27 and 3-28).
- The ligamentum teres is within the inferior free margin of the falciform ligament (see Figs. 3-29 and 3-30).
- The tail of the pancreas is the most superior and most posterior portion of the pancreas and is located next to the spleen (see Figs. 3-29 to 3-31).
- The quadrate lobe of the liver is between the gallbladder on the right and the ligamentum teres on the left (see Figs. 3-29 and 3-30).
- The left renal vein courses horizontally between the aorta posteriorly and the superior mesenteric artery anteriorly (see Figs. 3-30 and 3-31).
- The splenic vein joins with the superior mesenteric vein to form the hepatic portal vein posterior to the head and neck of the pancreas (see Figs. 3-12, 3-13, 3-50, and 3-59).
- The splenic flexure of the colon is posteriorly located on the left side (see Figs. 3-21 and 3-31).
- The head of the pancreas is limited by the second part of the duodenum on the right and by the fourth part of the duodenum on the left (see Figs. 3-18 and 3-31 to 3-34).
- The ascending colon is more anteriorly positioned than the descending colon and is on the right side (see Figs. 3-20, 3-21, 3-33, and 3-34).
- The third part of the duodenum is inferior to the head of the pancreas (see Figs. 3-18, 3-19, and 3-37).
- The ureter courses along the margin of the psoas muscle (see Figs. 3-33, 3-34 and 3-55).
- The abdominal aorta bifurcates into the right and left common iliac arteries at the L4 vertebral level (see Figs. 3-7, 3-56, and 3-57).
- The kidneys are located in the paravertebral grooves along the posterior abdominal wall (see Figs. 3-29 to 3-34).

Pathology

Hypertrophic Pyloric Stenosis

Hypertrophic pyloric stenosis is a congenital anomaly in which the pyloric canal is narrow because of a thickening of the pyloric sphincter. The initial sign is vomiting, at first mild then becoming more severe and projectile. The infant cries because of hunger, cramping, and constipation.

Intussusception

Intussusception is the prolapse of one part of the bowel into an adjacent distal region causing an obstruction. Most cases occur in children. If not treated, the bowel will become gangrenous because the blood supply is impeded.

Peptic Ulcers

A peptic ulcer is the erosion of the duodenal and/or gastric wall that is produced by gastric acid and proteolytic enzymes. The main symptom is pain that often radiates throughout the abdomen. If untreated, complications may occur, including peritonitis if the ulcer perforates into the abdomen, or life-threatening hemorrhage if blood vessels are involved in the perforation.

Gastritis

Gastritis is an inflammation of the stomach mucosa, which may be acute or chronic. Often related episodes of acute gastritis eventually lead to the chronic form. Etiologic agents include anything that irritates the stomach lining, such as alcohol, drugs, viruses, aspirin, and dietary irritants. If the condition becomes chronic, surgical intervention may be necessary.

Regional Enteritis

Regional enteritis, also known as Crohn's disease, is a chronic inflammation that may involve any part of the small intestine but usually affects the distal ileum and may extend into the proximal colon. The disease begins as an inflammation with regional scarring and thickening of the intestinal wall, which may lead to mechanical obstruction. Regional enteritis typically affects young adults and the initial symptoms may be similar to appendicitis. The etiology is unknown.

Ulcerative Colitis

Ulcerative colitis is an inflammatory disease that affects the mucosa of the colon, usually beginning in the rectal region and progressing into the sigmoid area. It is characterized by severe bloody diarrhea, which may lead to weight loss and electrolyte imbalances. The etiology is unknown, but some evidence suggests that it may have an autoimmune component.

Esophageal Varices

Esophageal varices are varicose veins of the esophagus. Conditions that create a resistance to blood flow through the liver result in a portal hypertension and inhibit normal venous drainage

Pathology—cont'd

through the portal system. The blood is directed through esophageal and gastric collateral veins and the increased blood flow through these vessels causes them to dilate.

Diverticulitis

A diverticulum is a protrusion of the mucosa and submucosa through the muscular layer at some point of weakness in the intestinal wall. The presence of diverticula is called *diverticulosis* and is usually asymptomatic. When inflammation occurs in the region of diverticula, the condition is called *diverticulitis*. Diverticula may occur in any portion of the intestine; however, they are more common in the sigmoid colon and may lead to bowel obstruction.

Adenocarcinoma of the Stomach

Adenocarcinoma is the most significant malignancy of the stomach. The symptoms are often vague but include bleeding, tiredness, loss of appetite, and weight loss. Blood tests may indicate anemia. Because the symptoms are vague, the individual may delay seeking medical intervention until the tumor is inoperable or has metastasized by way of lymphatic vessels or the bloodstream.

Adenocarcinoma of the Colon

Malignancies of the colon are typically adenocarcinomas, which are derived from the glandular epithelium in the lining of the wall. The majority of these tumors are in the rectum and sigmoid colon, which makes them fairly easy to detect with modern diagnostic techniques. Several predisposing factors have been proposed, including heredity, chronic ulcerative colitis, environment, and dietary habits.

Cystic Fibrosis

Cystic fibrosis is a hereditary disorder of the exocrine glands. The greatest threat is associated with the accumulation of excessively thick and adhesive mucus in the air passages, which obstructs bronchioles and restricts air movement, and from obstruction of the pancreatic ducts, which leads to inadequate enzymes for digestion and enzymatic necrosis of the pancreas with accompanying pancreatitis.

Cholelithiasis

Cholelithiasis is the presence or formation of gallstones, usually caused by the precipitation of substances out of the bile normally stored in the gallbladder. Generally, gallstones have a mixed composition, but most of them contain cholesterol, bilirubin, and calcium salts in varying proportions.

Cholecystitis

Cholecystitis is an acute inflammation of the gallbladder, often caused by obstruction of the cystic duct with gallstones. The condition is accompanied by a sudden onset of pain, fever, nausea, and vomiting. Repeated attacks of acute cholecystitis may damage the gallbladder and impair its function.

Pancreatitis

Pancreatitis is an inflammation of the pancreas resulting from autodigestion of pancreatic tissue by its own enzymes. The etiology is unknown, but it is associated with other conditions such as alcoholism, biliary tract obstruction, peptic ulcers, trauma, and certain drugs.

Cirrhosis

Cirrhosis is a liver condition characterized by the loss of normal liver tissue, which is replaced by fibrous bands of connective tissue. In its early stages it is asymptomatic, but as more and more liver tissue is replaced, functional impairments are evident, generally resulting in jaundice and portal hypertension. Cirrhosis of the liver is associated with chronic alcohol abuse, drugs, autoimmune disorders, metabolic and genetic disease, chronic viral infections, and chronic biliary tract obstructions.

Hepatitis

Hepatitis is a common condition characterized by inflammation of the liver tissue. It may be caused by alcoholism, toxic chemicals, parasites, and viruses. In a healthy individual, the liver will regenerate after hepatitis damage, but recurrent episodes may lead to permanent damage, including cirrhosis.

Jaundice

Jaundice is a yellowish discoloration of body tissues resulting from an accumulation of bile pigments (bilirubin), which are derived from the destruction of red blood cells and normally a component of bile. When bile is secreted into the small intestine, the pigments are eliminated in the feces. When a condition disturbs the normal flow of bile, the pigments accumulate in the blood and stain the tissues. The discoloration is most evident in the skin and eyes. Jaundice is not a disease entity but is evidence of a disease process.

Three general mechanisms can lead to jaundice. The first is obstructive jaundice, which is caused by an obstruction in the biliary system that impedes the flow of bile. The second mechanism is hemolytic jaundice, which is caused by excessive hemolysis of red blood cells, the source of the bile pigments. The third mechanism is hepatic jaundice, caused by liver disease, when the liver is unable to adequately process the bile pigments.

Pancreatic Carcinoma

Pancreatic carcinoma is a devastating malignancy of the pancreas, usually beginning in the head of the organ and progressing to the body and tail. It is rapidly progressive and often the symptoms are not apparent and diagnosed until the disease is in an advanced stage and has metastasized to other organs. Carcinoma in the head of the pancreas may impinge on the common bile duct and cause jaundice. Evidence indicates that smoking and high-fat diets increase the risk of pancreatic carcinoma.

Metastases

Primary tumors in abdominal organs, especially those that are drained by the hepatic portal system, frequently metastasize to the liver. Leukemias and lymphomas also affect the liver. Diffuse metastatic disease in the liver is not curable.

Polycystic Kidney Disease

Polycystic kidney disease is a hereditary disorder characterized by massive enlargement of the kidney and accompanied by the formation of cysts, which interferes with kidney function and

Continued

Pathology—cont'd

ultimately results in renal failure. Renal dialysis and kidney transplant during end-stage renal failure may prolong life.

Development and Position Anomalies
Agenesis, the congenital absence of an organ, and hypoplasia, a congenital abnormally small organ, of the kidney are relatively uncommon. Occasionally the lower poles of the two kidneys are fused resulting in a congenital abnormality called *horseshoe kidney*. Renal function usually is not impaired in the horseshoe kidney. Position anomalies are more common than the development anomalies. In position anomalies, the kidneys are in an abnormal location or rotation. These anomalies usually do not impair renal function unless the ureter is twisted or blocked to impede the flow of urine.

Acute Pyelonephritis
Acute pyelonephritis (commonly called *kidney infection*) is a bacterial infection of the renal parenchyma and renal pelvis usually caused by *Escherichia coli*. This represents probably the most common kidney disease. Kidney infections are more common in women than in men because women have a shorter urethra, making it possible for bacteria from the outside to enter the bladder and progress up the ureters to the kidney. Any condition that causes stagnation of urine or obstructs urine flow predisposes to kidney infection. Antibiotic therapy is usually successful.

Acute Glomerulonephritis
Glomerulonephritis is an inflammation of the capillary loops in the glomeruli of the kidney. This differs from pyelonephritis, which is an inflammation of the interstitial tissue rather than the parenchyma (nephrons) of the kidney. It appears that most cases are the result of an immune response to an inflammatory

agent. This may be an infection such as pyelonephritis, some other systemic disease, or toxic chemicals. The severity of the disorder depends on the number of glomeruli involved. Treatment is supportive to maintain electrolyte balance. In some cases, dialysis may be necessary.

Renal Calculi
Renal calculi, or kidney stones, precipitate from crystalline substances in the urine. Most often they form in the calyces or pelvis of the kidney but may occur in the urinary bladder. It is possible that those in the bladder actually developed in the kidney, passed down the ureter asymptomatically, and continued to grow in the bladder. Kidney stones are a common cause of urinary tract obstruction, particularly in adults. Predisposing factors include infections, inflammation, diet, metabolic disorders such as gout, and hyperactivity of the parathyroid gland.

Renal Cysts
Renal cysts are a common abnormality in the adult, particularly in those over the age of 50. Most cysts occur in the lower pole of the kidney and are asymptomatic.

Adenocarcinoma of the Kidney
Renal cell carcinoma (adenocarcinoma) is the most common malignant tumor of the kidney. It occurs twice as frequently in males as in females. Predisposing factors appear to be chronic inflammation, smoking, and exposure to hydrocarbons and other toxic chemicals. The tumors metastasize mainly through the bloodstream to the lungs, brain, bone, liver, and adrenal glands. The earliest symptom frequently is blood in the urine. If detected early enough, renal cell carcinomas are amenable to surgical treatment and may be cured.

Summary

- The abdominal cavity extends from the diaphragm to the superior pelvic aperture.
- The transpyloric plane is a horizontal plane midway between the xiphoid and umbilicus. It intersects the pyloric region of the stomach.
- The subcostal plane is a horizontal plane through the most inferior point of the rib cage. It marks the level of L3.
- The transumbilical plane passes horizontally through the umbilicus and generally marks the level of the disc between the L3 and L4 vertebrae.
- Two additional horizontal planes are the interiliac plane through the superior point of the iliac crest and the transtubercular plane through the tubercles of the iliac crests. The interiliac plane marks the level of L4 and the transtubercular plane marks the level of L5.
- The median and midclavicular planes are vertical planes. The right and left midclavicular planes extend vertically through the midpoint of the clavicle and the midinguinal point. The median plane, or midsagittal plane, passes through the umbilicus.

- The four quadrants of the abdomen are created by the horizontal transumbilical plane and the median plane.
- Horizontal subcostal and transtubercular planes intersecting with the vertical right and left midclavicular planes create nine abdominal regions. The central three regions, from superior to inferior, are the epigastric, umbilical, and hypogastric regions. Lateral to these on the right and left, from superior to inferior, are the hypochondriac, lumbar, and inguinal (iliac) regions.
- Lumbar vertebrae have large, bulky bodies, thick transverse processes, and short, thick, blunt spinous processes.
- The diaphragm is a musculotendinous partition between the thoracic cavity and the abdominopelvic cavity. The muscular fibers, which form two domes, converge on the central tendon.
- Three large and several small openings in the diaphragm allow passage of vessels from the thoracic cavity and the abdominal cavity. The caval hiatus, at T8, is an opening in the diaphragm for the inferior vena cava. The esophageal hiatus at T10 is for the esophagus, and the aortic hiatus at T12 is for the descending aorta.

- The rectus abdominis muscle, external oblique muscle, internal oblique muscle, and transverse abdominis muscle form the anterolateral abdominal wall.
- The psoas major muscle, the quadratus lumborum muscle, and the iliacus muscle form the posterior wall of the abdominopelvic cavity. The iliacus muscle does not appear in section of the abdomen because it is in the false pelvis.
- The lumbar vertebrae, normal lumbar lordosis, psoas major muscle, aorta, and inferior vena cava form an elevated ridge in the midline of the abdominal cavity. Any structure that crosses the midline is pushed anteriorly by this ridge. Fluids flow off the ridge and accumulate in the paravertebral grooves on either side of the ridge.
- The celiac trunk arises from the descending aorta at the upper L1 vertebral level. Its branches supply the liver, spleen, and a portion of the stomach. At the lower L2 vertebral level, the superior mesenteric artery branches from the descending aorta to supply the small intestine and two thirds of the large intestine. At the L3 level, the inferior mesenteric artery arises from the descending aorta to supply the distal one third of the large intestine.
- The paired branches from the descending aorta are the suprarenal arteries (lower L1) that supply the suprarenal glands, the renal arteries (upper L2) that supply the kidneys, and the gonadal arteries (lower L2) that supply the gonads.
- Two common iliac veins merge to form the inferior vena cava at the L5 vertebral level. Other visceral tributaries of the inferior vena cava are the right gonadal vein, right suprarenal vein, inferior phrenic veins, and hepatic veins.
- Blood from the digestive system flows through the portal veins and through the liver before the hepatic veins transport the blood to the inferior vena cava. The portal vein is formed by the splenic vein and the superior mesenteric vein. The inferior mesenteric vein usually drains into the splenic vein.
- The peritoneum is the double-layered, serous membrane of the abdominal cavity. If the peritoneum is associated with the intestines, it is called *mesentery*. Peritoneum associated with the stomach is called *omentum*. Anything that is not a mesentery or omentum usually is called a *peritoneal ligament*. In certain areas peritoneal folds form blind pouches called *cul-de-sacs*.
- The falciform ligament divides the parietal surface of the liver into a large right lobe and a smaller left lobe. The visceral surface shows two additional regions. The caudate lobe is between the ligamentum venosum and the inferior vena cava. The quadrate lobe is between the ligamentum teres and the gallbladder.
- Arterial blood supply to the liver is by the hepatic arteries. Blood from the digestive system is brought to the liver by the portal vein. Both the arterial blood and blood from the portal vein flow through the sinusoids of the liver lobules and enter the central veins. These small veins merge to form larger vessels and eventually form the hepatic veins that carry the blood to the inferior vena cava.
- The gallbladder is a saclike reservoir for bile that lies along the right edge of the quadrate lobe of the liver. The fundus usually protrudes from the inferior margin of the liver. In addition to its relationship to the liver, the gallbladder is anatomically related to the duodenum and transverse colon.
- The stomach is located in the upper left quadrant of the abdomen. It is divided into fundus, cardiac, body, and pyloric regions. Peritoneum associated with the stomach is called *omentum*.
- All the branches of the celiac trunk contribute to the arterial blood supply of the stomach. Venous blood flows through the portal system before it enters the inferior vena cava.
- The small intestine is divided into the duodenum, jejunum, and ileum. The shortest region, the duodenum, curves around the head of the pancreas. The middle region, the jejunum, is a tightly coiled tube that is located in the umbilical region of the abdomen. The final portion, the ileum, terminates at its junction with the ascending colon; this is the ileocecal valve.
- The large intestine is divided into the ascending colon, transverse colon, descending colon, sigmoid colon, and rectum. The transverse colon and sigmoid colon have a mesentery called the *mesocolon* and are relatively mobile.
- The ascending colon, descending colon, and rectum are retroperitoneal and are relatively fixed in position.
- The spleen is a highly vascular organ that is located in the left hypochondriac region, posterior to the stomach. In addition to the stomach, it is anatomically related to the tail of the pancreas, left kidney, and transverse colon.
- The retroperitoneal pancreas extends across the posterior abdomen from the duodenum to the spleen. It is divided into the head, neck, body, and tail.
- The head of the pancreas lies within the curve of the duodenum. The neck is a constricted portion to the left of the head. The portal vein is formed by the splenic vein and superior mesenteric vein posterior to the neck. The neck of the pancreas merges imperceptibly with the body, which extends to the left. The left extremity and most superior portion of the pancreas is the tail, which is in proximity to the hilus of the spleen.
- The kidneys are retroperitoneal along the posterior abdominal wall, just below the diaphragm, and adjacent to the vertebral column. A cushion of perirenal fat surrounds each kidney.
- The blood vessels and ureters enter and exit the kidney at the hilus, which generally is at the level of the transpyloric plane.
- The anterior and medial surface of the superior pole of each kidney is covered by a suprarenal (adrenal) gland.
- In addition to the suprarenal gland, the kidney is anatomically related to the diaphragm and the quadratus lumborum and psoas major muscles.
- The ureters are muscular ducts that transport urine from the kidneys to the urinary bladder. They descend retroperitoneally along the psoas major muscles.

• REVIEW QUESTIONS •

1. What is the superior boundary of the abdomen?
2. What vertebral level is indicated by each of the following planes?
   a. Transpyloric
   b. Subcostal
   c. Interiliac
   d. Transtubercular
3. What is the vertebral level for each of the following openings in the diaphragm?
   a. Aortic hiatus
   b. Caval hiatus
   c. Esophageal hiatus
4. What is the anterior abdominal wall muscle that is on either side of the linea alba?
5. What are the five features that contribute to the longitudinal ridge of the posterior abdominal wall?
6. What are the three unpaired visceral branches of the abdominal aorta and at what level does each one originate from the abdominal aorta?
7. Name six tributaries, in addition to the common iliac veins, that drain directly into the inferior vena cava.
8. What two vessels join to form the hepatic portal vein?
9. What term is used to denote an extension of the peritoneum that is associated with the stomach?
10. In addition to portions of the small and large intestines, name two organs and two vessels that are retroperitoneal.
11. What separates the caudate lobe of the liver from the following:
    a. Right lobe
    b. Left lobe
    c. Quadrate lobe
12. What are the four regions of the stomach, and which region is most superior?
13. What portion of the small intestine is retroperitoneal?
14. What portion of the duodenum is most inferior?
15. What portions of the colon are rather mobile because they have a mesentery?
16. What portion of the pancreas is related to the spleen?
17. What branch of the common hepatic artery is located in the head of the pancreas?
18. The ureters are usually associated with what large muscle?
19. What is the anterior relationship of the right suprarenal gland?
20. What is the most superior and posterior portion of the spleen?

• CHAPTER QUIZ •

Name the Following:

1. The superior abdominal region in the midline
2. The innermost muscle of the anterolateral abdominal wall
3. The structure or feature that separates the quadrate lobe of the liver from the right lobe
4. The most superior portion of the colon
5. The blood vessel that branches from the aorta just below the transpyloric line
6. The three structures in a portal triad
7. The portion of the stomach that is superior to the entrance of the esophagus
8. The portion of the duodenum that is at the L1 vertebral level
9. The three branches of the celiac trunk
10. The major blood vessel that is immediately anterior to the right suprarenal gland

True/False:

1. Portions of the liver, stomach, and spleen extend superiorly under the ribs and are protected by the thoracic cage.
2. The aortic hiatus is located at the level of the tenth thoracic vertebra.
3. The kidneys, the pancreas, and the stomach are retroperitoneal.
4. The celiac trunk arises from the aorta just above the transpyloric plane near the superior margin of the first lumbar vertebra.
5. The renal arteries are paired and arise from the aorta at the level of the third lumbar vertebra.
6. The hepatic veins, renal veins, and left gonadal vein drain directly into the inferior vena cava.
7. Blood normally flows from the inferior mesenteric vein into the superior mesenteric vein.
8. The greater curvature of the stomach is directed inferiorly and to the right, and the greater omentum is attached to it.
9. The third part of the duodenum is horizontal and is related to the inferior margin of the head of the pancreas.
10. The head of the pancreas is the most superior portion and is located on the right side of the midline, adjacent to the spleen.

Answers to the Review Questions and Chapter Quiz questions can be found at http://evolve.elsevier.com/Applegate/SAlearning/

CHAPTER FOUR

The Pelvis | 4

Anatomical Review of the Pelvis
Pelvic Cavity
Osseous Components
Muscular Components
Vascular Components
Nerve Supply to the Pelvis
Viscera of the Pelvis

Sectional Anatomy of the Pelvis
Sections of the Female Pelvis
Sections of the Male Pelvis
Working with Images of the Pelvis
**Important Anatomical Relationships
in the Pelvis**

OBJECTIVES

Upon completion of this chapter, the student should be able to do the following:
• Define the term *pelvis*.
• Differentiate between the greater, or false, pelvis and the lesser, or true, pelvis.
• Describe the features of the sacrum and coccyx.
• Name the three bones that form the os coxa and describe the features of the os coxa.
• Compare the structure of the os coxa in the child and in the adult.
• Identify the two principal muscles that line the wall of the true pelvis.
• Describe the structures that support the pelvic viscera and prevent them from falling through the pelvic outlet.
• Identify and compare the three muscles in the urogenital region of the perineum in the male and in the female.
• Describe the vascular supply to the pelvis.
• Name two nerves that emerge from the sacral plexus and state the importance of each.
• Describe the anterior relationships of the rectum both in the male and in the female.
• Compare the relationships of the urinary organs both in the male and in the female.
• Describe the normal location and attachments of the ovaries and factors that may alter the location.
• Identify the largest ligament that supports the uterus and name three smaller supporting ligaments.
• Describe the normal position and relationships of the uterus.
• Describe the relationships of the fornix of the vagina to the cervix.
• Describe the structure and location of the testes and the epididymis.
• Describe the structure of the scrotum and the spermatic cord.
• Identify three accessory glands of the male reproductive system and describe the location of each gland.
• Discuss the relationships of the seminal vesicles and prostate glands.
• Compare the dorsal and ventral columns of erectile tissue in the body and the root of the penis.
• Compare vessel and muscle relationships in transverse sections through the sacroiliac joint and in transverse sections through the lower part of the sacrum.
• Distinguish between the rectovesical pouch, the vesicouterine pouch, and the rectouterine pouch.
• Identify the muscles, viscera, blood vessels, and skeletal components of the female pelvis in transverse, sagittal, and coronal sections.
• Identify the muscles, viscera, and blood vessels, as well as skeletal components, of the male pelvis in transverse, sagittal, and coronal sections.

Key Terms, Structures, and Features to Be Identified and/or Described

Ascending colon	Labia majora	Rectouterine pouch
Broad ligament	Labia minora	Rectovesical pouch
Bulbourethral gland	Levator ani muscle	Rectum
Cervix	Lumbosacral angle	Sacral hiatus
Clitoris	Lumbosacral trunk	Sacral promontory
Coccyx	Membranous urethra	Sacroiliac joint
Common iliac arteries	Obturator externus muscle	Sciatic nerve
Common iliac veins	Obturator internus muscle	Scrotum
Corpus cavernosum	Os coxae	Seminal vesicles
Corpus spongiosum	Ovarian ligament	Seminiferous tubules
Descending colon	Ovary	Sigmoid colon
Ductus deferens	Pectineal line	Spermatic cord
Epididymis	Pectineus muscle	Suspensory ligament
External iliac arteries	Pelvic diaphragm	Symphysis pubis
External iliac veins	Pelvis major	Testes
Femoral arteries	Pelvis minor	Transverse colon
Femoral nerve	Penile (spongy) urethra	Trigone
Femoral veins	Piriformis muscle	Ureters
Great saphenous veins	Posterior fornix	Urethra
Iliacus muscle	Prostate gland	Urinary bladder
Iliopsoas muscle	Prostatic urethra	Urogenital diaphragm
Ilium	Psoas muscle	Uterine tube
Internal iliac arteries	Pubic arch	Uterus
Internal iliac veins	Pubis	Vagina
Ischiopubic ramus	Pudendal nerve	Vesicouterine pouch
Ischium	Pudendum	Vestibule

Anatomical Review of the Pelvis

The term *pelvis* is ambiguous and confusing, because it has a variety of meanings in modern usage. First of all, *pelvis* is used to describe a loosely defined region of the body where the trunk meets the lower limbs. The term also is applied to the bony ring formed by the sacrum, the coccyx, and the two hip bones; this structure is sometimes referred to as the *bony pelvis*. The *pelvis* also can describe the cavity enclosed by the bony pelvis; this is the *pelvic cavity*. Generally, the context of the discussion clarifies the meaning.

Pelvic Cavity

The bony pelvis encloses a funnel- or basin-shaped cavity that is the inferior portion of the larger abdominopelvic cavity. The pelvic cavity is divided into a **pelvis major,** or false pelvis, and a **pelvis minor,** or true pelvis. The cavity of the pelvis major is the space between the iliac fossae, and its inferior boundary is defined by the pelvic brim. It is considered a part of the abdominal cavity, and it contains abdominal viscera, such as portions of the small intestine and the **sigmoid colon.** The iliac crest is such an obvious dividing point on transverse sections that the pelvis major is included in the discussion of the pelvis rather than with the abdomen. The pelvis minor is the space below the pelvic brim and is enclosed by the sacrum, the ischium, the

pubis, and the pelvic portions of the ilium. It contains the urinary bladder, the rectum, the internal reproductive organs, and portions of the mobile intestinal tract that may be able to reach it.

Osseous Components

The bony framework of the pelvis is formed by the sacrum, the coccyx, and the paired os coxae, or hip bones.

Sacrum. The sacrum and the coccyx (Fig. 4-1) make up the posterior midline portion of the bony pelvis. The sacrum transmits the weight of the body to the hip bones and then to the lower extremities. Normally, five sacral vertebrae fuse into one triangular mass, called the *sacrum*, that articulates with the fifth lumbar vertebra superiorly, the coccyx inferiorly, and the os coxae laterally. Where the sacrum meets the fifth lumbar vertebra, the sacrum is tilted posteriorly to form a **lumbosacral angle.** In some individuals the first sacral vertebra remains separate from the other four, or the fifth lumbar vertebra may fuse with the sacrum. Both conditions put a strain on the nearest intervertebral articulation, which may result in joint degeneration and cause low back pain.

When the five sacral vertebrae fuse together, they form a normal curvature so that the anterior, or pelvic, surface is concave. Anteriorly, the upper margin of the first sacral

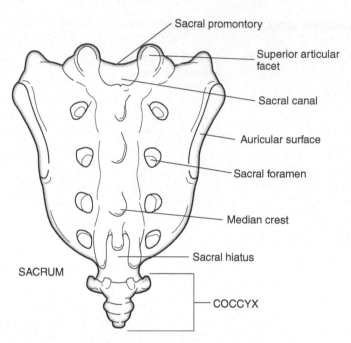

FIG. 4-1. Sacrum and coccyx.

vertebra forms the **sacral promontory,** which marks the posterior portion of the true pelvic inlet, or pelvic brim. Both the anterior and posterior surfaces of the sacrum have two bilateral columns of four openings called **sacral foramina.** Branches of the sacral nerves pass through the sacral foramina. On the posterior surface, between the sacral foramina, poorly defined and fused spinous processes form the **median crest.** The fifth sacral vertebra has no spinous process or lamina. This deficiency in the neural arch leaves a midline opening, called the **sacral hiatus.** Local anesthetics may be injected through the sacral hiatus; this procedure is called ex*tradural, epidural,* or *caudal anesthesia.*

On each side of the upper portion of the sacrum is a rather large **auricular surface** for articulation with the iliac bones to form the sacroiliac (iliosacral) joint. The connection between the bones is further enhanced by strong **interosseous ligaments,** which act as cords to bind the bones together.

Coccyx. The most inferior portion of the vertebral column is the **coccyx,** or tailbone, which is joined to the sacrum by cartilage. It usually consists of four rudimentary vertebrae with no processes or foramina, although the number varies from three to five. During adulthood, the bones of the coccyx usually fuse to form a single structure. The coccyx offers no support for the vertebral column but does provide attachment for a portion of the gluteus maximus muscle and some of the muscles of the pelvic floor. Sometimes, such as during childbirth or a fall, the sacrum and coccyx may separate, resulting in pain, especially when sitting.

Os Coxae. The **os coxae** (innominate bones) are commonly called the *hip bones.* Each os coxa consists of an **ilium,** a **pubis,** and an **ischium.** In the child these are three separate bones joined together by hyaline cartilage, and

each bone has its own ossification center in the cartilage. Ossification continues during childhood until the cartilage is replaced by bone. By puberty, only a small amount of cartilage remains as a Y-shaped region where the three bones meet in the acetabulum. When ossification is complete, the ilium, the ischium, and the pubis are fused together to form a single unit, called the *os coxa* (Fig. 4-2).

The **ilium** is the largest of the three bones of the os coxa. The superior part of the ilium presents a large, flaring, winglike surface called the **ala.** The inner aspect of the ala is the **iliac fossa,** which is the origin of the iliacus muscle. The **iliac crest,** the most superior portion of the hip bone, is the superior margin of the ala. The crest terminates both anteriorly and posteriorly in short projections, the **superior** and **inferior iliac spines.** Posteriorly, the ilium articulates with the sacrum at the **sacroiliac joint.**

The bodies of the two **pubic bones** meet in the anterior midline at the **symphysis pubis.** A small projection that is just lateral to the body forms the **pubic tubercle,** and from this point the **superior pubic ramus** extends laterally to meet the ilium. The pelvic surface of the superior margin of the superior pubic ramus is sharp and forms the **pectineal line,** which is continuous with the arcuate line of the ilium and the sacral promontory to mark the pelvic brim. The **inferior pubic ramus** extends inferiorly from the body to connect with the ischium. The inferior rami of the two pubic bones meet at the symphysis pubis to form the **pubic arch,** or **subpubic angle.** This angle is usually less than 70 degrees in the male and greater than 80 degrees in the female. The difference in the subpubic angle contributes to the variation in the contour of the pelvic cavity between the sexes. The male pelvis is deep and conical; the female pelvis is shallow and broad. In this way, the female pelvis is adapted for childbearing.

The inferior portion of the os coxa is formed by the **ischium.** Anteriorly, the ramus of the ischium meets the inferior pubic ramus at an indistinct point; together they often are

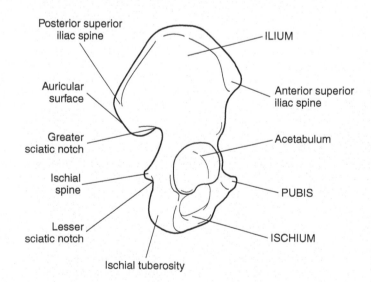

OS COXA (right, lateral view)

FIG. 4-2. Os coxa.

called the **ischiopubic ramus.** The posterior and inferior border of the ischium is formed by a bulky, rough area called the **ischial tuberosity.** A sharp, pointed **ischial spine** divides the space between the ischial tuberosity and the ilium into the **lesser sciatic notch,** which is between the ischial tuberosity and the ischial spine, and the **greater sciatic notch,** which is between the ischial spine and the ilium. The notches are made into foramina by ligaments and are closed by muscles.

The ilium, ischium, and pubis meet in the **acetabulum,** which is a deep fossa for articulation with the head of the femur. The three bones also surround an opening called the **obturator foramen,** which is directed inferiorly. This foramen is closed by the obturator membrane and muscles. The **pelvic outlet** (inferior pelvic aperture) must also be covered to give support and maintain the pelvic viscera in position. The features of the os coxa are summarized in Table 4-1; see Figs. 4-2 and 4-3 to identify the features.

QUICK CHECK

4.1 What is the inferior boundary of the pelvis major?
4.2 What articulates with the auricular surface of the sacrum?
4.3 What bones form the os coxa?
4.4 Where do the three bones of the os coxa meet?

Muscular Components

Functionally, the muscles of the pelvic wall are associated with movements of the thigh. Other muscles, such as the gluteal muscles and the anterior thigh muscles, are external to the pelvis but are seen in pelvic sections. These muscles are mentioned here and described in greater detail with the lower extremity. Table 4-2 summarizes the pelvic muscles.

Muscles in the Wall of the Greater (False) Pelvis. The muscles in the wall of the greater, or false, pelvis are actually abdominal muscles. The two principal muscles, the **psoas major muscle** and the **iliacus muscle,** extend

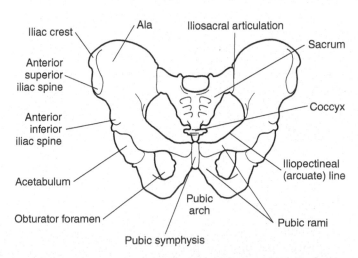

FIG. 4-3. Bones of the pelvis: sacrum, coccyx, and os coxae.

throughout the whole pelvic region and continue into the anterior thigh. The computed tomography (CT) image in Fig. 4-4 illustrates these two muscles in a transverse plane.

The long, fleshy **psoas major muscle** appears as a muscle mass lateral to the vertebral bodies as it continues from the abdomen into the pelvis. The muscle passes deep to the inguinal ligament as it continues from the pelvis into the thigh, where it inserts on the lesser trochanter of the femur. The psoas major muscle acts with the iliacus muscle as a powerful flexor of the thigh. Lumbar nerves provide the innervation.

The **iliacus muscle** is a fan-shaped muscle that originates along the crest and fossa of the ilium and lines the iliac fossa. In the pelvis it appears lateral to the psoas major muscle. Fibers of the iliacus muscle insert on the femur with the psoas major muscle. Because the iliacus muscle and psoas major muscle appear to merge into one muscle and they have a close functional relationship, the two muscles often are referred to as the single **iliopsoas muscle.** The iliacus muscle is innervated by the femoral nerve, which is a branch of the lumbar plexus.

Muscles in the Wall of the True Pelvis. Most of the inner surface of the bony true pelvis is lined with muscle. The **obturator internus** and **piriformis** muscles are the principal muscles that make up the wall of the true pelvis and form this lining. The line drawing in Fig. 4-5 illustrates the two muscles, and Fig. 4-6 is a CT image of these muscles.

The **obturator internus muscle** is a fan-shaped muscle that covers most of the lateral wall of the true pelvis. It originates on the inner surface of the pelvic bones, crosses over the **obturator foramen** to close off the opening, and then leaves the pelvis through the lesser sciatic notch. As it passes through the **lesser sciatic notch,** it becomes tendinous and makes a sharp turn to insert on the medial surface of the greater trochanter. The obturator internus muscle is innervated by branches from the L5 and S1 spinal nerves. This muscle rotates the thigh.

The **piriformis muscle** is located partially on the posterior wall of the true pelvis and partially external to the pelvis, posterior to the hip joint. It originates on the anterior surface of the sacrum and passes through the **greater sciatic notch** to insert on the greater trochanter of the femur. The piriformis muscle is closely associated with the sacral nerve plexus and is innervated by sacral nerves. It rotates and abducts the thigh.

Muscles of the Pelvic Outlet. The pelvic outlet (inferior pelvic aperture) must be covered to give support to and maintain the position of the pelvic viscera. The floor of the pelvis includes all structures that contribute to this support; specifically, these are the peritoneum, pelvic diaphragm, urogenital diaphragm, and muscles of the perineum.

The principal structure supporting the pelvic viscera is the **pelvic diaphragm,** which forms a muscular pelvic floor. It is a hammock-like structure consisting primarily of the **levator ani** and **coccygeus** muscles. Of the two

TABLE 4-1   Important Markings on the Coxal Bones

Marking	Description	Purpose
Acetabulum	Deep depression on lateral surface of coxal bone	Socket for articulation with head of femur (thigh bone)
Obturator foramen	Large opening between the pubis and ischium	Passageway for blood vessels, nerves, muscle tendons; largest foramen in the body
Ilium	Large flaring region that forms the major portion of the coxal bone	
Alae (wings)	Large flared portions of the ilium	Large area for numerous muscle attachments; forms false pelvis
Iliac crest	Thickened superior margin of the ilium	Muscle attachment; forms prominence of hips
Anterior superior iliac spine	Blunt projection at anterior end of the iliac crest	Attachment for muscles of trunk, hip, thigh; can be easily palpated
Posterior superior iliac spine	Blunt projection at posterior end of the iliac crest	Attachment for muscles of trunk, hip, thigh
Anterior inferior iliac spine	Projection on ilium inferior to the anterior superior iliac spine	Attachment for muscles of trunk, hip, thigh
Posterior inferior iliac spine	Projection on ilium inferior to the posterior superior iliac spine	Attachment for muscles of trunk, hip, thigh
Greater sciatic notch	Deep indentation inferior to the posterior inferior iliac spine	Passageway for sciatic nerve and some muscle tendons
Iliac fossa	Slight concavity on medial surface of alae	Attachment for iliacus muscle
Auricular surface	Large, rough region at posterior margin of iliac fossa	Articulates with sacrum to form the sacroiliac joint
Iliopectineal (arcuate) line	Sharp curved line at inferior margin of iliac fossa	Attachment for muscles; marks the pelvic brim
Ischium	Lower, posterior portion of the coxal bone	
Ischial spine	Projection near junction of ilium and ischium; projects into pelvic cavity	Attachment for a major ligament; distance between the two spines tells the size of the pelvic cavity
Ischial tuberosity	Large rough inferior portion of ischium	Muscle attachment; portion on which we sit; strongest part of the coxal bones
Lesser sciatic notch	Indentation below the ischial spine	Passageway for blood vessels and nerves
Pubis	Most anterior part of coxal bone	
Pubic symphysis	Anterior midline where two pubic bones meet	
Pubic rami	Armlike portions that project from the pubic symphysis	Form margins of the obturator foramen
Pubic arch	V-shaped arch inferior to the pubic symphysis formed by the inferior pubic rami	Broadens or narrows the dimensions of the true pelvis

muscles that form the pelvic diaphragm, the **levator ani muscle** is the larger and more important. The integrity of the pelvic floor depends on the appropriate function of the levator ani muscles. In females, these muscles are particularly vulnerable during a strenuous delivery. If the muscles are damaged, support for the pelvic viscera is weakened, and urinary incontinence and prolapse of the uterus may result. The levator ani muscles originate on the pelvic surface of the pubis and the spine of the ischium. The fibers converge to insert on the coccyx, and some fibers insert on the muscle of the opposite side. The levator ani muscles are innervated by the pudendal nerve.

The **coccygeus** muscle is the smaller of the two muscles that form the pelvic diaphragm. From its origin on the spine of the ischium, the fibers fan out to form a triangular sheet that inserts on the sacrum and coccyx. Branches of the pudendal nerve innervate the coccygeus muscle.

The **urogenital diaphragm** lies immediately deep to the external genitalia. It consists of the sheetlike **transversus perinei** muscle and the **external anal sphincter.**

External to the pelvic and urogenital diaphragms are the muscles of the perineum. The outline of this region is roughly diamond shaped (Fig. 4-7). Anteriorly to posteriorly, the region extends from the pubic arch to the tip of the coccyx. The two ischial tuberosities form the two lateral points. A line drawn between the ischial tuberosities divides the perineum into two regions: a posterior anal region and an anterior urogenital region.

TABLE 4-2   Pelvic Muscles

Muscle	Origin	Insertion	Action	Innervation
Iliacus	Iliac fossa	Lesser trochanter of femur	Flexes thigh	Femoral nerve
Psoas	Lumbar vertebrae	Lesser trochanter of femur	Flexes thigh	Ventral rami of lumbar nerves
Obturator internus	Inner surface of pelvis	Greater trochanter of femur	Rotates thigh	Branches of L5 and S1
Piriformis	Anterior surface of sacrum	Greater trochanter of femur	Rotates and abducts thigh	Branches of S1 and S2
Levator ani	Inside pelvis from pubis to sacrum	Coccyx and levator ani on opposite side	Supports pelvic viscera	Pudendal nerve
Coccygeus	Spine of ischium	Supports pelvic viscera	Sacrum and coccyx	Branches of pudendal nerve

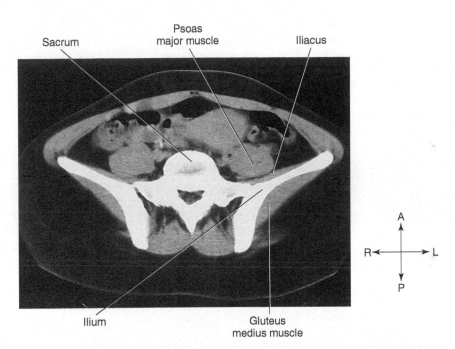

FIG. 4-4. CT image of the muscles in the wall of the false pelvis.

The arrangement of the muscles in the anal region is the same in both sexes; however, the muscles in the urogenital region are arranged differently in the male and female.

The muscles found in the anal region are the **levator ani** and the **sphincter ani.** The levator ani muscle has been described previously as a primary muscle of the pelvic diaphragm. The sphincter ani muscle is part of the urogenital diaphragm and surrounds the anal canal. The musculature of the urogenital region consists of the **bulbospongiosus, ischiocavernosus,** and **transversus perinei** muscles. Fig. 4-8 illustrates the arrangement in the female, and Fig. 4-9 shows the arrangement in the male. The **transversus perinei** muscles are horizontal, arising on the ischial tuberosities and passing medially to insert on

the central perineal tendon. In other words, they pass along the line that divides the perineum into the urogenital and anal regions. The **ischiocavernosus** muscles also arise on the ischial tuberosities but pass forward to insert on the pubic arch and the crus of the penis in the male or the clitoris in the female. The **bulbospongiosus** muscle is in the median line of the urogenital region. In the female, the two parts of this muscle are separated by the urethra and the vagina. In the male, the fibers of the two muscles unite in the midline and encircle the corpus spongiosum of the penis.

Extrapelvic Muscles Seen in Pelvic Sections.   Numerous muscles, such as the gluteal muscles and the thigh muscles, are external to the pelvis but are apparent in sections

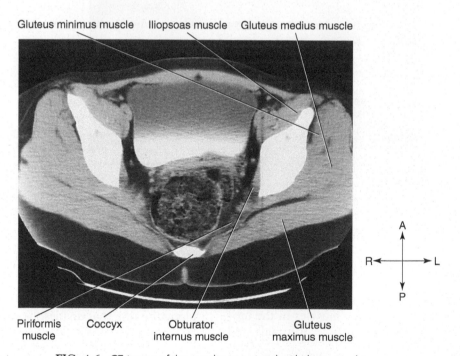

External iliac artery and vein

Rectus abdominis muscle

Ilium

Iliopsoas muscle

Sartorius muscle

Tensor fasciae latae muscle

Femoral nerve

Gluteus medius muscle

Obturator internus muscle

Gluteus minimus muscle

Ureter

Gluteus maximus muscle

Internal iliac artery and vein

Rectum

Piriformis muscle

A / R ← → L / P

FIG. 4-5. Muscles associated with the true pelvis.

Gluteus minimus muscle Iliopsoas muscle Gluteus medius muscle

Piriformis muscle Coccyx Obturator internus muscle Gluteus maximus muscle

A / R ← → L / P

FIG. 4-6. CT image of the muscles associated with the true pelvis.

through the pelvis. These muscles are associated with the hip joint and movement of the lower extremity. Some of the more important and obvious extrapelvic muscles are named and described briefly in Table 4-3. They are discussed in more detail with the lower extremity. Some of these muscles are illustrated with the pelvic wall muscles in Figs. 4-5 and 4-6.

QUICK CHECK

4.5 What muscle forms the lateral wall of the pelvis minor?

4.6 What muscle fills the greater sciatic notch?

4.7 What are the two muscle of the pelvic diaphragm?

4.8 What muscle of the perineum extends from the ischial tuberosity to the central tendon?

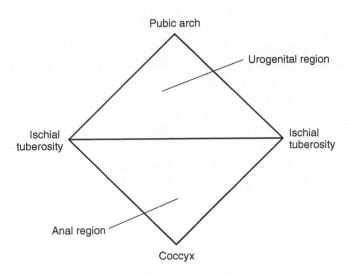

FIG. 4-7. Regions of the perineum.

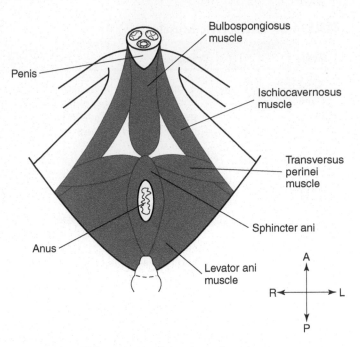

FIG. 4-9. Muscles in the male perineum.

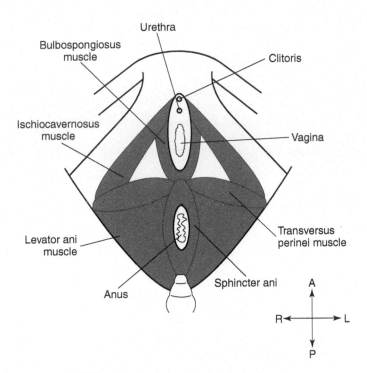

FIG. 4-8. Muscles in the female perineum.

Vascular Components

At the level of the fourth lumbar vertebra, the abdominal aorta divides into the right and left **common iliac arteries.** These vessels descend to the pelvic brim, where they pass over the sacroiliac joint at the level of the disc between the fifth lumbar vertebra and the sacrum. At this point, the common iliac arteries divide into the **external** and **internal iliac arteries.** The external iliac artery follows the pelvic brim, then passes under the inguinal ligament to become the femoral artery, which continues through the thigh. The internal iliac artery, a short vessel that is only 4 cm long, branches profusely. Parietal branches supply blood to the pelvic wall, and the visceral branches supply blood to the pelvic organs. Blood is drained from the pelvis primarily by the **internal iliac veins** and their tributaries.

Lymph vessels from the pelvic viscera generally pass through lymph nodes associated with the iliac arteries and their branches. These include the common iliac lymph nodes, external iliac lymph nodes, and internal iliac lymph nodes. Efferent vessels from the external and internal iliac lymph nodes pass to the common iliac lymph nodes. From there, efferent vessels transport lymph to the lateral aortic lymph nodes. Efferent vessels from these nodes form left and right lumbar trunks that drain into the cisterna chyli, which is the beginning of the thoracic duct.

Nerve Supply to the Pelvis

Portions of the fourth and fifth lumbar nerves unite to form a thick, cordlike **lumbosacral trunk,** which descends obliquely over the sacroiliac joint to enter the pelvis. In the pelvis, the lumbosacral trunk joins with the first four sacral nerves to form the **sacral plexus,** which lies on the piriformis muscle. Numerous nerves emerge from the sacral plexus to supply pelvic structures, the buttocks, and the lower limb. Two of these nerves, the sciatic nerve and the pudendal nerve, are included in this discussion. With a few exceptions, branches of the sacral plexus leave the pelvis through the greater sciatic notch (foramen).

TABLE 4-3   Extrapelvic Muscles

Muscle	Description
Gluteus maximus	The largest and most superficial muscle of the gluteal region; forms most of the mass of the buttocks
Gluteus medius	A thick, broad muscle of the gluteal region; located deep to the gluteus maximus but originating more superiorly, which results in the covering of the inferior one third by the gluteus maximus
Gluteus minimus	The smallest and deepest muscle of the gluteal region; underlies both the gluteus maximus and the gluteus medius
Gemelli	Two small muscle masses inferior to the piriformis muscle and deep to the lower part of the gluteus maximus; associated with the obturator internus tendon
Quadratus femoris	A short, flat, rectangular muscle that is located inferior to the gemelli and the extrapelvic portions of the obturator internus muscles
Tensor fasciae latae	A superficial muscle of the superior lateral thigh; overlies the superior lateral portion of the gluteus medius
Sartorius	A long, straplike muscle that courses obliquely and inferiorly across the anterior thigh; most superficial muscle of the anterior thigh
Rectus femoris	A large ropelike muscle mass that extends the length of the anterior thigh; one of the quadriceps femoris muscle group
Vastus lateralis	A large muscle that forms the lateral portion of the thigh; partially covered by the iliotibial fascia; one of the quadriceps femoris muscle group
Vastus medialis	A large muscle that forms the medial portion of thigh; one of the quadriceps femoris muscle group
Vastus intermedius	An elongated muscle next to the shaft of the femur; deep to the rectus femoris, between the other two vastus muscles; one of the quadriceps femoris group
Pectineus	A flat muscle, medial to the iliopsoas, in the floor of the femoral triangle; apparent anterior to the pubic bone in transverse sections
Adductor longus	A superficial, flat muscle that extends obliquely from the pubis to the femur; medial to the pectineus
Adductor brevis	A flat muscle deep to the adductor longus on the medial aspect of the thigh
Adductor magnus	The largest of the adductor muscles in the medial compartment of the thigh; deep to the adductor longus and adductor brevis
Obturator externus	A relatively small, fan-shaped muscle that covers the obturator foramen; closely associated with the adductor muscles
Gracilis	A thin, straplike, superficial band of muscle that extends down the medial aspect of the thigh from the pubis to the tibia
Biceps femoris	A large, elongated muscle on the posterior and lateral aspects of the thigh; the superior portion is deep to the gluteus maximus; one of the hamstring muscles
Semitendinosus	A superficial muscle medial to the biceps femoris; the superior portion is deep to the gluteus maximus; one of the hamstring muscles
Semimembranosus	A fleshy muscle, deep and medial to the semitendinosus; one of the hamstring muscles

Sciatic Nerve.   The **sciatic nerve,** one of the branches of the sacral plexus, is the largest nerve in the body. The sciatic nerve passes through the greater sciatic notch (foramen) at the lower border of the piriformis muscle to enter the gluteal region and then descends in the posterior compartment of the thigh. Its branches supply the flexor muscles of the thigh and all the muscles of the leg and foot. Because of its location, the sciatic nerve may be injured in dislocations and fractures of the hip. This nerve also is vulnerable when intramuscular injections are given into the buttock.

Pudendal Nerve.   The **pudendal nerve,** another branch of the sacral plexus, leaves the pelvis through the lesser sciatic notch (foramen) to supply the perineum, the external anal sphincter, and the sensory fibers of the external genitalia. This is the nerve that is anesthetized in a pudendal nerve block during childbirth and during surgical procedures on the female genitalia.

Obturator Nerve.   The **obturator nerve** does not arise from the sacral plexus but from the lumbar plexus of nerves in the abdomen. It enters the pelvis, runs along the lateral pelvic wall, and then leaves through the obturator foramen. The obturator nerve supplies the **obturator externus muscle** and the adductor muscles of the thigh. It also sends branches to the hip and knee joints. Because of its proximity to pelvic lymph nodes, it is vulnerable to injury during surgery for malignant disease in the pelvis. It also may be affected by changes in the ovary, which is near the nerve. Because the nerve supplies both the hip and knee joints, pain from the hip may be referred to the knee, making it difficult to locate the cause.

QUICK CHECK

4.9   What blood vessel provides the drainage from the pelvic viscera?

4.10   What branch of the sacral plexus innervates the perineum and external anal sphincter?

Viscera of the Pelvis

Gastrointestinal Organs   Most of the length of the gastrointestinal tract is located in the abdomen. Loops of the mobile small intestine, especially the ileum, may extend into the pelvis. Portions of the colon normally are located within the false pelvis, and if the mobile transverse colon is particularly pendulous, it may extend down into the true pelvis. Because of the mobility of the portions of the gastrointestinal tract that have a mesentery, the amount in the pelvis varies.

The cecum and ascending colon normally are found within the greater (or false) pelvis on the right side. The descending colon on the left side becomes continuous with the sigmoid colon at the pelvic brim. In contrast to the descending colon, which is retroperitoneal, the sigmoid colon is surrounded by peritoneum and has a mesentery, which allows considerable mobility. At its junction with the rectum, the sigmoid colon becomes fixed to the posterior pelvic wall.

The rectum begins near the middle of the sacrum and follows the curvature of the sacrum and coccyx onto the pelvic floor. The levator ani muscle supports the rectum on the pelvic floor. The rectum penetrates the levator ani muscle to become the anal canal. In the female, the peritoneum over the anterior surface of the rectum extends to the surface of the uterus and forms the **rectouterine pouch.** Inferior to the rectouterine pouch, the rectum is related anteriorly to the vagina. In the male, the upper portion of the rectum is separated from the urinary bladder by peritoneum, which forms the **rectovesical pouch.** Inferior to this, the rectum is related anteriorly to the urinary bladder, the seminal vesicles, and the prostate gland without the intervening peritoneum.

Urinary Organs.   The upper half of each **ureter** is located in the abdomen, but the lower half enters the pelvis. The ureter crosses over the pelvic brim near the bifurcation of the common iliac artery. As it enters the pelvis, the ureter is anterior to the internal iliac artery and follows a course similar to that of the vessel. Retroperitoneally located and closely adherent to the peritoneum over it, the ureter descends along the lateral pelvic wall to a point near the ischial spine, where it turns medially to enter the urinary bladder on its posterior surface.

The **urinary bladder** is a distensible, muscular organ that, when empty, lies entirely within the true pelvis. As it fills, the bladder may extend into the abdomen. In the female, the urinary bladder rests on the pelvic floor posterior to the symphysis pubis. In the male, the prostate gland is between the urinary bladder and the pelvic floor. The superior surface is covered by peritoneum and is related to the sigmoid colon and coils of the ileum. In the female, the peritoneum reflects from the superior surface of the bladder onto the anterior wall of the uterus to form the **vesicouterine pouch.** In the male, the peritoneum reflects from the superior surface of the bladder over the ductus deferens and the seminal vesicles onto the rectum to form the **rectovesical pouch.** Held in place by peritoneal ligaments, the bladder is relatively movable except in the inferior neck region, where it is firmly anchored. In the female, the neck is attached to the pelvic diaphragm. In the male, the neck rests on the prostate gland. Urine is conveyed from the bladder to the exterior through the **urethra.**

Internally, the mucosal lining of the bladder is arranged in irregular folds, which allow for expansion. The oblique openings of the two ureters, which convey urine from the kidneys to the bladder, are in the base of the bladder. These two openings plus the **internal urethral orifice** form a triangular region, called the **trigone,** in the base (Fig. 4-10). The trigone is the region of the bladder that is most sensitive to pain.

The **female urethra** (see Fig. 4-10) is a short, muscular tube about 4 cm long that conveys urine from the bladder to the exterior. The external urethral orifice opens into the vestibule just anterior to the vagina. About five times as long as the female urethra, the **male urethra** opens to the exterior at the tip of the glans penis. For descriptive purposes, it may be divided into three regions. The **prostatic urethra** passes through the substance of the prostate gland, and the ejaculatory duct and ducts from the prostate gland open into this portion. The **membranous urethra,** the shortest and narrowest portion, penetrates the urogenital diaphragm to enter the penis. The final portion is the **penile (spongy) urethra.** This is the longest part, extending the full length of the corpus spongiosum of the penis. The ducts of the bulbourethral glands open into the proximal region of the spongy urethra. Fig. 4-11 illustrates the three parts of the male urethra.

QUICK CHECK

4.11   In the male, the rectovesical pouch is a peritoneal cul-de-sac between what two organs?

4.12   In the female, the urinary bladder rests on the pelvic floor, but in the male another organ is between the bladder and the pelvic floor. What is this organ?

4.13   What three openings form the corners of the trigone in the urinary bladder?

4.14   What is the most proximal portion of the male urethra?

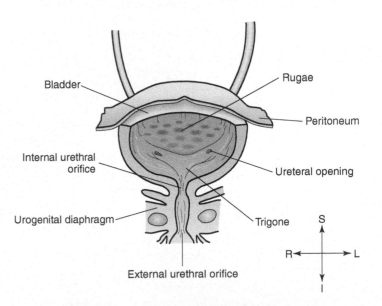

FIG. 4-10. Urinary bladder and female urethra.

FIG. 4-11. Three regions of the male urethra.

Female Reproductive Organs and Accessory Structures. The female reproductive organs located in the pelvic cavity are the ovaries, uterine tubes, uterus, and a portion of the vagina (Fig. 4-12).

To visualize the relationships of these organs and their peritoneal ligaments, one must understand the nature of the primary peritoneal fold in the female pelvis. The peritoneum projects upward in a fold over the midline uterus and then drapes from the uterine tubes that extend laterally from the uterus. To visualize this, imagine an individual standing with arms outstretched at the sides with a sheet draped over the head and arms. The sheet illustrates the peritoneum, the body represents the uterus, and the arms portray the uterine tubes. This large fold of peritoneum, called the **broad ligament,** divides the pelvic cavity into two compartments. One compartment contains the urinary bladder, and the other compartment contains the rectum.

A girl is born with about 250,000 primary oocytes, each capable of developing into a mature ovum. This multitude of potential ova is contained in a pair of **ovaries.** Each **ovary** is a small, solid, oval structure about 3 cm long. It resembles an almond in size and shape. After menopause the ovaries gradually become smaller.

Each ovary is located in an ovarian fossa, a shallow depression in the lateral wall of the pelvis, on either side of the uterus. Three peritoneal ligaments loosely anchor the ovary in place. The **mesovarium** attaches the ovary to the posterior layer of the broad ligament of the uterus. The **ovarian ligament,** a cordlike thickening in the broad ligament, attaches the ovary to the lateral wall of the uterus. An extension of the broad ligament, the **suspensory ligament,** carries the ovarian vessels and attaches the ovary to the lateral pelvic wall. The position of the ovaries varies considerably, especially during pregnancy, when they are moved upward by the expanding uterus. Loops of intestine may also displace the ovaries.

The outer ovarian tissue is granulated in appearance because of the presence of the numerous ovarian follicles. Each month an ovarian follicle matures into a graafian follicle. At ovulation, the mature follicle ruptures to release an oocyte, with some surrounding follicular cells, into the peritoneal cavity.

The two slender **uterine tubes,** also called **fallopian tubes** or **oviducts,** are about 10 or 12 cm long. They are in the upper border of the broad ligament and extend from the upper lateral angle of the uterus to the region of the

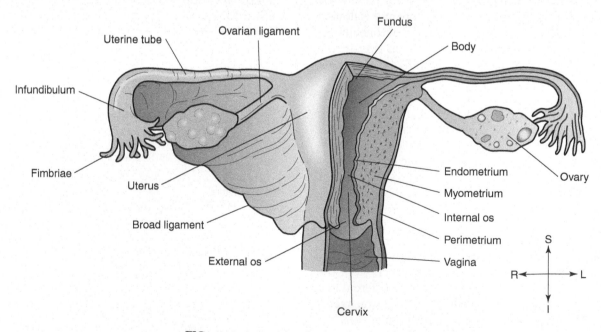

FIG. 4-12. Internal female reproductive organs.

ovary. The lumen of the tube is continuous with the cavity of the uterus. Near the ovary, the tube expands to form a funnel-shaped **infundibulum,** which is edged with finger-like extensions called **fimbriae.**

The ovary and the uterine tube are not directly connected; however, some of the fimbriae may touch the ovary. The ovulated oocyte is swept into the tube by a current set up in the peritoneal fluid by the beating motion of the fimbriae. Once inside the tube, the oocyte is propelled by the cilia that line the tube and by the contraction of smooth muscle in the walls. Passage through the uterine tube takes about 3 days.

If fertilization occurs, it usually takes place while the oocyte is moving through the uterine tube. The fertilized ovum, or zygote, continues the passage into the uterus for implantation and subsequent development. Occasionally something interferes with the passage into the uterus, and implantation occurs in the uterine tube; this results in an ectopic tubal pregnancy. The uterine tube cannot expand sufficiently to accommodate the growing embryo, consequently it is likely to rupture. This may result in a severe, life-threatening hemorrhage that necessitates immediate surgery to control the bleeding.

The proximal end of each uterine tube opens into the uterine cavity. The infundibular, or distal, end opens into the peritoneal cavity. These openings in the uterine tubes permit communication between the external environment and the peritoneal cavity and provide a pathway for pathogens to enter the abdominopelvic cavity.

The **uterus,** a hollow muscular organ shaped somewhat like a pear, functions to receive the embryo that results from a fertilized egg and to sustain its life during development. Although its size and shape change greatly during pregnancy, the typical, nonpregnant, premenopausal uterus is about 7 or 8 cm long and 5 cm across at its widest part. It is located in the anterior portion of the pelvic cavity, superior to the vagina. The uterus usually is tilted forward relative to the vagina (anteverted) and is bent forward over the upper surface of the urinary bladder (anteflexed). Occasionally, the uterus tilts posteriorly in a retroverted position.

The wall of the uterus is relatively thick and is composed of three layers. The lining, called the **endometrium,** is a special type of mucous membrane that is covered with columnar epithelium and contains numerous glands. It also contains blood vessels and connective tissue. The middle layer, or **myometrium,** is a thick layer of interlaced smooth muscle fibers. Contraction of the myometrium helps expel the fetus from the uterus during childbirth. A layer of serous peritoneum, called the **perimetrium,** covers the outside of the uterus. The perimetrium is continuous with the broad ligament.

The upper two thirds of the uterus, called the *body*, has a bulging superior surface known as the **fundus.** When the uterus is anteverted and anteflexed, the fundus is directed anteriorly. The **uterine tubes,** or oviducts, enter the uterus at its broadest part, between the fundus and the body. The lower one third of the uterus is a tubular **cervix** that extends downward into the upper portion of the **vagina.** The opening of the cervix into the vagina is called the *external os*. When the uterus is in its normal anteflexed position, it is bent forward on its own axis so that the body is at an angle to the cervix. Fig. 4-13 illustrates some of the relationships of the uterus.

Folds of peritoneum anchor and support the uterus in the pelvic cavity. Laterally the peritoneum extends from the anterior and posterior uterine surfaces to the lateral pelvic wall. This peritoneal extension is the **broad ligament,** which not only supports the uterus but also encloses the uterine tubes. A pair of **round ligaments** extend from the lateral walls of the uterus, near the uterine tubes, to the anterior pelvic wall. The round ligaments pass through the inguinal canal on each side and attach to the subcutaneous tissue of the labia majora. The **uterosacral ligaments** extend from the uterus to attach on the sacrum. The **lateral cervical (cardinal) ligaments** extend from the lateral walls of the cervix to the pelvic floor and primarily stabilize the cervix.

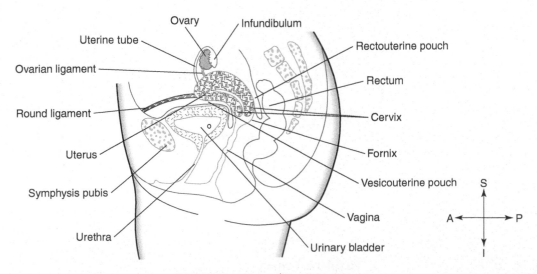

FIG. 4-13. Relationships of the uterus.

Even with the support of the various ligaments, the body of the uterus is relatively mobile, and the muscles of the pelvic floor and pelvic viscera are its principal support.

Peritoneum is reflected from the superior surface of the bladder onto the uterus, forming the **vesicouterine pouch.** This pouch, or space, usually is empty but may contain a loop of small intestine. The peritoneum continues over the surface of the uterus as the perimetrium and then is reflected onto the rectum; this forms the **rectouterine pouch,** or pouch of Douglas. The vesicouterine and rectouterine spaces are sometimes called *cul-de-sacs.*

> **QUICK CHECK**
> 4.15   What is the largest peritoneal ligament that supports the uterus?
> 4.16   When the uterus is in normal position, in what direction is the fundus pointed?

The **vagina** plays a key role in both the beginning and the end of the reproductive process. In addition to receiving the erect male penis during coitus, it functions as the birth canal during parturition, or childbirth. The vagina is a muscular tube 10 to 15 cm long that extends from the cervix of the uterus to the vestibule on the exterior. It is situated between the urethra and the bladder anteriorly and the rectum posteriorly.

The cervix of the uterus projects into the vagina at an angle, which makes the anterior wall of the vagina shorter than the posterior wall. The vagina forms recesses, or spaces, around the cervix, which are called **fornices** (singular, **fornix**). The posterior fornix is longer than the anterior fornix because of the angle at which the cervix enters the vagina. The posterior fornix is related to the rectouterine pouch of the peritoneum;

consequently, instruments inserted into the vagina may inadvertently penetrate the peritoneum of the rectouterine pouch, possibly resulting in hemorrhage and peritonitis.

The muscular walls of the vagina are lined with stratified squamous epithelium that is arranged in transverse folds, called **rugae,** which allow for expansion during coitus and parturition.

> **QUICK CHECK**
> 4.17   What portion of the uterus projects downward into the vagina?
> 4.18   Which of the two fornices of the vagina is closely related to the rectouterine pouch?

The external accessory structures of the female genital system are closely associated with the perineum. The term **vulva,** or **pudendum,** is a collective term that refers to all the female external genitalia, which includes the mons pubis, labia majora, labia minora, vestibule, clitoris, and vestibular glands (Fig. 4-14).

The **mons pubis** is a subcutaneous pad of fatty tissue that is covered with skin and forms a rounded elevation anterior to the symphysis pubis. During puberty, the mons pubis becomes covered with coarse pubic hairs.

Passing posteriorly from the mons pubis, the **labia majora** are large folds of skin filled with subcutaneous fat. The skin on the lateral surface has sweat glands and sebaceous (oil) glands, and after puberty it is covered by pubic hair. Embryologically, the labia majora are homologous with the scrotum in the male; this means that they have a similar structure and are derived from the same undifferentiated tissue. The labia majora are the lateral margins of the vulva.

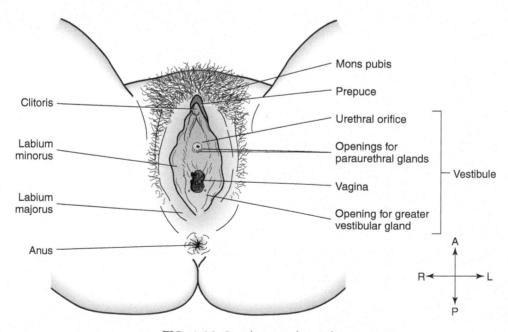

FIG. 4-14. Female external genitalia.

The **labia minora** are two thin, delicate folds of skin located between the labia majora. Although devoid of fat and hair, the labia minora are richly supplied with blood vessels, nerves, and sebaceous glands. The labia minora lie on either side of the urethra and the vaginal openings and enclose the vestibule. Anteriorly, the folds of the labia minora unite to form a prepuce over the clitoris.

The **clitoris,** which is homologous to the penis in the male, is located posterior and inferior to the mons pubis and is between the anterior ends of the labia minora. Although only 2 to 3 cm long, it is composed of two columns of erectile corpora cavernosa and is anchored to the os coxae by two crura. Like the male penis, it is capable of enlargement when stimulated.

The **vestibule** is the narrow cleft between the two labia minora. The clitoris is at the anterior end of the vestibule and posterior to the clitoris; the urethra opens into the anterior portion of the vestibule. The vaginal orifice is posterior to the urethra. Two elongated masses of corpora spongiosa lie along the lateral margins of the vestibule, deep to the bulbospongiosus muscle, to form the bulb of the vestibule. Vestibular glands, so named because they are located within the vestibule, include the **paraurethral glands** and the **greater vestibular glands.** The paraurethral glands, homologous to the prostate gland of the male, are located on the either side of the external urethral orifice and secrete mucus for lubrication. The greater vestibular glands, also called Bartholin's glands, are homologous to the bulbourethral glands of the male and are located on either side of the vaginal orifice. They secrete a mucoid substance for lubrication. Normally vestibular glands are not palpable, but they may become enlarged and irritating when they are infected.

QUICK CHECK

4.19 What is another term for the vulva?

4.20 What glands are included as vestibular glands?

Male Reproductive Organs and Accessory Structures. The male genital organs include the testes in the scrotum, ductus deferens, ejaculatory duct, seminal vesicles, prostate, bulbourethral glands, and penis. All of these are located in the pelvic cavity except the testes and penis. The anatomical relationships of the male reproductive organs are illustrated in Fig. 4-15.

The primary reproductive organs of the male are the paired **testes** (Fig. 4-16). These ovoid structures are suspended in a sac of skin called the *scrotum.* Each testis is covered by a tough, fibrous connective tissue, the **tunica albuginea.** Extensions of the tunica albuginea project inward, dividing each testis into about 300 lobules. Each lobule contains one to three tightly coiled **seminiferous tubules.** Spermatogenesis, the production of sperm, takes place in the seminiferous tubules.

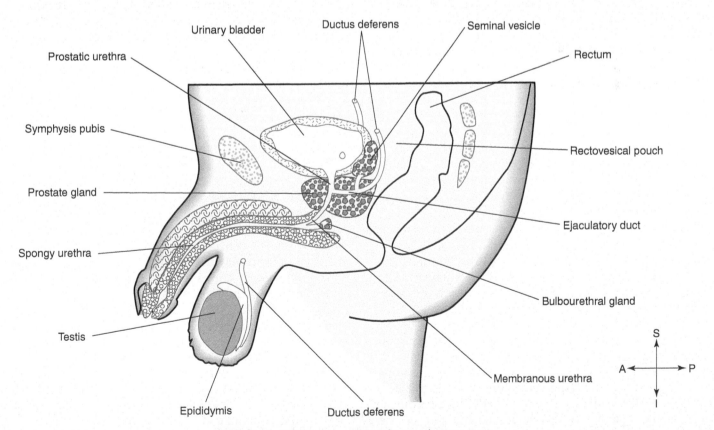

FIG. 4-15. Relationships of the male reproductive organs.

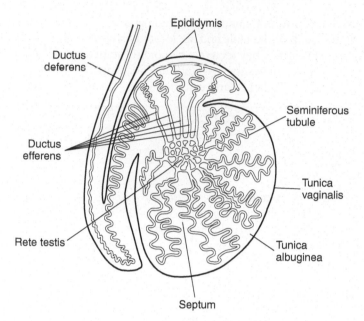

Epididymis

Ductus
deferens

Seminiferous
tubule

Ductus
efferens

Tunica
vaginalis

Tunica
albuginea

Rete testis

Septum

FIG. 4-16. Sagittal section of a testis and epididymis.

In addition to the tunica albuginea, the testes are covered by a thin, serous sac, the **tunica vaginalis,** which is derived from peritoneum. Because this is a serous membrane, it has two layers: a parietal layer, which lines the scrotum, and a visceral layer, which covers the testes. The testes develop in the lumbar region of the abdomen, near the kidneys, and usually descend into the scrotum through the inguinal canal shortly before birth. Because the testes develop in the abdomen, their arterial blood supply is from the abdomen, and venous drainage returns to the abdomen. An extension or diverticulum of peritoneum precedes the testes during the descent into the scrotum. This peritoneum becomes the tunica vaginalis. It is important that the testes descend into the scrotum, because spermatozoa cannot survive the warmer temperatures of the abdominal cavity.

The **epididymis** is a flattened, tightly coiled, tubular structure on the posterior surface of each testis. The spermatids produced by spermatogenesis in the seminiferous tubules pass through efferent ducts into the epididymis for maturation and storage. The epididymis is continuous with the ductus deferens, which transports sperm to the ejaculatory duct.

The **scrotum** is a saclike structure that contains the testes, their coverings, or tunics, and the epididymis. The scrotum consists of a layer of skin, which covers a thin layer of connective tissue that is interspersed with smooth muscle fibers, called the **dartos muscle.** Contraction of the dartos muscle gives a wrinkled appearance to the scrotum. Internally, the scrotum is divided by a **median raphe,** or septum, into two compartments, each containing a testis that is suspended by the **spermatic cord.** Each **ductus deferens** is a thick-walled, muscular tube that is a continuation of the epididymis. Beginning in the tail of the

epididymis at the inferior border of the testis, the ductus deferens ascends in the spermatic cord and passes through the inguinal canal. As the ductus deferens enters the pelvis, it crosses over the external iliac vessels. From the inguinal canal, the ductus deferens descends retroperitoneally along the lateral wall of the pelvis and then crosses the ureter to pass between the ureter and the bladder. The ductus deferens descends posterior to the bladder and medial to the ureter and the seminal vesicles. The terminal portion, near the base of the bladder, is joined by the duct from the seminal vesicles to form the **ejaculatory duct,** which opens into the prostatic urethra.

A **spermatic cord** extends from each testis to the inguinal canal on the same side. Structures passing to and from the testis make up the contents of the spermatic cord. These structures include the ductus deferens, the testicular artery, a venous plexus (pampiniform plexus), lymph vessels, nerves, and connective tissue. This bundle of structures is surrounded by connective tissue and muscle fibers to make a cord that suspends the testis in the scrotum. The **cremaster muscle,** derived from the internal oblique muscle of the abdomen, extends through the spermatic cord to the testes. This muscle functions with the dartos muscle to alter the position of the testes to maintain optimum temperature for the production and maturation of spermatozoa.

The **seminal vesicles** are paired accessory glands that consist of coiled tubes that appear to be twisted to form small pouches or vesicles. The glands are located between the posterior surface of the bladder and the rectum. The duct of each seminal vesicle joins with the associated ductus deferens to form an **ejaculatory duct,** which opens into the prostatic urethra. The secretion of the seminal vesicles has a high fructose content, which provides an energy source for the sperm.

The largest accessory gland of the male reproductive system is the **prostate gland.** It is composed partially of glandular parenchyma and partially of connective tissue stroma. Located inferior to the bladder, this chestnut-shaped gland surrounds the prostatic urethra. About 20 to 30 small prostatic ducts empty into the urethra. The secretion of the prostate gland aids the motility and fertility of the sperm. Because of the prostate's close relationship to the urethra, hypertrophy of the prostate frequently interferes with the passage of urine. Subsequent problems related to the stasis of urine may then develop. Surgery may be indicated if urination becomes too difficult or impossible.

Each **bulbourethral gland,** also known as a Cowper's gland, is about 1 cm in diameter. The glands, one on either side of the urethra, are located posterior and lateral to the membranous urethra. Their relatively long ducts pass through the membranous urethra to empty into the proximal portion of the spongy urethra. In response to sexual stimulation, the bulbourethral glands secrete a small amount of an alkaline, mucoid substance that neutralizes the acidity of the spongy urethra and lubricates the tip of the penis.

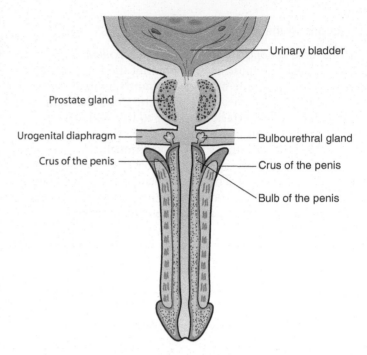

FIG. 4-18. Root of the penis.

The **penis** is a copulatory organ used to introduce spermatozoa into the vagina of the female. It is cylindrical and is divided into a root and a body. Structurally, the penis consists of three cylindrical masses of erectile tissue, each surrounded by a connective tissue tunica albuginea. The two dorsal cylinders of erectile tissue are the **corpora cavernosa,** and the smaller, midventral cylinder, which encircles the spongy urethra, is the **corpus spongiosum.** Fig. 4-17 illustrates this arrangement. Distally, the corpus spongiosum expands to form the **glans penis.**

The **root** of the penis (Fig. 4-18) is the attached portion and consists of a bulb and two crura. The **bulb** is the expanded proximal end of the corpus spongiosum. It is anchored to the tissue of the urogenital diaphragm in the pelvic floor and is enclosed by the bulbospongiosus muscle of the perineum. The two **crura** are the tapered proximal ends of the corpora cavernosa that diverge to attach to the ischiopubic rami. The ischiocavernosus muscle of the perineum envelops the crura.

The **body** of the penis is the free portion that is pendulous in the flaccid condition. The three cylindrical columns of erectile tissue are surrounded by connective tissue fascia and skin. Facing anteriorly when flaccid, the dorsum of the penis is continuous with the anterior abdominal wall. The ventral, or urethral, aspect faces poste-

riorly in the flaccid condition and anteriorly when erect. The **glans penis,** at the distal end of the body, is corpus spongiosum and has the opening for the urethra. The skin covering the body of the penis continues over the glans penis as the **prepuce.** The prepuce, or foreskin, is sometimes removed shortly after birth in a surgical procedure called *circumcision.*

During sexual stimulation, parasympathetic reflexes cause dilation of the arteries that supply the penis, and the sinuses of the erectile tissue fill with blood. At the same time, the pressure of the dilated arteries and the filled sinuses compresses the veins leaving the penis, so that the blood is retained. These vascular changes result in an erection. The penis returns to its flaccid state when the arteries constrict and pressure on the veins is reduced.

Sectional Anatomy of the Pelvis

For convenience, this discussion of the sectional anatomy of the pelvis includes the false pelvis. In other words, transverse sections begin with the iliac crest. In these more superior sections of the false pelvis, the organs seen will be familiar, because they are continuous with those studied in the abdomen.

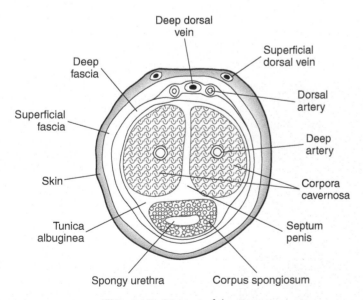

FIG. 4-17. Structure of the penis.

Sections of the Female Pelvis

Transverse Section Through the Sacroiliac Joint. A line through the most superior point of the two iliac crests usually intersects the body of the fourth lumbar vertebra. This is the level of the aortic bifurcation into the **right** and **left common iliac arteries.** Inferior to this, at level L5, the two **common iliac veins** join to form the inferior vena cava. Fig. 4-19 illustrates a section through the sacroiliac joint. Common iliac arteries and common iliac veins are present at this level. The lower portions of the **ascending colon** and the **cecum** are located in the right iliac fossa. The smaller **descending colon** is in the left iliac fossa.

Because of the variable nature of the **transverse colon,** it is impossible to state specifically when it will or will not be seen. It drapes inferiorly and anteriorly between the right and left colic flexures. In some individuals, it is pendulous and extends down into the pelvis. Transverse sections through the false pelvis of these individuals show two regions of the transverse colon. One region is on the right side as the transverse colon descends and the other on the left as it ascends toward the left colic (splenic) flexure. More commonly, sections at this level are inferior to the transverse colon.

As in the abdomen, the **psoas muscles** are on either side of the vertebral column. The **ureters** descend anterior to the psoas muscle. The **iliacus muscle** lines the iliac fossa, and the **gluteal muscle** originates on the lateral surface of the ilium. The CT image in Fig. 4-20 is near the same level as Fig. 4-19 and illustrates many of the same structures.

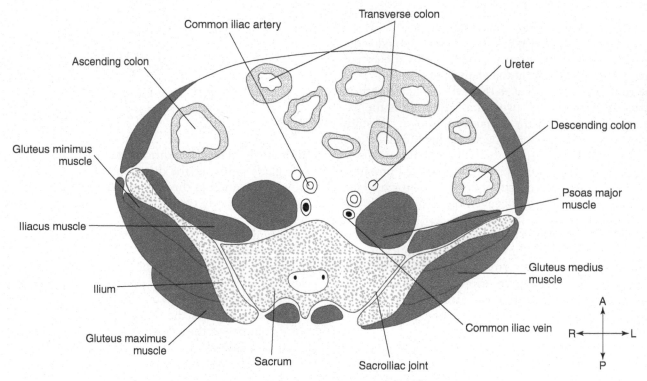

FIG. 4-19. Transverse section through the sacroiliac joint.

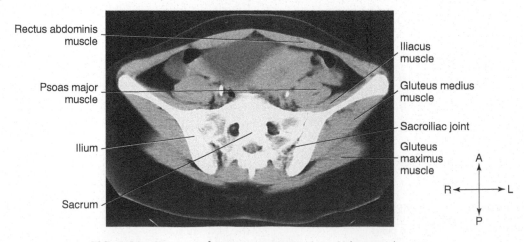

FIG. 4-20. CT image of a transverse section through the sacroiliac joint.

Transverse Section Through the Lower Part of the Sacrum. The relationships of structures in the lower part of the sacrum, primarily muscles, are illustrated in Fig. 4-21. The fibers of the psoas and iliacus muscles merge to form the **iliopsoas muscle.** Observe the close relationship of the **femoral nerve** to this muscle. All three gluteal muscles are evident lateral and posterior to the ilium. The **gluteus maximus** is the most superficial, and the **gluteus minimus** is the deepest, next to the ilium. The **piriformis muscle** is in the **greater sciatic foramen** (notch) between the ilium and the sacrum. The **obturator internus** muscle,

which lines the cavity of the true pelvis, is medial to the ilium. The common iliac vessels generally have bifurcated at this level, with the **external iliac vessels** associated with the iliopsoas muscles as they proceed to the upper thigh region. The **ureter** is more closely associated with the **internal iliac vessels** in the true pelvis. The CT image in Fig. 4-22 is near this level and shows many of the same structures.

Transverse Section Through the Uterus. Fig. 4-23 and the transverse CT image in Fig. 4-24 illustrate a transverse

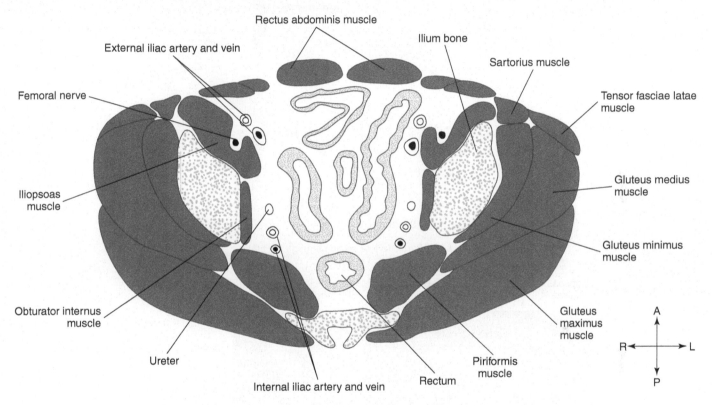

FIG. 4-21. Transverse section through the lower part of the sacrum.

FIG. 4-22. CT image of a transverse section through the lower part of the sacrum.

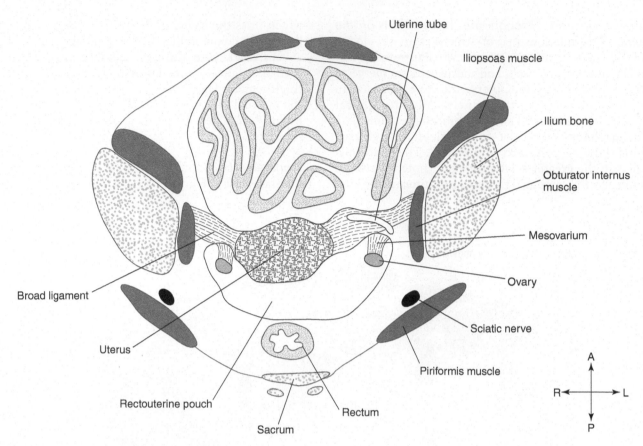

FIG. 4-23. Transverse section through the uterus.

FIG. 4-24. Transverse CT image through the uterus. (Modified from Bo WJ et al: *Basic atlas of sectional anatomy: with correlated imaging,* ed 4, St Louis, 2007, Elsevier/Saunders.)

section through the **uterus.** This section shows the **broad ligament,** which extends from the uterus to the lateral pelvic wall. The **ovaries** are attached to the posterior portion of the broad ligament by the mesovarium, and the **uterine tube** is in the upper margin of the ligament but may be difficult to see. The space between the uterus and the rectum is the **rectouterine pouch** (pouch of Douglas), which may contain loops of bowel. The **obturator internus** muscle originates on the inner surface of the ilium and covers most of the lateral wall of the true pelvis.

Transverse Section Through the Urinary Bladder. Fig. 4-25 illustrates a transverse section through the superior surface of the urinary bladder. This shows the **ureters** posterior to the bladder as they are about to penetrate the bladder wall. The **cervix** is interposed between the bladder and the rectum. The **obturator internus** and **levator ani** muscles form the lateral walls and floor of the pelvic cavity. Anteriorly, the **pectineus muscle** originates on the pubis. The CT image in Fig. 4-26 is near this level and illustrates some of the same structures.

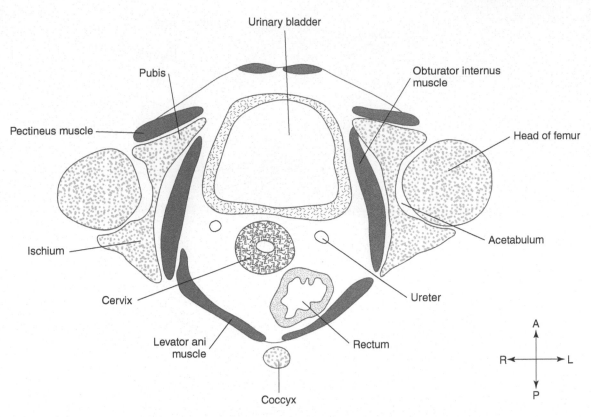

FIG. 4-25. Transverse section through the urinary bladder.

FIG. 4-26. CT image of a transverse section through the urinary bladder.

QUICK CHECK

4.26 In transverse sections through the sacroiliac joint, which is present: the inferior vena cava or the common iliac veins?

4.27 In transverse sections through the uterus, what is the space between the uterus and the rectum?

4.28 In transverse sections through the urinary bladder in the female, what portion of the reproductive system may be present between the bladder and the rectum?

Midsagittal Section Through the Female Pelvis. The line drawing in Fig. 4-27 illustrates a midsagittal section through the female pelvis. The magnetic resonance (MR) image in Fig. 4-28 is from a similar region. Posteriorly, the **rectum** follows the curvature of the sacrum. Anteriorly, the **urinary bladder** is in a position immediately posterior to the symphysis pubis. The **fundus** and **body** of the uterus are anteverted over the superior surface of the bladder and are anteflexed with the **cervix**. The peritoneum forms two cul-de-sacs related to the uterus that are nicely illustrated

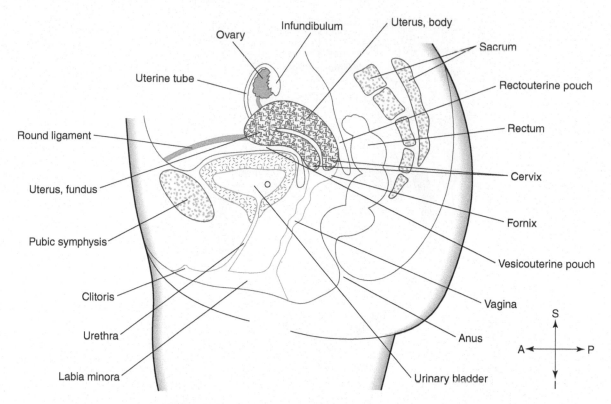

FIG. 4-27. Midsagittal section through the female pelvis.

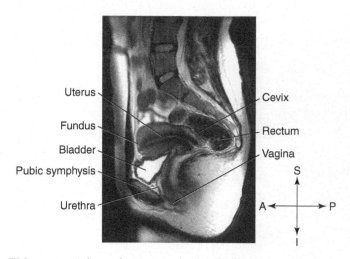

FIG. 4-28. Midsagittal MR image through the female pelvis. (Modified from Weir J, Abrahams PH: *Imaging atlas of human anatomy,* ed 3, St Louis, 2003, Elsevier/Mosby.)

in midsagittal sections. Posteriorly, the **rectouterine pouch** extends between the rectum and the uterus; then, as the peritoneum continues from the fundus of the uterus to the superior surface of the bladder, it forms the **vesicouterine pouch.** The **vagina** slants posteriorly as it ascends to the cervix of the uterus, where the vagina surrounds the cervix to form the **fornices.** The **posterior fornix** is longer than the anterior fornix. The **urethra** extends from the bladder and through the urogenital diaphragm to open into the **vestibule,** anterior to the vaginal orifice and posterior to

the **clitoris.** The **labia minora** form the lateral margins of the vestibule.

Coronal Section Through the Body of the Uterus.   Fig. 4-29 illustrates a coronal section through the anterior part of the pelvis, showing the **body** of the uterus and the **urinary bladder. Uterine tubes** extend from the uterus toward the lateral pelvic wall. The urinary bladder is inferior to the uterus and separated from it by the **vesicouterine** space. **Obturator internus** muscles form the lateral walls of the cavity and the hammock-like **levator ani** muscles form the pelvic floor. Two **crura** of the clitoris, composed of corpus cavernosum, are associated with the ischiopubic ramus. The **labia majora,** which are homologous to the scrotum in the male, enclose the smaller **labia minora,** which form the lateral margins of the vestibule. Fig. 4-30 is an MR image from a similar region.

QUICK CHECK

4.29   In a midsagittal section through the female pelvis, what structure is bent over the superior surface of the urinary bladder?

4.30   In coronal sections through the uterus, what is the space between the uterus and the urinary bladder?

Sections of the Male Pelvis

Transverse Section Through the Seminal Vesicles.   The line drawing in Fig. 4-31 illustrates the relationships of the **ureters, seminal vesicles,** and **ductus deferens.** The ureters

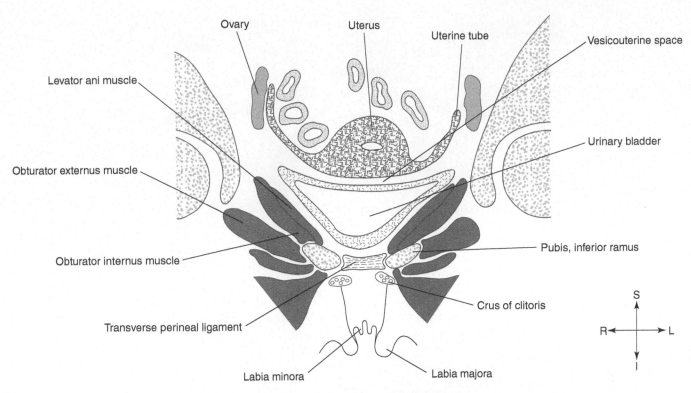

FIG. 4-29. Coronal section through the female pelvis.

FIG. 4-30. Coronal MR image through the female pelvis. (Modified from Weir J, Abrahams PH: *Imaging atlas of human anatomy,* ed 3, St Louis, 2003, Elsevier/Mosby.)

are shown as they penetrate the wall of the bladder. The **seminal vesicles** are glandular structures between the rectum and urinary bladder. The **ductus deferens** are medial to both the ureters and the seminal vesicles. The space between the bladder and the rectum is the **rectovesical space,** a peritoneal cul-de-sac in the male. Anteriorly, between the iliopsoas and pectineus muscles, the femoral triangle contains the femoral artery, vein, and nerve. The spermatic cord, anterior and medial to the margin of the pectineus muscle, contains the testicular artery, ductus deferens, and

pampiniform venous plexus. The CT image in Fig. 4-32 is from a similar region.

Transverse Section Through the Prostate Gland. The **prostate gland** is inferior to the bladder and posterior to the symphysis pubis. It surrounds the **prostatic urethra** (Fig. 4-33). A **prostatic venous plexus** surrounds the gland. The **rectum** is posterior to the prostate. Because the prostate rests on the curved pelvic floor, a portion of the floor, specifically the **levator ani** muscle, is evident. The pelvic walls are lined

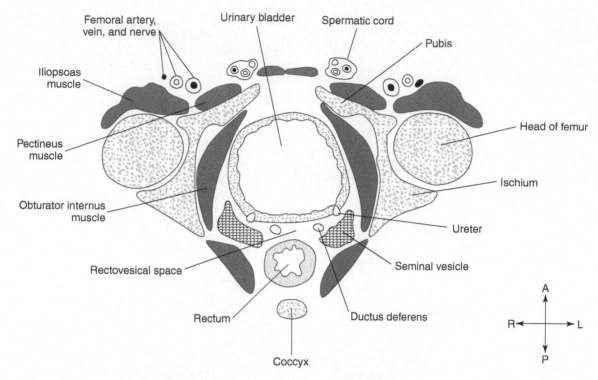

FIG. 4-31. Transverse section through the seminal vesicles.

FIG. 4-32. Transverse CT image through the seminal vesicles.

with the **obturator internus** muscle. The CT image in Fig. 4-34 also shows the prostate gland.

Transverse Section Through the Root of the Penis. The line drawing in Fig. 4-35 and the CT image in Fig. 4-36 illustrate the root of the penis, which consists of a bulb and two crura. The **bulb** portion of the root is **corpus spongiosum** and surrounds the urethra. The **transverse perinei muscle** extends horizontally between the two ischial rami with the bulb anterior and the anal canal posterior to the muscle. The **bulbospongiosus muscle** is associated with the bulb of the penis. Lateral to the bulb, the two **crura** of

corpus cavernosum diverge to attach to the ischial rami. The **ischiocavernosus muscle** is related to the crura.

QUICK CHECK

4.31 In transverse sections through the seminal vesicles, which is more medial: the ureters or the ductus deferens?

4.32 In transverse sections through the prostate gland, what portion of the urinary tract is present?

4.33 In transverse sections through the root of the penis, what muscle is associated with the bulb?

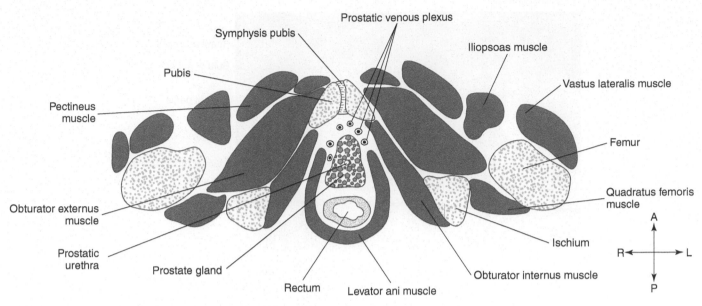

FIG. 4-33. Transverse section through the prostate gland.

FIG. 4-34. Transverse CT image through the prostate gland.

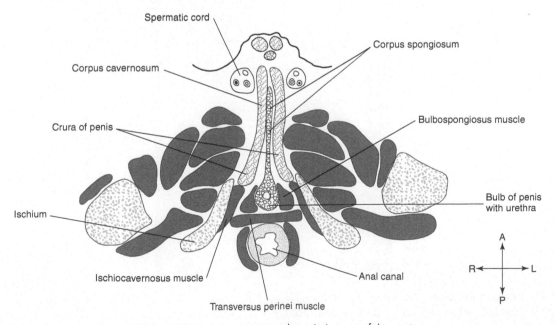

FIG. 4-35. Transverse section through the root of the penis.

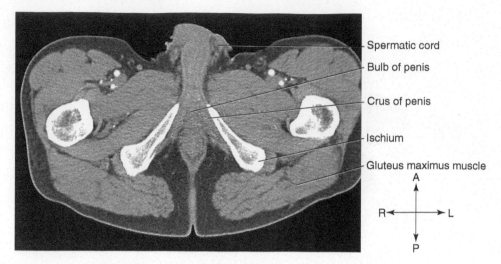

FIG. 4-36. Transverse CT image through the root of the penis.

Midsagittal Section of the Male Pelvis. Midsagittal sections of the male pelvis show the typical relationships of the male reproductive organs discussed previously and illustrated by the line drawing in Fig. 4-15. Refer to this figure while reviewing the relationships discussed in this paragraph. The sagittal MR image in Fig. 4-37 also illustrates some of these relationships. Fig. 4-15 shows how the rectum follows the curvature of the sacrum. The peritoneum continues down the posterior wall and then curves over the seminal vesicles and urinary bladder. The seminal vesicles are between the bladder and the rectum, just inferior to the peritoneal rectovesical pouch. The prostate gland is inferior to the bladder and rests on the pelvic floor. The duct from the seminal vesicles joins the ductus deferens to form the ejaculatory duct, which penetrates the prostate gland to empty into the prostatic urethra. The urethra continues through the urogenital diaphragm as the membranous urethra and then enters the corpus spongiosum of the penis to become the penile, or spongy, urethra. The duct from the bulbourethral gland empties into the spongy urethra.

Coronal Section Through the Prostate Gland and the Root of the Penis. The line drawing in Fig. 4-38 and the MR image in Fig. 4-39 illustrate a coronal section of the male pelvis through the prostate gland and root of the penis. **Obturator internus muscles** line the pelvic wall and fill the space of the obturator foramen. **Levator ani muscles** form the hammock-shaped pelvic floor, and the **transverse perinei muscle** extends between the two ischial tuberosities. The **prostate gland,** inferior to the **urinary bladder,** rests on the pelvic floor and encircles the **prostatic urethra.** The urethra continues through the muscle and fascia of the **urogenital diaphragm** as the **membranous urethra**

FIG. 4-37. Sagittal MR image through the male pelvis. (Modified from Weir J, Abrahams PH: *Imaging atlas of human anatomy,* ed 3, St Louis, 2003, Elsevier/Mosby.)

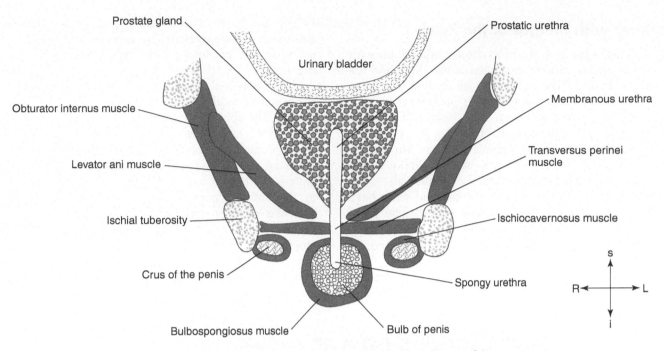

FIG. 4-38. Coronal section through the prostate gland and the root of the penis.

FIG. 4-39. MR image of a coronal section through the prostate gland and the root of the penis.

and then penetrates the corpus spongiosum in the bulb of the penis to become the **spongy urethra.** The components of the root of the penis, the bulb and the two crura, are also represented. The **bulb,** which consists of **corpus spongiosum,** is surrounded by the **bulbospongiosus muscle** and anchored to perineal membrane. It encircles the spongy urethra. The two crura of **corpus cavernosum** are surrounded by **ischiocavernosus muscle** and are anchored to the ischial tuberosities.

QUICK CHECK

4.34   In midsagittal sections of the male pelvis, what glandular structure is posterior to the urinary bladder?

4.35   In coronal sections through the prostate gland and root of the penis, what portions of the root are on both sides of the bulb?

Working with Images of the Pelvis

The CT image in Fig. 4-40 shows the sacroiliac joint with the gluteus medius muscle superficial to the ilium and the iliacus muscle lining the wall of the false pelvis. The aorta and inferior vena cava are no longer present; they have been replaced by the common iliac vessels. The psoas muscles are lateral to the sacrum. Numerous loops of bowel fill the cavity. The rectus abdominis muscles form the anterior wall. The external oblique, internal oblique, and transversus abdominis muscles form the lateral wall.

In Fig. 4-41, the common iliac arteries and veins have bifurcated into external and internal vessels. The psoas muscle is merging with the iliacus to form the iliopsoas. Posteriorly, the gluteus maximus muscle is superficial to the gluteus medius.

The CT image in Fig. 4-42 shows the greater sciatic notch with the piriformis muscle in the space created by the notch. All three gluteal muscles are present in this image. The **external iliac arteries** and **veins** are adjacent to the iliopsoas muscle with the artery anterior to the vein.

The region depicted in Fig. 4-43 shows the urinary bladder posterior to the symphysis pubis and anterior to the rectum. The obturator internus muscle lines the wall of the true pelvis. The muscle between the femur and the spine of the ischium is the gemellus muscle. The sciatic nerve and pudendal vessels are between the gemellus muscle and the gluteus maximus muscle. Several features should be noted in the anterior portion of this section. The pectineus muscle is adjacent to the pubic bone and forms one side of a triangle that contains the femoral artery and vein. Other muscles in the region are the iliopsoas, sartorius, rectus femoris, and tensor fasciae latae.

The CT image in Fig. 4-44 shows the superior portion of the urinary bladder and the cervix of the uterus posterior to

Common iliac artery

Gluteus medius muscle

Sacroiliac joint

FIG. 4-40. Transverse CT image through the sacroiliac joint.

External iliac artery

Internal iliac artery

FIG. 4-41. Transverse CT image showing external and internal iliac arteries.

FIG. 4-42. Transverse CT image through the greater sciatic notch.

— External iliac vein

— Piriformis muscle

FIG. 4-43. Transverse CT image through the symphysis pubis.

— Urinary bladder

— Obturator internus muscle

— Rectum

FIG. 4-44. Transverse CT image through the cervix.

— Urinary bladder

— Cervix

it. In this case, the urinary bladder is empty and small. The obturator externus muscle is lateral to the obturator internus. Anteriorly, the femoral artery has given off a deep femoral branch, and the great saphenous vein has branched from the femoral vein.

The CT image in Fig. 4-45 shows the bottom of the urinary bladder with the urethral orifice. Some of the adductor group of muscles are apparent adjacent to the inferior ischiopubic ramus.

The CT image in Fig. 4-46 shows the fat-filled labia majora lateral to the labia minora and the vestibule. The clitoris is at the anterior end of the vestibule. Posteriorly, the bulb of the vestibule diverges on either side of the vagina.

The ultrasound image in Fig. 4-47 is a sagittal image of an ovary with follicular cysts. The asterisks indicate the outline of the ovary, with the follicular cysts in the

parenchyma. A portion of the echogenic tunica is evident.

The ultrasound image in Fig. 4-48 was done transvaginally and shows a retroverted uterus. The fundus is at the right side of the image. The uterine cavity is the dark line in the center. The asterisks indicate the basal layer of the endometrium. The remaining tissue, between the endometrium and the margin (serosa) of the uterus, is myometrium.

The procedure used to obtain the image in Fig. 4-49 was a transvaginal ultrasound. It shows the same features as Fig. 4-48; however, this one is a normal anteverted uterus so the fundus is on the left side of the image, and it has a thicker endometrium.

The ultrasound image in Fig. 4-50 shows an embryo in the amniotic sac at approximately 7 weeks of development. The head is to the left, and the rump is to the right. The

FIG. 4-45. Transverse CT image through the urinary bladder.

FIG. 4-46. Transverse CT image through the vagina and bulb of vestibule.

FIG. 4-47. Sagittal ultrasound image of an ovary with follicular cysts.

FIG. 4-48. Ultrasound image of a retroverted uterus.

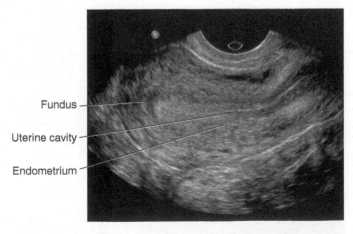

FIG. 4-49. Ultrasound image of a normal anteverted uterus.

FIG. 4-50. Ultrasound image of an embryo at approximately 7 weeks of development.

umbilical cord attaches the embryo to the placenta, which is in a very early stage of development.

The ultrasound image in Fig. 4-51 shows a fetal arm with the radius and ulna. The carpals, metacarpals, and phalanges are also evident. The "hump" in the lower part of the image is a myometrial contraction. The placenta is at the top of the image.

The ultrasound image in Fig. 4-52 shows a fetal spine and head at approximately 20 weeks of development. The head is at the right side of the image, and the spine curves to the left. The placenta is at the top of the image.

The transverse CT image of the male pelvis in Fig. 4-53 is inferior to the urinary bladder and shows the prostate gland. The symphysis pubis is anterior to the prostate, and the rectum is posterior. Numerous familiar muscle relationships are evident. Identify the obturator internus, obturator externus, pectineus, iliopsoas, sartorius, tensor fasciae latae, rectus femoris, gemellus, and gluteus maximus. The femoral artery and vein are present in the femoral triangle.

The transverse CT image in Fig. 4-54 shows the right and left testicles in the scrotum. The section is through the femur and shows the adductor group of muscles and the gracilis muscle. Anteriorly the muscles of the quadriceps femoris are evident.

The sonogram in Fig. 4-55 shows the two seminal vesicle glands in the male pelvis with the right and left ductus deferens between them. The urinary bladder is anterior to the seminal vesicles, and the rectum is posterior.

The sonogram in Fig. 4-56 shows a sagittal view of the left testicle and a portion of the epididymis in the scrotum. The head of the epididymis is on the left side of the image. The asterisks outline a small epididymal cyst. The top of the image shows the wall of the scrotum.

The sonogram in Fig. 4-57 shows the right and left testicles in the scrotum. The wall of the scrotum is at the top of the image, and the raphe separates the two testicles. The asterisks denote the small space between the tunica albuginea of the testicles and the wall of the scrotum.

FIG. 4-51. Ultrasound image of a fetal arm and hand.

FIG. 4-52. Ultrasound image of a fetal spine and head at approximately 20 weeks of development.

Placenta

Head

Sartorius muscle

Tensor fasciae latae muscle

Rectus femoris muscle

Femoral artery

Femoral vein

Pectineus muscle

Greater trochanter

Obturator externus muscle

Obturator internus muscle

Prostate gland

Rectum

FIG. 4-53. Transverse CT image through the prostate gland.

Adductor longus muscle

Adductor brevis muscle

Gracilis muscle

Adductor magnus muscle

FIG. 4-54. Transverse CT image through the testicles.

FIG. 4-55. Ultrasound image of the seminal vesicles and ductus deferens.

FIG. 4-56. Ultrasound image of the left testicle.

FIG. 4-57. Transverse ultrasound image of the testicles.

Important Anatomical Relationships in the Pelvis

- The common iliac veins join to form the inferior vena cava at the L5 vertebral level (see Chapter 3).
- The common iliac arteries are anterior to the common iliac veins (see Figs. 4-19 and 4-20).
- The iliacus muscle lines the iliac fossa of the false pelvis (see Figs. 4-19 and 4-20).
- The fibers of the psoas and iliacus muscles merge to form the iliopsoas muscle (see Figs. 4-21 and 4-22).
- The femoral nerve is located near the junction of the iliacus and psoas muscles (see Figs. 4-21 and 4-22).
- External iliac arteries are anterior to internal iliac arteries (see Fig. 4-21).
- External iliac veins are anterior to internal iliac veins (see Fig. 4-21).
- External iliac arteries are anterior to external iliac veins (see Fig. 4-21).
- Internal iliac arteries are anterior to internal iliac veins (see Fig. 4-21).
- The piriformis muscle passes through the greater sciatic notch (see Figs. 4-21 and 4-22).
- The rectouterine space is the peritoneal pouch between the uterus and the rectum (see Figs. 4-13 and 4-27).
- The sciatic nerve is anterior (deep) to the piriformis muscle (see Fig. 4-23).
- The obturator internus muscle lines the lateral walls of the true pelvis (see Figs. 4-21, 4-23, and 4-26).
- The broad ligament extends laterally from the uterus to attach to the lateral pelvic wall (see Figs. 4-12, 4-24, and 4-30).
- The posterior fornix of the vagina is between the cervix and the rectum and is inferior to the rectouterine space (see Figs. 4-13 and 4-27).
- The urinary bladder is inferior to the body of the uterus (see Figs. 4-13, 4-27, and 4-30).
- The peritoneal space between the uterus and the urinary bladder is the vesicouterine space (see Figs. 4-13 and 4-27).
- The pectineus muscle is anterior to the pubic bone (see Figs. 4-25, 4-26, 4-31, and 4-43).
- The urethra is anterior to the vagina (see Figs. 4-13 and 4-27).
- The clitoris is at the anterior end of the vestibule (see Fig. 4-14).
- The labia minora enclose the vestibule (see Fig. 4-14).
- The ductus deferens descend posterior to the urinary bladder, along the medial margin of the seminal vesicles and medial to the ureters (see Figs. 4-15 and 4-31).
- The seminal vesicles are posterior to the urinary bladder (see Figs. 4-15, 4-31, and 4-32).
- The prostate gland surrounds the prostatic urethra and is inferior to the urinary bladder (see Figs. 4-15, 4-33, and 4-34).
- The two dorsal columns of erectile tissue in the penis are the corpora cavernosa (see Figs. 4-17, 4-35, and 4-36).
- The single ventral column of erectile tissue in the penis is the corpus spongiosum, which surrounds the urethra (see Figs. 4-17, 4-35, and 4-37).

Pathology

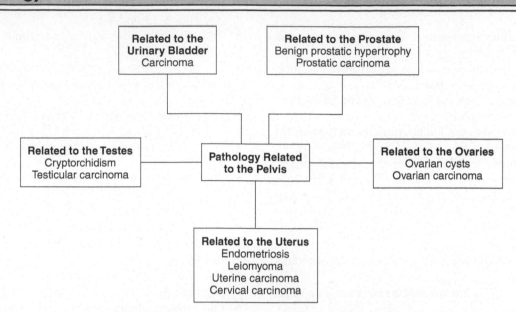

**Related to the
Urinary Bladder**
Carcinoma

Related to the Prostate
Benign prostatic hypertrophy
Prostatic carcinoma

Related to the Testes
Cryptorchidism
Testicular carcinoma

**Pathology Related
to the Pelvis**

Related to the Ovaries
Ovarian cysts
Ovarian carcinoma

Related to the Uterus
Endometriosis
Leiomyoma
Uterine carcinoma
Cervical carcinoma

Bladder Carcinoma

Bladder carcinoma occurs in the transitional epithelium of the mucosa, or lining, of the urinary bladder. The incidence of bladder carcinoma in males is three times the incidence in females and it usually appears after the age of 50. Smoking is the most significant risk factor. Excessive coffee drinking and exposure to certain industrial chemicals have also been implicated as possible risk factors.

Benign Prostatic Hypertrophy

Benign prostatic hypertrophy is a nonmalignant hyperplasia of the prostate gland and is common in men over the age of 50. Because the prostate surrounds the urethra, the enlargement may obstruct the flow of urine from the bladder.

Prostatic Carcinoma

Carcinoma of the glandular tissue in the prostate ranks third in the leading causes of cancer in men. Early detection is important because metastasis soon involves the regional lymph nodes, bones, and lungs.

Cryptorchidism

Cryptorchidism is the failure of one or both of the testes to descend into the scrotum. During prenatal development, the testes first appear in the abdomen. About the seventh month, they descend into the groin area, then pass through the inguinal canal into the scrotum. If this does not occur in a normal manner, cryptorchidism results. Viable sperm are not produced if the testes do not completely descend; consequently, if both testes are involved and untreated, sterility results.

Testicular Carcinoma

The incidence of malignant tumors of the testes is fairly uncommon; however, they usually occur at a relatively young age, between the ages of 18 and 40. There are two primary groups, seminoma and teratoma. The seminoma appear to arise from the seminiferous tubules of the testes and are quite radiosensitive, which makes the prognosis good with early detection. The

teratoma appear to arise from primitive germ cells and are associated with a poor prognosis. Both types are malignant and metastasize through the lymphatic and blood vessels.

Ovarian Cysts

Numerous types of benign cysts may occur in the ovary, including cysts in the ovarian follicles, corpus luteum, and glandular tissue. The most common is a cystadenoma, a cyst originating from the glandular tissue. Polycystic ovaries consist of enlarged ovaries with numerous small cysts and characterized by amenorrhea and sterility. Fibroid cysts arise from unfertilized ova and often contain hair, fat, and possibly even bone and teeth.

Serous carcinoma from the surface epithelium of the ovary is the most common type of ovarian cancer. Although ovarian carcinomas are less common than other carcinomas of the female reproductive system, they are usually asymptomatic until late in the development of the disease, which greatly reduces the chance for a cure. These malignant tumors readily invade their capsule and release tumor cells all around the pelvis and abdomen.

Endometriosis

Endometriosis is a condition in which an area of endometrial tissue grows outside the uterus. The cause is unknown but it is thought to be due to retrograde menstruation or hormonal disturbances. The symptoms vary but may include pelvic pain, dysmenorrhea, and infertility.

Leiomyoma

The most common benign tumor in women is the leiomyoma, also referred to as a fibroid tumor. It develops from the smooth muscle layer of the uterus and grows during the reproductive years, then typically shrinks after menopause. The tumors may be small or large, single or numerous. Symptoms and treatment vary with the severity of the disease. A small tumor may be asymptomatic and require no treatment. Large tumors may put pressure on the bladder causing frequent urination, compress the rectum resulting in obstruction and constipation, and cause infertility.

Pathology—cont'd

Uterine Cancer

Adenocarcinoma of the uterus is one of the most common malignancies in the female reproductive system, usually occurring in postmenopausal women. It usually arises from the basal cells of the epithelial lining, the endometrium, and may cause postmenopausal bleeding. Uterine cancer may be detected by dysplasia of the epithelial cells in a Pap smear. It then progresses to carcinoma in situ and finally to an invasive malignant carcinoma. With early detection, before the carcinoma becomes invasive, the prognosis is good and the cure rate is fairly high.

Cervical Carcinoma

Cervical carcinoma arises from epithelial tissue around the neck of the uterus. The most common symptom is vaginal bleeding. The treatment and prognosis for survival depend on the stage of the disease when it is diagnosed. With regular gynecologic examinations with Pap smear analysis, leading to early detection, the prognosis is good.

Summary

- The term *pelvis* is used to describe the lower portion of the abdominopelvic cavity, which is the cavity enclosed by the sacrum, coccyx, and os coxae.
- The greater, or false, pelvis is the space between the alae of the ilium bones; the pelvis minor, or true pelvis, is the space below the pelvic brim.
- The sacrum consists of five fused vertebrae with sacral foramina, a median sacral crest, and a sacral hiatus. The coccyx consists of four rudimentary vertebrae fused together.
- Each os coxa is formed by the ilium, ischium, and pubis. The most noticeable features are the acetabulum, obturator foramen, and greater sciatic notch.
- In the child, the three bones of the os coxa are separate. In the adult, they are fused into one piece.
- The muscles that line the wall of the true pelvis are the obturator internus and the iliacus.
- The pelvic viscera are supported by a pelvic diaphragm, a urogenital diaphragm, and the muscles of the perineum.
- The muscles in the urogenital region of the perineum are the bulbospongiosus, ischiocavernosus, and transversus perinei.
- The common iliac arteries enter the pelvis and then divide into external and internal branches. The internal iliac artery branches profusely and supplies the pelvic viscera. Veins follow the same pattern.
- The sciatic nerve and pudendal nerve emerge from the sacral plexus. The sciatic nerve supplies the thigh, leg, and foot. The pudendal nerve supplies the perineum, external anal sphincter, and the external genitalia.
- In the female, the rectum is separated from the uterus by the rectouterine pouch. In the male, the rectovesical pouch is between the rectum and the urinary bladder.
- In the female, the urinary bladder is inferior to the uterus and separated from it by the vesicouterine pouch.
- In the male, the seminal vesicles are posterior to the bladder, and the prostate gland is inferior to the bladder.
- The ovaries are located in the lateral wall of the pelvis and are held in place by the mesovarium, the ovarian ligament, and the suspensory ligament.
- The largest ligament that supports the uterus is the broad ligament. Other ligaments are the round ligament, the uterosacral ligament, and the lateral cervical ligament.
- The uterus normally is anteverted and anteflexed.
- The fornix is the vaginal space that surrounds the cervix. The posterior fornix is larger than the anterior fornix.
- The testes and epididymis are located within the scrotum. Each testis contains seminiferous tubules, where sperm are produced. The epididymis is a coiled, tubular structure along the margin of the testes.
- The scrotum consists of a layer of skin, a thin layer of connective tissue, and smooth muscle fibers, called *dartos muscle*. The spermatic cord suspends the testes in the scrotum and contains the ductus deferens, testicular vessels, lymphatics, and connective tissue.
- The seminal vesicles are posterior to the bladder, the prostate gland is inferior to the bladder, and the bulbourethral glands are lateral to the membranous urethra.
- The dorsal columns of erectile tissue in the penis are the corpora cavernosa, which diverge to form the crura in the root of the penis. The ventral column is the corpus spongiosum, which enlarges to form the bulb in the root.
- The rectovesical pouch is the peritoneal cul-de-sac between the rectum and the urinary bladder in the male. The vesicouterine pouch is between the uterus and the bladder in the female, and the rectouterine pouch is between the rectum and the uterus.

• REVIEW QUESTIONS •

1. What is the difference between the true pelvis and the false pelvis?
2. What feature marks the posterior portion of the pelvic brim?
3. What are the three bones that make up an os coxa?
4. What is the large opening surrounded by the three bones of the os coxa?
5. What two muscles form the wall of the false pelvis?
6. What are the two principal muscles that make up the wall of the true pelvis?
7. What is the larger and more important muscle of the pelvic diaphragm?
8. What is the principal artery that supplies blood to the pelvis, including the wall and contents?
9. What branch of the sacral plexus innervates the perineum and external genitalia?
10. What is the name of the peritoneal space that is anterior to the rectum in males? In females?
11. What is the name of the peritoneal space that is inferior to the uterus?
12. What structure is between the urinary bladder and the pelvic floor in males?
13. What are the three parts of the male urethra and where are they located?
14. What are the three peritoneal ligaments that are attached to the ovaries?
15. What are the four peritoneal ligaments that are attached to the uterus?
16. What are the three parts of the uterus and which part projects into the vagina?
17. Describe the normal position of the uterus.
18. What is the relationship of the epididymis to the testes?
19. What are the components of the spermatic cord?
20. Name and state the location of three glands associated with the male reproductive system.
21. Name two muscles in the anal region of the perineum and three muscles in the urogenital region.
22. What are two types of vestibular glands in the female, where are they located, and what are they homologous to in the male?
23. What are the two components of the root of the penis, what is their composition, where are they attached, and what muscle is associated with each one?
24. What are the three columns of erectile tissue in the penis? What is their relative location? Which one contains the urethra?

• CHAPTER QUIZ •

Name the Following:

1. The feature on the pubic bones that marks the pelvic brim
2. The pelvic wall muscle that closes the greater sciatic notch
3. The larger muscle of the pelvic diaphragm
4. The muscle that lines the lateral wall of the true pelvis
5. The triangular-shaped region that is outlined by the openings of the two ureters and the urethra
6. The large fold of peritoneum that extends from the sides of the uterus
7. The vaginal space around the cervix of the uterus
8. The extension of the internal oblique muscle that is found in the spermatic cord
9. The male accessory gland that is between the posterior surface of the urinary bladder and the rectum
10. The female accessory gland that is homologous to the male prostate

True/False:

1. The urogenital diaphragm is superficial to the pelvic diaphragm.
2. Sperm pass from the epididymis into the ejaculatory duct.
3. Ovaries usually are displaced inferiorly during pregnancy.
4. The uterus normally is retroverted and anteflexed.
5. Two dorsal columns of corpus spongiosum are present in the body of the penis.
6. The crura of the penis are associated with the ischiocavernosus muscle.
7. The psoas muscle is more medial than the iliacus muscle.
8. The sciatic nerve is associated with the iliopsoas muscle.
9. Both males and females have an ischiocavernosus muscle, but only males have a bulbospongiosus muscle.
10. The prostate gland is between the urinary bladder and the pelvic diaphragm.

Answers to the Review Questions and Chapter Quiz questions can be found at http://evolve.elsevier.com/Applegate/SAlearning/

CHAPTER FIVE

The Head | 5

Anatomical Review of the Head
Osseous Components
Muscular Components
Salivary Glands
Brain
Orbital Cavity and Contents

Sectional Anatomy of the Head
Transverse Sections
Sagittal Sections
Coronal Sections
Working With Images of the Head
Important Anatomical Relationships in the Head

OBJECTIVES

Upon completion of this chapter, the student should be able to do the following:
- Name the bones of the cranium and face.
- Identify the four paranasal sinuses.
- Name five muscles of facial expression, describe the location of each, and state the insertion and innervation of this group.
- Name four muscles of mastication, describe the location of each muscle, and state the insertion and innervation of this muscle group.
- Compare the location and relationships of the three salivary glands.
- Identify the five lobes of the cerebrum.
- Describe the relationships of the basal ganglia.
- Describe the location and structure of the diencephalon.
- Locate the components of the brainstem.
- Compare the cerebrum and cerebellum with respect to size, appearance, location, and structure.
- Trace the flow of cerebrospinal fluid through the ventricles in the brain.
- Describe the three layers of meninges.
- Identify six subarachnoid cisterns by describing their location and significance.
- Describe the arterial blood supply to the brain.
- Identify the major venous sinuses that return blood from the brain to the internal jugular vein.
- Name the 12 cranial nerves and the foramen that serves as a passageway for each and the functions of each nerve.
- Describe the structure of the eye, including the bulbus oculi, musculature, vascular supply, and protective features.
- Discuss the relationships of the internal jugular vein, external jugular vein, internal carotid artery, and external carotid artery to each other and to other surrounding structures, such as the parotid gland and the sternocleidomastoid muscle.

Key Terms, Structures, and Features to Be Identified and/or Described

Anterior cerebral arteries
Aqueous humor
Arachnoid
Basal ganglia
Basilar artery
Brainstem
Bulbus oculi
C1 and C2
Calvaria
Caudate nucleus
Cavernous sinus
Cerebellar peduncles
Cerebellomedullary cistern

Cerebellum
Cerebral aqueduct
Cerebral peduncles
Cerebrospinal fluid
Cerebrum
Choroid plexus
Circulus arteriosus cerebri
Cisterna ambiens
Condyle of the mandible
Corpora quadrigemina
Corpus callosum
Diencephalon
Dura mater

Epicranial aponeurosis
Ethmoid sinus
External auditory canal
Falx cerebelli
Falx cerebri
Fourth ventricle
Frontal bones
Frontal lobe
Frontal sinus
Hypophysis
Inferior sagittal sinus
Insula
Internal capsule

Internal carotid arteries
Internal jugular vein
Interventricular foramen
Lateral fissure (sulcus)
Lateral ventricle
Lentiform nucleus
Longitudinal fissure
Mammillary bodies
Mandible
Masseter muscle
Mastoid process
Maxillae
Maxillary sinus
Medulla oblongata
Meninges
Middle cerebral arteries
Nasal conchae
Nasal septum
Occipital bone

Occipital lobe
Optic chiasma
Optic nerves
Optic tracts
Paranasal sinuses
Parietal bones
Parietal lobe
Parotid gland
Petrous ridge
Pharynx
Pia mater
Pineal body
Pons
Pontine cistern
Ramus of the mandible
Septum pellucidum
Sigmoid sinus
Sphenoid bone
Sphenoid sinus

Spinal cord
Sternocleidomastoid muscle
Straight sinus
Subarachnoid space
Sublingual gland
Submandibular (submaxillary) gland
Superior cistern
Superior sagittal sinus
Temporal bones
Temporal lobe
Temporalis muscle
Tentorium cerebelli
Thalamus
Third ventricle
Transverse sinus
Trigeminal nerve
Vertebral arteries
Vitreous humor
Zygoma and zygomatic arch

Anatomical Review of the Head

The principal bony structure of the head is the skull, which is especially adapted to house and protect the brain and pituitary gland, the two organs that integrate body activities. The head is the location of the special sensory organs of vision, hearing, equilibrium, taste, and smell, which provide information concerning our surroundings. The digestive and respiratory systems begin with openings in the head and continue as passageways in the neck. The intricate structure of the head is an appropriate complement to the functional complexity of this region.

Osseous Components

The bony framework of the head is called the skull. This is the most complex osseous structure of the body, and it consists of 22 bones connected by immovable joints, called *sutures*. For descriptive purposes, these bones are divided into the cranium and the facial skeleton, although no distinct line of demarcation separates the two parts. Some of the bones surround a large cranial cavity that contains the brain. The superior surface of this region is covered by the scalp. Some skull bones adjacent to the nasal cavity contain air-filled spaces, called *paranasal sinuses*. Many of the bones in the skull have holes or openings, called *foramina*, that serve as passageways for nerves and blood vessels. In addition to the skull, seven other bones are associated with the head; these are the auditory ossicles and the hyoid bone. The osseous components of the head are summarized in Table 5-1.

Cranium.   The eight bones of the cranium surround the cranial cavity, which houses the brain. The single **frontal bone** forms the forehead and superior part of the orbit of the eye. It contains the frontal sinuses, which communicate with the nasal cavity. Two **parietal bones** form most of

TABLE 5-1   Summary of Bones Associated With Head

Bone	Number	Total
Bones of the Cranium		8
Frontal	1	
Parietal	2	
Occipital	1	
Temporal	2	
Sphenoid	1	
Ethmoid	1	
Bones of the Face		14
Maxillae	2	
Nasal	2	
Zygomatic	2	
Lacrimal	2	
Mandible	1	
Vomer	1	
Inferior nasal conchae	2	
Palatine	2	
Middle Ear Bones		6
Malleus	2	
Incus	2	
Stapes	2	
Hyoid Bone		1

the top of the cranium. Two **temporal bones** form a portion of the sides and base, or floor, of the cranium. Each temporal bone has a thin, flat, squamous portion that forms the inferior-lateral part of the cranium. The posterior portion of the temporal bone is the **mastoid process.** The **external auditory canal** (meatus), the tympanic membrane, the middle ear, and the inner ear are located in the **petrous portion,** which extends medially to form part of the base of the cranium. The **zygomatic process** of the temporal bone extends anteriorly to join the zygomatic bone to form the zygomatic arch. The single **ethmoid bone** is located between the eyes and forms most of the medial wall of each orbit. The superior surface of the ethmoid bone forms a part of the base of the cranial cavity and the roof of the nasal cavities. A thin, perpendicular plate of the ethmoid bone extends inferiorly to form part of the **nasal septum.** The superior and middle conchae (turbinates) in the nasal cavity are part of the ethmoid bone. The single **sphenoid bone** lies at the base of the skull anterior to the temporal bones. Often described as bat shaped, the sphenoid bone has "wings" that form the anterior-lateral portion of the cranium and the lateral walls of the orbits. The sella turcica is found in the center of the bone and is the location of the pituitary gland. The single **occipital bone** forms the posterior portion and part of the base of the cranium. It has a large hole, the foramen magnum, for passage of the spinal

cord and the vertebral vessels. The bones of the cranium are illustrated in Figs. 5-1 to 5-4.

The domelike superior portion of the cranium is the **calvaria,** or skullcap. It is composed of the superior portions of the frontal, parietal, and occipital bones. The calvaria is covered by the scalp, which extends from the eyebrows to the superior nuchal line on the occipital bone. Structurally, the scalp has five layers. The outer layer, the **skin,** covers the second layer, which is composed of highly vascularized **subcutaneous connective tissue.** The third layer, or epicranium, consists of two thin muscles connected by a broad, flat tendon, or aponeurosis. This musculoaponeurotic sheet has the frontalis muscle at the anterior end and the occipitalis muscle at the posterior end. The strong aponeurosis that connects the two muscles is known as the **epicranial aponeurosis,** or **galea aponeurotica.** These three layers of the scalp are bound tightly together and move as

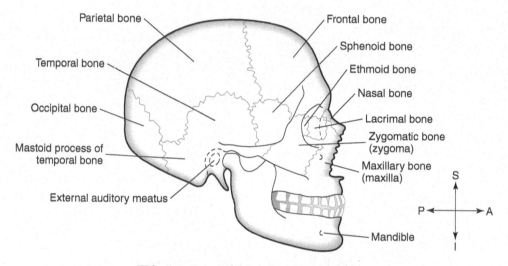

FIG. 5-1. Bones of the skull (cranium and face).

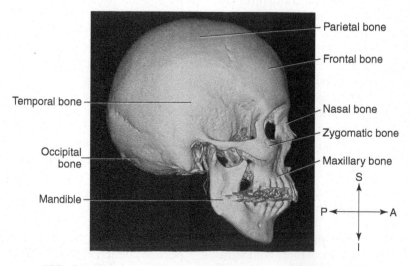

FIG. 5-2. Reconstructed CT image of the lateral surface of the skull.

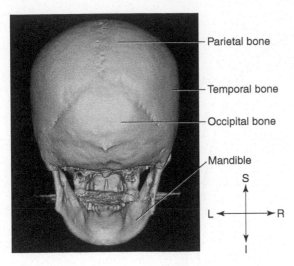

FIG. 5-3. Reconstructed CT image of the skull, posterior aspect.

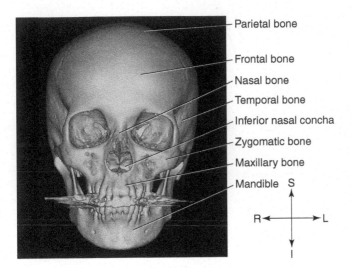

FIG. 5-4. Reconstructed CT image of the skull, anterior aspect.

a unit. Collectively, they often are referred to as the *scalp proper*. A fourth layer that consists of **loose connective tissue** separates the scalp proper from the fifth layer, the **periosteum,** or pericranium. The loose connective tissue layer permits mobility of the scalp proper, but it is also considered a potentially dangerous area, because it allows scalp infections to spread easily. Lacerations of the scalp typically bleed profusely because of the extensive vascularization of the subcutaneous connective tissue. The acronym SCALP serves as a useful mnemonic tool for remembering the five layers of the scalp.

S = Skin
C = Connective tissue
A = Aponeurosis
L = Loose connective tissue
P = Periosteum

The cranial cavity, a large space formed by the eight cranial bones, contains the brain. The floor of the cranial cavity is subdivided into anterior, middle, and posterior cranial fossae (Fig. 5-5). The **anterior cranial fossa** is formed by portions of the ethmoid, sphenoid, and frontal bones. This fossa houses the frontal lobes of the brain. The floor of the **middle cranial fossa** is composed of the body and greater wings of the sphenoid and the squamosal and petrous portions of the temporal bones. This region contains the temporal lobes of the brain. The **posterior cranial fossa** comprises the remainder of the cranial cavity and is formed by parts of the sphenoid, temporal, and occipital bones. This region contains the cerebellum, the pons, and the medulla oblongata. The inferior-most portion of the posterior cranial fossa shows the large **foramen magnum,** through which the spinal cord passes.

Face. The facial portion of the skull consists of 14 bones. Some of these bones are illustrated in Figs. 5-1, 5-2, and 5-4. The two **maxillae** (singular, **maxilla**) unite in the midline to form the upper jaw. A horizontal piece of each maxilla, the **palatine process,** forms the anterior portion of the roof of the mouth, which is the hard palate. If the palatine processes of the two maxillae fail to join during prenatal development, a cleft palate results. Each maxilla contains a maxillary sinus, which is a large air space that communicates with the nasal cavity. Two **palatine bones** form the posterior portion of the hard palate. Two **zygomatic bones,** one on each side, form the prominence of the cheek and the lateral margin of the orbit. A process of the zygomatic bone extends posteriorly and unites with the temporal bone to form the **zygomatic arch.** Two small, rectangular **nasal bones** join in the midline to form the bridge of the nose. Fractures of these bones are common facial injuries.

The anterior part of the medial wall of each orbital cavity consists of a small, thin **lacrimal bone.** Each bone has a groove that helps to form the nasolacrimal canal, which allows the tears of the eye to drain into the nasal cavity. The single **vomer** is a thin bone shaped like the blade of a plow. It forms the inferior portion of the nasal septum. The two **inferior nasal conchae** are scroll-like bones that project horizontally from the lateral walls of the nasal cavities. The **superior** and **middle** conchae are part of the ethmoid bone, but the inferior nasal conchae are separate bones. The conchae are covered by a mucous membrane, which warms and moistens the air that enters the nasal cavities. The single **mandible** forms the lower jaw. The posterior ends of the mandible extend vertically to form the **rami** (singular, **ramus**). Each ramus has a knoblike condyle and a pointed coronoid process. The mandibular condyle articulates with the temporal bone to form the temporomandibular joint, which is the only movable joint in the skull.

QUICK CHECK

5.1 Which bones of the cranium are paired?
5.2 What muscles are in the middle layer of the scalp?
5.3 Which facial bones are present as single bones (not paired)?

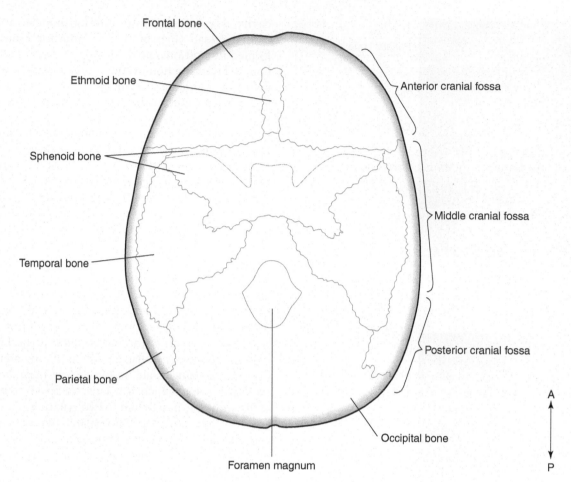

Frontal bone

Ethmoid bone

Sphenoid bone

Temporal bone

Parietal bone

Foramen magnum

Anterior cranial fossa

Middle cranial fossa

Posterior cranial fossa

Occipital bone

A

P

FIG. 5-5. Cranial fossae (floor of the cranial cavity).

Paranasal Sinuses.   The **paranasal sinuses** are air-filled spaces in some of the bones adjacent to the nasal cavity. The four sets of paranasal sinuses are named according to the bone in which they are located; they are the **frontal sinus, ethmoid sinus, sphenoid sinus,** and **maxillary sinus.** Usually developing after birth as outgrowths of the nasal cavity, the sinuses retain their original openings so that their secretions drain into the nasal cavity. The mucous membrane that lines the sinuses is continuous with the mucosa of the nasal cavity, but it is thinner and less vascular than the nasal mucosa. Fig. 5-6 illustrates the paranasal sinuses.

The **frontal sinuses** are located in the frontal bone near the midline. They develop in the child and are usually visible on radiographs by the time the child is 7 years of age; however, the sinuses continue to enlarge throughout adolescence. The frontal sinuses drain into the **middle meatus** of the nasal cavity, between the middle and inferior nasal conchae, by way of a frontonasal duct.

The **ethmoid sinuses** consist of numerous air spaces in the ethmoid bone between the orbit of the eye and the upper part of the nasal cavity. Although a few ethmoidal air cells are present in the neonate, they are not readily visible on radiographs until the infant is 2 years old, and they do

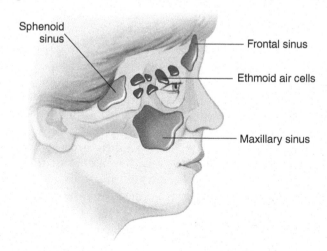

Sphenoid sinus

Frontal sinus

Ethmoid air cells

Maxillary sinus

FIG. 5-6. The paranasal sinuses. (Modified from Thibodeau GA, Patton KT: *Anatomy & physiology,* ed 6, St Louis, 2007, Elsevier/ Mosby.)

not enlarge significantly until later in the childhood years, usually around 6 to 8 years of age. The ethmoid sinuses have numerous openings into the **superior meatus** between the superior and middle conchae and into the **middle meatus** between the middle and inferior conchae.

The **sphenoid sinuses** are located in the body of the sphenoid bone just posterior to the ethmoid sinuses and the nasal cavity. The sinuses occupy most of the volume of the sphenoid body, so that only a thin plate of bone separates the sinuses from the pituitary gland, the optic nerve, the optic chiasma, the internal carotid artery, and the cavernous sinus. Tiny sphenoid sinuses may be present in the newborn, but their development is more likely to occur in a child of about 2 years of age, with additional growth during late childhood and adolescence. The sphenoid sinuses drain into the **sphenoethmoidal recess** above the superior nasal conchae.

Small **maxillary sinuses,** which are located in the bodies of the maxillae, are present in the newborn and grow slowly until the child reaches puberty. The accelerated development of the maxillary sinuses during adolescence contributes to the apparent change in facial features that typically occurs during this period. When fully developed, the maxillary sinuses are the largest of the paranasal sinuses. The maxillary sinus drains into the nasal cavity by way of a relatively long **hiatus semilunaris,** which opens into the **middle meatus.** A couple of factors hinder the drainage of this sinus: the hiatus traverses a superior direction when the body is erect, thus necessitating drainage "against gravity," and the opening from the sinus into the hiatus is in a superior location. The drainage problem is further complicated because the maxillary sinus is the most inferiorly located of the paranasal sinuses, and communicating channels allow the other sinuses to drain into the maxillary sinus. For these reasons, the maxillary sinus is the sinus most often involved in infections. The frontal, ethmoid, and sphenoid sinuses are innervated by branches of the ophthalmic division of the **trigeminal nerve,** which is the fifth cranial nerve. The maxillary sinus is innervated by branches of the maxillary division of the fifth cranial nerve. (The cranial nerves are discussed later in the chapter.) Sinuses and other features of the skeleton of the head are illustrated by the radiographs in Figs. 5-7 and 5-8.

Foramina of the Skull. **Foramina** are openings in bones that serve as passageways for nerves and blood vessels. The vessels that transport blood and the nerves that carry impulses must pass through the sutured, helmetlike bones of the skull on their way to and from the brain; therefore these bones have numerous foramina. Table 5-2 provides a summary of the foramina of the skull.

Additional Bones Associated With the Skull. Six auditory ossicles (three pairs) and a single hyoid bone are associated with the head, in addition to the eight bones of the cranium and the 14 bones of the facial skeleton.

The ear has three chambers: the inner ear, the middle ear, and the external ear. The ear ossicles, the **malleus, incus,** and **stapes,** are located in the middle ear chamber in the petrous portion of the temporal bone. The ossicles transmit and amplify sound waves through the middle ear. The single **hyoid bone** is located in the neck just superior to the larynx. The hyoid is unique because it does not attach directly to any other bone; instead, it is suspended by ligaments. Muscles associated with the hyoid bone are described in Chapter 6.

> **QUICK CHECK**
> 5.4 Which of the paranasal sinuses is/are usually present in the newborn?
> 5.5 Which paranasal sinus drains into the space above the superior nasal conchae?
> 5.6 What foramen of the skull transmits the vertebral arteries and accessory nerves?

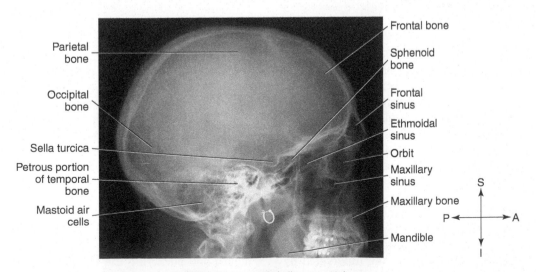

FIG. 5-7. Lateral skull radiograph.

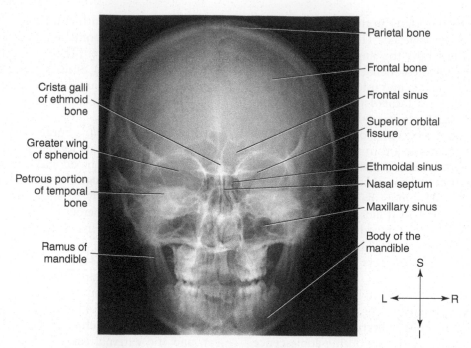

FIG. 5-8. Radiograph, skull, posteroanterior (PA) projection, frontal view.

Crista galli of ethmoid bone
Greater wing of sphenoid
Petrous portion of temporal bone
Ramus of mandible
Parietal bone
Frontal bone
Frontal sinus
Superior orbital fissure
Ethmoidal sinus
Nasal septum
Maxillary sinus
Body of the mandible

TABLE 5-2   Major Foramina of the Skull

Foramen	Location	Structures Transmitted
Carotid canal	Temporal bone	Internal carotid artery; sympathetic nerves
Hypoglossal canal	Occipital bone	Hypoglossal nerve
Infraorbital	Maxilla	Maxillary branch of trigeminal nerve; infraorbital nerve and artery
Internal auditory meatus	Temporal bone	Vestibulocochlear nerve
Jugular	Temporal bone	Internal jugular vein; vagus, glossopharyngeal, and spinal accessory nerves
Magnum	Occipital bone	Medulla oblongata/spinal cord; accessory nerves; vertebral arteries
Nasolacrimal canal	Lacrimal bone	Nasolacrimal (tear) duct
Olfactory	Ethmoid bone	Olfactory nerves
Optic	Sphenoid bone	Optic nerve; central artery and vein of retina
Ovale	Sphenoid bone	Mandibular branch of trigeminal nerve
Rotundum	Sphenoid bone	Maxillary branch of trigeminal nerve
Stylomastoid	Temporal bone	Facial nerve

Muscular Components

Numerous muscles are located in the head, many of them small and difficult to separate from adjacent muscles. They are even more difficult to isolate by imaging techniques. These muscles have functional significance because they deal with facial expression and the chewing of food. Only the larger and more significant muscles are presented in this text (Table 5-3).

Muscles of Facial Expression.   The muscles of facial expression are located in the subcutaneous tissue of the face. They originate in the fascia or on the underlying bone, and they insert on the skin of the face. All are innervated by cranial nerve VII, the facial nerve. Many of these muscles

are small and thin and are difficult to dissect or to distinguish on sections. Actions of the facial muscles are easily observed, however, because they are used to express feelings. Five of the more prominent facial muscles are mentioned here. The **frontalis** muscle is part of the scalp. Originating from the aponeurosis, which is located on the top of the head, the frontalis inserts on the skin of the eyebrow and forehead. When it contracts, this muscle elevates the eyebrows and produces transverse wrinkles in the skin of the forehead. The **orbicularis oris** muscle is an important sphincter that encircles the mouth and forms the muscular bulk of the lips. This muscle's function involves closing the mouth and puckering the lips, as in whistling. It plays an important role in the enunciation of words. A similar

TABLE 5-3   Muscles Associated With Facial Expression and Mastication

Muscle	Origin	Insertion	Action	Innervation
Muscles of Facial Expression				
Frontalis	Aponeurosis of scalp	Skin of eyebrow and forehead	Elevates eyebrows; wrinkles forehead	Facial (cranial nerve VII)
Orbicularis oris	Maxillae and mandible	Lip mucosa and skin at corner of mouth	Closes mouth and puckers lips, as in whistling	Facial (cranial nerve VII)
Orbicularis oculi	Frontal bones and maxillae around orbit	Eyelid	Closes eye, as in winking and blinking	Facial (cranial nerve VII)
Buccinator	Buccinator ridge of mandible, alveolar processes of maxillae, pterygomandibular ligament	Orbicularis oris at angle of mouth	Compresses cheeks when blowing, as when playing a musical instrument	Facial (cranial nerve VII)
Platysma	Fascia of the cervical region	Mandible, the skin of the neck, and the orbicularis oris	Depresses lower jaw, forms ridges on neck	Facial (cranial nerve VII)
Muscles of Mastication				
Temporalis	Temporal bone	Mandible	Elevates mandible to close mouth	Trigeminal (cranial nerve V), mandibular division
Masseter	Zygomatic arch	Mandible	Elevates mandible	Trigeminal (cranial nerve V), mandibular division
Lateral pterygoid	Sphenoid	Mandible	Pulls mandible forward (protracts)	Trigeminal (cranial nerve V), mandibular division
Medial pterygoid	Sphenoid	Mandible	Protracts mandible and moves mandible laterally	Trigeminal (cranial nerve V), mandibular division

sphincter, the **orbicularis oculi** muscle, surrounds the eye. Contraction of these muscle fibers reduces the orbital opening, as in winking and blinking. The **buccinator** muscle is an accessory muscle in mastication and compresses the cheeks when blowing, as in playing a musical wind instrument. It inserts on the orbicularis oris at the angle of the mouth. The **platysma** muscle is a broad, flat muscle in the subcutaneous tissue of the neck. It inserts on the mandible, the skin of the neck, and the orbicularis oris muscle. When it contracts, it depresses the lower jaw and forms ridges in the skin of the neck.

Muscles of Mastication.   The four muscles of mastication provide chewing movements by acting on the temporomandibular joint to move the mandible (see Table 5-3). All insert on the mandible and are innervated by the mandibular division of the fifth cranial nerve. They are quite readily seen on transverse sections. The fan-shaped **temporalis** muscle covers the squamosal portion of the temporal bone and is a powerful muscle used to close the mouth by elevating the mandible. The **masseter muscle,** or chewing muscle, is located on the lateral aspect of the **ramus of the mandible.** Both the **lateral** and **medial pterygoid** muscles originate on the

lateral pterygoid plate of the sphenoid bone and insert on the medial surface of the mandible. When these muscles are observed in transverse sections, the temporalis is seen in the more superior sections. In lower sections, starting at the lateral surface and in sequence, the masseter, the ramus of the mandible, the lateral pterygoid, and the medial pterygoid are seen.

QUICK CHECK

5.7   What cranial nerve innervates the orbicularis oris and orbicularis oculi muscles?

5.8   Which muscle of mastication is the most superior and what nerve innervates it?

Salivary Glands

Three pairs of salivary glands are located in the region of the face. These glands are usually considered part of the digestive system, because they secrete a fluid to moisten food particles for taste and swallowing. They also secrete an enzyme, salivary amylase, that initiates digestion of carbohydrates. All of the salivary glands are easily seen in sectional views.

Parotid Gland.   The largest of the glands is the **parotid gland,** wedged between the ramus of the mandible and the mastoid portion of the temporal bone. The parotid gland occupies the space just anterior and inferior to the auricle of the ear, and a portion of the gland overlies the masseter muscle in the cheek. The well-defined duct of the parotid gland, Stensen's duct, extends across the masseter muscle, then turns to penetrate the buccinator muscle, and opens into the vestibule of the mouth near the upper second molar tooth.

Submandibular Gland.   The **submandibular (submaxillary) gland** is located medial to the body and angle of the mandible. The gland can be felt as a small lump along the inferior border of the posterior half of the mandible. The secretions of this gland reach the oral cavity by means of the submandibular (Wharton's) duct, which opens near the midline beneath the tongue.

Sublingual Gland.   The third salivary gland is the **sublingual gland.** It is the smallest and most deeply situated of the salivary glands. Located under the mucous membrane in the floor of the mouth, the two sublingual glands unite anteriorly to form a glandular mass around the lingual frenulum. These glands open into the floor of the mouth by means of a major sublingual duct (Bartholin's duct) and numerous small sublingual ducts (ducts of Rivinus) along the midline. Sometimes ducts from the sublingual glands may open into the submandibular duct.

QUICK CHECK
5.9   Which salivary gland is the most superior?

Brain

The predominant structure in the cranial cavity is the brain, a rather unimpressive looking mass of tissue that weighs approximately 3 pounds. It is composed of organized regions of white matter and gray matter. The **white matter** consists of nerve fibers that are covered with a white, fatty substance called *myelin.* The **gray matter** consists of nerve cell bodies and unmyelinated fibers. Some of the gray matter is grouped together to form regions called **basal ganglia.** Generally, the gray areas are regions of *synapse*, or electrical communication between neurons. Fluid-filled spaces, called **ventricles,** are located within the brain and are surrounded by brain tissue. The brain is separated from the cranial bones by layers of connective tissue, called **meninges,** that help protect the surface of the brain. Further protection is provided by cerebrospinal fluid, which circulates through the ventricles and around the brain. Although the brain accounts for only about 2% of body weight, it is metabolically very active; consequently, it receives 15% to 20% of the cardiac output through its arterial blood supply. After the blood circulates through the capillaries to provide oxygen for the brain tissue, it is returned to the heart by veins. Another feature of the brain involves the 12 pairs of cranial nerves that emerge from the inferior surface. These nerves provide pathways for incoming sensory impulses, which are processed and interpreted by the brain, and for outgoing motor impulses, which travel from the brain to a muscle or gland and effectuate an action.

Regions of the Brain.   For descriptive purposes, the brain may be divided into the **cerebrum, diencephalon, brainstem,** and **cerebellum.**

Cerebrum.   The largest portion of the brain is the **cerebrum,** which consists of two cerebral hemispheres connected by a mass of white matter called the **corpus callosum.** The anterior end of the corpus callosum is called the **genu,** and the posterior end is called the **splenium.** The deep cleft between the two cerebral hemispheres is the **longitudinal fissure.** The surface of the cerebrum has numerous convolutions, which greatly increase the surface area of the cerebral cortex. The ridges are called **gyri** (singular, **gyrus**), and the furrows between them are called **sulci** (singular, **sulcus**).

Superficially, the cerebrum is divided into lobes. A **central sulcus** separates the **frontal lobe** from the **parietal lobe.** Posteriorly, the **parieto-occipital sulcus** separates the parietal lobe from the **occipital lobe.** Laterally, the **temporal lobe** is situated below the **lateral fissure (sulcus).** A fifth lobe, called the **insula,** or island of Reil, is located deep within the lateral fissure. The lobes and fissures of the brain are illustrated in Fig. 5-9.

The surface layer of the cerebrum is **gray matter,** which consists of nerve cell bodies and unmyelinated fibers; this is called the *cerebral cortex.* It is 2 to 4 mm thick. Lying beneath the cerebral cortex is the lighter colored **white matter,** which is made up of myelinated nerve fibers.

Scattered throughout the white matter are distinct regions of gray matter called **basal ganglia.** Two of the larger basal ganglia are the **caudate nucleus** and the **lentiform nucleus,** or **lenticular nucleus.** In sectional anatomy, the caudate nucleus is usually visualized in association with the lateral ventricle. The lentiform nucleus is rather centrally located in each cerebral hemisphere. It is subdivided into the lateral, or external, **putamen,** and the medial, or internal, **globus pallidus.** The **claustrum,** another of the basal ganglia, is a thin layer of gray matter just lateral to the lentiform nucleus and deep to the cortex of the insula. A band of white matter that is medial to the lentiform nucleus is called the **internal capsule.** The white matter that is present between the lentiform nucleus and the claustrum is the **external capsule.** The claustrum is separated from the insula by the **extreme capsule.** Because of their appearance, the caudate nucleus, the internal capsule, and the lentiform nucleus are sometimes referred to as the **corpus striatum.** Fig. 5-10 illustrates the arrangement of the basal ganglia in a transverse section. The axial computed tomography (CT) image in Fig. 5-11 shows some of the features of the cerebrum and basal ganglia.

Diencephalon.   The **diencephalon** is centrally located and is nearly hidden from view by the large cerebral hemispheres.

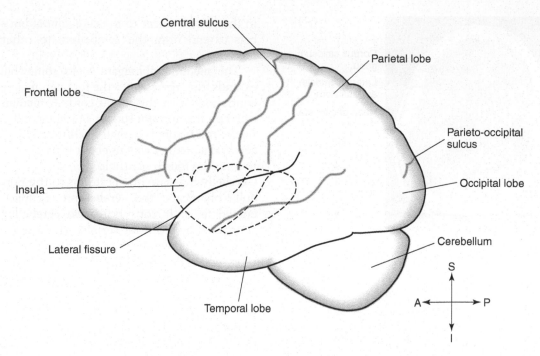

FIG. 5-9. Surface of the brain with lobes and fissures.

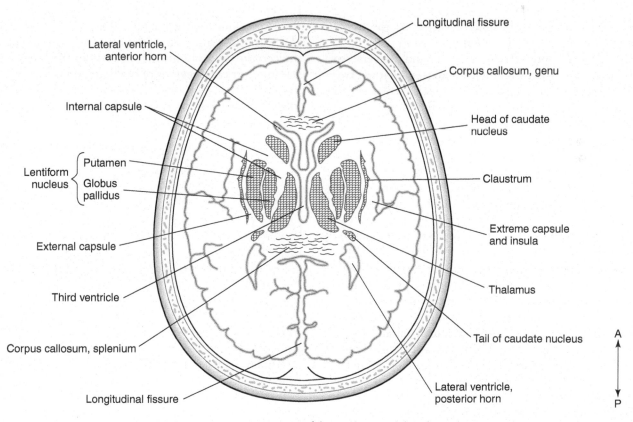

FIG. 5-10. Transverse section of the cerebrum with basal ganglia.

Corpus callosum, genu

Lateral ventricle, anterior horn

Head of caudate, nucleus

Thalamus

Septum pellucidum

Third ventricle

FIG. 5-11. Axial CT of the cerebrum.

It surrounds the midline third ventricle and consists of the **epithalamus, thalamus,** and **hypothalamus.** The largest portion, the thalamus, is a mass of gray matter that lies on either side of the third ventricle and forms its lateral walls. This is a major relay station of the afferent, or sensory, pathway that carries impulses to the cerebral cortex. The epithalamus forms the roof of the third ventricle. A midline projection of the epithalamus forms the **pineal gland.** The hypothalamus forms the floor of the third ventricle. The following structures are located on the inferior aspect of the hypothalamus: the **infundibulum,** or **pituitary stalk;** the **optic chiasma,** where the **optic nerves** cross over and then emerge as optic tracts; and the **mammillary bodies,** which are two spherical masses of gray matter surrounded by a layer of white matter. The mammillary bodies function in some swallowing reflexes.

Brainstem.   The **brainstem** is subdivided into the midbrain, the pons, and the medulla oblongata. The smallest division is the **midbrain,** which is located between the diencephalon and the pons. The midbrain surrounds the **cerebral aqueduct,** a long, slender channel for the passage of cerebrospinal fluid from the third to the fourth ventricle. Four rounded protuberances, the **corpora quadrigemina,** are visible on the dorsal aspect of the midbrain. The upper pair, **superior colliculi,** functions in the visual pathway, whereas the lower pair, the **inferior colliculi,** functions in the auditory pathway. Just above the corpora quadrigemina is a small glandular structure projecting from the diencephalon. This is the **pineal body,** or **pineal gland.** On the ventral aspect of the midbrain are two ropelike bundles called **cerebral peduncles.** These are composed of motor fibers that extend from the cerebral cortex to the spinal cord. A narrow band of darkly pigmented cells crosses each cerebral peduncle; this is the **substantia nigra.** The dark color is due to the presence of melanin in the cells. The substantia nigra seems to be involved in the production of dopamine in the brain and also functions in muscle tone reflexes.

The **pons** appears as a prominent band of fibers between the midbrain and the medulla oblongata. Most of the fibers

in the pons connect to the cerebellum, but some of the fibers extend from the cerebellum to other parts of the brain.

The **medulla oblongata** looks somewhat conical and extends from the pons to the foramen magnum, where it is continuous with the spinal cord. A **median fissure** is located on the anterior surface of the medulla, and on either side of this fissure is a small swelling called a **pyramid.** The **cerebral aqueduct** widens about halfway along the medulla to form the fourth ventricle.

Cerebellum.   Situated posterior to the pons and the medulla oblongata, the **cerebellum** occupies the posterior cranial fossa. It consists of two **cerebellar hemispheres** connected by a central **vermis,** which resembles a coiled-up worm. The word *vermis* is derived from the Latin word *verm,* which means worm. The surface of the cerebellum is covered by a layer of gray matter, the **cerebellar cortex.** Deep to the cortex is the white matter. Because the gray matter and white matter are laminated or foliated in appearance, the arrangement is sometimes called **arbor vitae.** **Cerebellar peduncles** connect the cerebellum with other portions of the brain. There are three pairs of cerebellar peduncles. The **superior cerebellar peduncles** connect the cerebellum to the midbrain. Fibers of the **middle cerebellar peduncles** connect the cerebellum and the pons. The **inferior cerebellar peduncles** consist of fibers passing between the cerebellum and the medulla oblongata. The cerebellum plays an important role in the control of muscle tone and the coordination of muscular activity of the body. Some of the structures and regions of the brain are illustrated by the line drawing in Fig. 5-12. The magnetic resonance (MR) image in Fig. 5-13 also shows features of the brain in a midsagittal plane.

QUICK CHECK

5.10   What is the name of the mass of white fibers that connect the two cerebral hemispheres?

5.11   What is the largest portion of the diencephalon?

5.12   What are the three regions of the brainstem and which is most superior?

5.13   What structures connect the cerebellum to other regions of the brain?

Ventricles of the Brain.   Ventricles are fluid-filled cavities in the brain. These ventricles include the two lateral ventricles, the third ventricle, and the fourth ventricle. The ventricles and their communicating channels are illustrated in Fig. 5-14.

Lateral Ventricles.   Within each cerebral hemisphere is a large **lateral ventricle.** The major portion of each lateral ventricle is located in the parietal lobe. These ventricles extend into the frontal lobes as the anterior horns, into the occipital lobes as the posterior horns, and into the temporal lobes as the inferior horns. The lateral ventricles are separated from each other medially by a thin vertical partition called the **septum pellucidum.** Each lateral ventricle

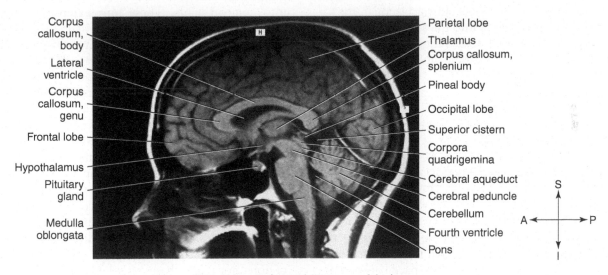

FIG. 5-12. Midsagittal section of the brain.

FIG. 5-13. Midsagittal MR image of the brain.

communicates with the third ventricle by a small opening called the **interventricular foramen,** or the foramen of Monro.

Third Ventricle. The **third ventricle** is a narrow midline chamber enclosed by the diencephalon. The lateral walls of the third ventricle are formed by the right and left masses of the thalamus. The epithalamus and hypothalamus form the ventricle's roof and floor, respectively. A small band of white fibers, called the **intermediate mass,** passes through the ventricle between the right and left

thalami. The third ventricle communicates with the fourth ventricle by means of a relatively long **cerebral aqueduct,** also called the **aqueduct of Sylvius,** which passes through the midbrain.

Fourth Ventricle. The **fourth ventricle** lies internal to the pons and the medulla oblongata at the level of the cerebellum. Two openings, called the **foramina of Luschka,** are present in the lateral walls of the fourth ventricle. In the medial aspect of the dorsal wall is a single opening called the **foramen of Magendie.** The

FIG. 5-14. Ventricles of the brain.

ventricles communicate with the subarachnoid space through these three openings. The fourth ventricle is continuous with the narrow central canal that extends throughout the length of the spinal cord.

Choroid Plexus.   The **choroid plexus** is a group of specialized vascular structures located in the lateral, third, and fourth ventricles. The choroid plexus produces the **cerebrospinal fluid** by filtration and secretion. Originating in the ventricles, the fluid circulates outward through the foramina in the fourth ventricle into the subarachnoid space around the brain and spinal cord. From there the fluid is reabsorbed into the venous system and returned to the heart as part of the blood.

QUICK CHECK

5.14   What channel for cerebrospinal fluid passes through the midbrain?

5.15   Which ventricle of the brain is located in the region of the diencephalon?

Meninges.   Three distinct connective tissue membranes, called *meninges*, cover the brain. These meninges are the dura mater, the arachnoid, and the pia mater. Cerebrospinal fluid circulates in the subarachnoid space between the arachnoid and the pia mater. In certain areas the arachnoid and the pia mater are widely separated, which creates spaces called *cisterns*.

Dura Mater.   The outermost layer of the meninges is the **dura mater,** which is composed of tough, fibrous connective tissue. This forms a strong outer covering that serves as a supportive and protective structure for the brain. Although the dura mater is sometimes described as consisting of two layers, it is important to realize that what is called the outer layer of the dura mater is actually the endosteum (internal periosteum) of the calvaria. This outer layer is continuous with the external periosteum at the sutures and foramina. The inner, or meningeal, layer is the true dura

mater, and it is continuous with the spinal dura at the foramen magnum. It also provides tubular sheaths for the cranial nerves as they pass through the foramina in the floor of the cranial fossa. The endosteum and true meningeal dura are closely adherent, except where there are venous sinuses.

The meningeal, or true, dura mater forms four inward-projecting folds that partially divide the cranial cavities into compartments. These four extensions of the dura mater are the **falx cerebri,** which is located between the cerebral hemispheres; the **falx cerebelli,** which is found between the cerebellar hemispheres; the **tentorium cerebelli,** which is between the cerebrum and cerebellum; and the **diaphragma sellae,** which forms a bridge over the sella turcica and covers the hypophysis.

Arachnoid.   The middle layer of the meninges is an extremely thin and delicate **arachnoid.** This layer is separated from the dura mater by a small subdural space that contains just enough fluid to keep the adjacent surfaces moist. The arachnoid is separated from the innermost pia mater by the **subarachnoid space,** which contains the cerebrospinal fluid and the larger blood vessels of the brain. Samples of cerebrospinal fluid may be withdrawn from the subarachnoid space and examined for evidence of infections or subarachnoid bleeding. This is usually done in the lumbar region of the vertebral column to minimize danger to the brain or spinal cord. From the inner surface of the arachnoid, minute trabeculae extend across the subarachnoid space to become continuous with the pia mater. This presents a cobweblike appearance and is the basis of the name *arachnoid.* In the vicinity of the venous sinuses are numerous outgrowths, or diverticula, of the arachnoid that penetrate the dura and project into the venous sinuses. The interior of these **arachnoid villi** is continuous with the subarachnoid space and contains cerebrospinal fluid; this permits reabsorption of the fluid into the venous system. Arachnoid villi are illustrated in Fig. 5-15.

Arachnoid villi in
superior sagittal sinus

Bone of cranium

Arachnoid

Cerebral cortex

Dura mater

Pia mater

Falx cerebri

FIG. 5-15. Meninges and arachnoid villi.

Pia Mater. The **pia mater** is the innermost layer of the meninges. It is a thin, highly vascular layer intimately adherent to the cortical tissue of the brain surface and closely follows the contours of the brain. The arachnoid and pia mater together are frequently referred to as the **leptomeninges.** These two layers of meninges are in close contact at the crests of the gyri, but as the pia mater follows the dips of the sulci and the arachnoid bridges over the top of the gyri, they become separated and triangular subarachnoid spaces are formed.

Subarachnoid Cisterns. In addition to the subarachnoid spaces described previously, in certain other areas around the base of the brain the arachnoid and the pia mater are widely separated. This creates spaces called **cisterns,** which contain relatively large amounts of cerebrospinal fluid. Some of the cisterns are illustrated in Figs. 5-16 and 5-17. The **cerebellomedullary cistern,** or cisterna magna, is formed by the arachnoid as it bridges the interval between the medulla oblongata and the inferior surface of the cerebellum. The foramen of Magendie (median aperture) from the fourth ventricle opens into this cistern. When it is especially difficult or dangerous to perform a lumbar puncture to obtain samples of cerebrospinal fluid, the fluid may be taken from the cerebellomedullary cistern by a cisternal puncture. The **pontine cistern** is a space on the ventral surface of the pons. This cistern contains the basilar artery and receives cerebrospinal fluid from the fourth ventricle through the foramina of Luschka (lateral apertures). As the arachnoid bridges the gap from the temporal lobe to the frontal lobe, it forms the **cistern of the lateral sulcus,** which contains the middle cerebral artery. Between the two temporal lobes, the arachnoid is separated from the cerebral peduncles by an interpeduncular cistern, which contains the circle of Willis. Anteriorly and superiorly, the **interpeduncular cistern** continues as the **chiasmatic cistern.** The **cisterna ambiens** occupies the interval between the splenium of the corpus callosum and the superior surface of the cerebellum. It contains the great cerebral vein

and the pineal gland. The cisterna ambiens is also called the *cistern of the great cerebral vein,* **superior cistern,** or *quadrigeminal cistern.* The pineal gland, which is located in this cistern, usually becomes calcified after adolescence and can be visualized on normal radiographs. This characteristic makes it an important landmark in neuroradiography and neurosurgery.

> **QUICK CHECK**
>
> **5.16** Between which two layers of meninges does the cerebrospinal fluid circulate?
>
> **5.17** What is the extension of dura mater that is between the cerebral hemispheres?

Arterial Blood Supply. Blood is supplied to the brain by two pairs of arteries, the **internal carotid arteries** and the **vertebral arteries.** The **circulus arteriosus cerebri** is also discussed in this section.

Internal Carotid Artery. The cerebral portion of the internal carotid artery extends to the medial end of the lateral cerebral fissure, where it divides into the anterior cerebral and middle cerebral arteries. The two **anterior cerebral arteries** pass forward and medially toward the longitudinal fissure, where they are connected by a small **anterior communicating artery.** The two arteries then run parallel in the longitudinal fissure and give off numerous branches to supply much of the frontal and parietal lobes. The **middle cerebral artery** passes through the lateral fissure to spread out over the lateral surface of the brain. A third branch of the internal carotid artery, the **posterior communicating artery,** runs posteriorly to anastomose with the posterior cerebral arteries.

Vertebral Arteries. The right and left vertebral arteries, which are branches of the subclavian arteries, course superiorly through the transverse foramina of the cervical vertebrae beginning at C6. As they pass through the foramen magnum, they pierce the dura mater to enter the cerebellomedullary

FIG. 5-16. Midsagittal section of the brain showing cisterns.

FIG. 5-17. Midsagittal CT image showing cisterns of the brain.

cistern of the subarachnoid space. The right and left vertebral arteries join to form the **basilar artery,** which passes over the anterior surface of the pons. The basilar artery then divides to form two **posterior cerebral arteries,** which supply the occipital lobes.

Circulus Arteriosus Cerebri. The typical configuration at the base of the brain shows the vessels anastomosing to form a "circle," called the **circulus arteriosus cerebri,** or **circle of Willis.** This circle (Fig. 5-18) is formed by the internal carotid arteries, the anterior cerebral arteries, the anterior communicating artery, the posterior cerebral arteries, and the posterior communicating artery. Berry aneurysms often occur in the vessels of the circle of Willis. The circle of Willis, which is located in the interpeduncular cistern, encloses the optic chiasma, infundibulum, and mammillary bodies. The angiogram in Fig. 5-19 shows some of the vessels in the circle of Willis, and the reconstructed CT image in Fig. 5-20 shows the circle of Willis in situ.

Venous Drainage. Venous channels that drain blood from the brain and the meninges are called *sinuses*. They are generally located between the endosteum of the calvaria and the meningeal dura or between two layers of dura mater. Unlike other veins, venous sinuses have no valves. The **superior sagittal sinus** is triangular in cross section, occupies the entire length of the superior portion of the falx cerebri, and increases in size as it passes posteriorly. At the internal occipital protuberance, it usually continues as the right lateral sinus. The smaller **inferior sagittal sinus** occupies the free inferior edge of the falx cerebri. At the junction of the falx cerebri with the tentorium cerebelli, the inferior sagittal sinus receives the great cerebral vein and becomes the **straight sinus,** which courses along the tentorium cerebelli. At the internal occipital protuberance, the straight sinus usually continues as the left lateral sinus. The **lateral sinuses** are continuations of either the superior sagittal sinus or the straight sinus, but at their origin they may form a common space called the *confluence of sinuses*. The lateral sinuses are subdivided into

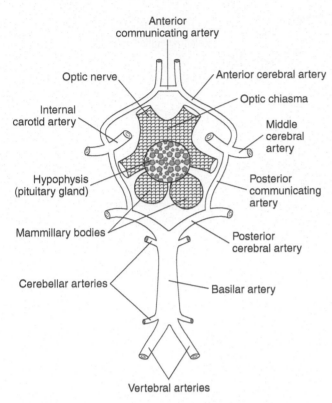

FIG. 5-18. Circulus arteriosus cerebri (circle of Willis).

FIG. 5-19. Angiogram of portions of the circle of Willis.

FIG. 5-20. Reconstructed CT image showing the circle of Willis.

transverse and sigmoid portions. The **transverse sinus** passes from the internal occipital protuberance (confluence of sinuses) to the junction of the petrous and mastoid portions of the temporal bone. The **sigmoid sinus,** which is a continuation of the transverse sinus, follows an S-shaped path that loops over the petrous and mastoid portions to the jugular foramen, where it becomes the **internal jugular vein.** The venous sinuses are illustrated in Fig. 5-21. In addition to these main sinuses, numerous smaller ones drain specific portions of the brain and empty into one of the larger sinuses.

A rather large **cavernous sinus** is located on each side of the body and sella turcica of the sphenoid bone (see Fig. 5-21). These sinuses receive venous blood from the ophthalmic and middle cerebral veins and are drained by small petrosal sinuses that empty into the sigmoid sinus or into the internal jugular vein. The internal carotid artery enters the cavernous sinus through the foramen lacerum, makes a hairpin turn at the end of the sinus, and leaves the sinus to enter the subarachnoid space. The angiogram in Fig. 5-22 shows the internal carotid artery in the cavernous sinus. The abducens nerve is closely related to the internal carotid artery as it traverses the cavernous sinus. Associated with the lateral wall of the cavernous sinus, superior to inferior, are the oculomotor (III), trochlear (IV), and ophthalmic and maxillary divisions of the trigeminal (V) nerves. The relationships of the vessels and nerves in the cavernous sinus are illustrated in Fig. 5-23. Injuries in the region of the cavernous sinus exhibit a variety of signs, because an intimate relationship exists between the vessels and nerves within the sinus. Some of these signs may be detected in the orbit of the eye. The proximity of the cavernous sinus to the sphenoidal paranasal sinus contributes to the development of meningitis as a sequela to sinusitis.

QUICK CHECK

5.18 What two pairs of arteries supply oxygenated blood to the brain?

5.19 What venous sinus loops over the petrous portion of the temporal bone and then drains into the internal jugular vein?

FIG. 5-21. Venous sinuses.

FIG. 5-22. Angiogram showing the internal carotid artery in the cavernous sinus, lateral projection.

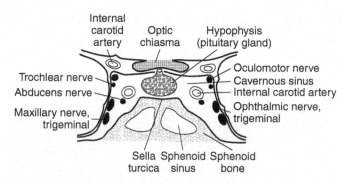

FIG. 5-23. Relationships within the cavernous sinus.

Cranial Nerves.   Twelve pairs of cranial nerves emerge from the inferior surface of the brain. These nerves pass through foramina of the skull to innervate structures in the head and neck Head in the viscera in the body. The cranial nerves are designated by name and by Roman numerals, according to the order in which they appear on the inferior surface of the brain. Fig. 5-24 illustrates the cranial nerves.

Cranial Nerve I (Olfactory).   The olfactory nerves provide the body with the sense of smell. They begin in the mucous membrane of the olfactory region of the nasal cavity and continue through the olfactory foramina in the cribriform plate of the ethmoid bone to enter the olfactory bulb on the inferior surface of the brain. From the olfactory bulb, the olfactory tract proceeds posteriorly to the olfactory cortex on the medial side of the temporal lobe of the brain.

Cranial Nerve II (Optic).   Mediating visual function, the optic nerve originates in the nerve cells of the retina. From there the two nerves, one for each eye, are directed posteriorly and medially through the optic foramen of the sphenoid bone into the cranial cavity, where they meet at the optic chiasma on the inferior surface of the hypothalamus. In the optic chiasma, the fibers from the medial part of the retina of each eye cross to the opposite side, whereas

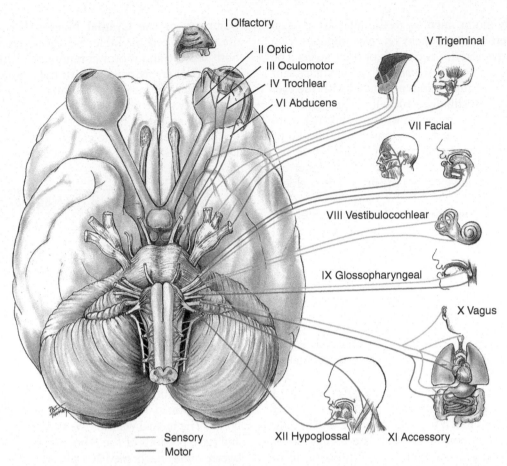

I Olfactory

II Optic
III Oculomotor
IV Trochlear
VI Abducens

V Trigeminal

VII Facial

VIII Vestibulocochlear

IX Glossopharyngeal

X Vagus

Sensory
Motor

XII Hypoglossal   XI Accessory

FIG. 5-24. Cranial nerves. (From Applegate E: *The anatomy and physiology learning system,* ed 3, St Louis, 2006, Elsevier/Saunders.)

the fibers from the lateral portions of the retinas remain on the same side. After this partial decussation, or crossing over, in the chiasma, the fibers continue as the optic tract to the visual area of the occipital lobe.

Cranial Nerve III (Oculomotor). Cranial nerve III is a motor nerve to the superior, inferior, and medial rectus muscles and to the inferior oblique muscle of the eye. These muscles are responsible for a variety of eye movements. In addition to these four extrinsic muscles, the nerve also has fibers innervating the levator palpebrae superioris muscle, which elevates the upper eyelid to open the eye. Some parasympathetic fibers supply the ciliary muscle, which changes the shape of the lens in accommodation, and the sphincter muscle of the iris, which changes the size of the pupil. In passing from the cranial cavity to the orbital cavity, the oculomotor nerve passes through the superior orbital fissure.

Cranial Nerve IV (Trochlear). The trochlear nerve is motor in function and supplies the superior oblique muscle of the eye. In passing from the cranial cavity to the orbital cavity, the trochlear nerve passes through the superior orbital fissure with the oculomotor nerve.

Cranial Nerve V (Trigeminal). The largest of the cranial nerves is the trigeminal nerve, which contains motor fibers for the muscles of mastication and sensory fibers from the

head. After emerging from the lateral side of the pons, the nerve divides into three branches. The ophthalmic branch passes through the superior orbital fissure to receive sensory impulses from the conjunctiva and cornea of the eye, the upper eyelid, the forehead, the nose, and the scalp. The maxillary branch first passes through the foramen rotundum, then curves around to enter the orbital cavity through the inferior orbital fissure. It leaves the cavity through the infraorbital foramen to receive sensory impulses from the skin of the cheek, the lateral nose, the upper lip, and the teeth. The mandibular branch emerges through the foramen ovale. It receives sensory impulses from the skin over the mandible and temporal region, the tongue, the floor of the mouth, the lower teeth and gingivae, and the buccal surface of the cheek. It also has motor fibers that stimulate the muscles of mastication.

Cranial Nerve VI (Abducens). The abducens nerve emerges from the inferior surface of the brain at the junction of the pons and the medulla. It enters the orbital cavity through the superior orbital fissure to supply motor impulses to the lateral rectus muscle of the eye.

Cranial Nerve VII (Facial). The seventh cranial nerve, the facial nerve, contains both sensory and motor fibers. After leaving the skull through the stylomastoid foramen, it passes through the substance of the parotid gland, where it branches to supply motor impulses to the muscles of facial expression. The sensory component receives impulses from the taste buds on the anterior two thirds of the tongue. The nerve also stimulates the sublingual and submaxillary salivary glands and the lacrimal glands associated with the eye.

Cranial Nerve VIII (Vestibulocochlear).   The eighth cranial nerve is a special sensory nerve with two distinct components. The vestibular branch functions in equilibrium by receiving sensory impulses from the semicircular canals, the utricle, and the saccule. These structures of the inner ear detect the position and movement of the head. The cochlear branch functions in hearing by receiving impulses from the organ of Corti in the cochlear duct, also in the inner ear. Both branches enter the cranial cavity through the internal auditory meatus. The vestibulocochlear nerve is sometimes referred to as the *acoustic,* or *auditory, nerve.*

Cranial Nerve IX (Glossopharyngeal).   As the name implies, the chief distribution of the glossopharyngeal nerve is to the tongue and **pharynx.** It is a mixed nerve, with both sensory and motor functions. This nerve supplies motor impulses to muscles that aid in swallowing and to the parotid salivary gland. The sensory component may be divided into three functional groups. Some of the fibers convey the sensation of taste from the posterior one third of the tongue. Others transmit the general sensations of pain, temperature, and touch from the pharynx and middle ear. The third group is concerned with the regulation of respiration and blood pressure by receiving impulses from the chemoreceptors and pressure receptors associated with the carotid arteries in the neck. The ninth cranial nerve exits the cranial cavity through the jugular foramen.

Cranial Nerve X (Vagus).   The word *vagus* is derived from the Latin word meaning wandering. This is an appropriate name for the tenth cranial nerve, which has the most extensive distribution of all the nerves. It leaves the cranial cavity through the jugular foramen. The fibers of this mixed nerve may be divided into four groups: (1) somatic motor fibers, which supply the skeletal muscles of the pharynx and larynx; (2) visceral motor fibers, which carry impulses to the thoracic and abdominal viscera; (3) somatic sensory fibers, which convey impulses concerned with pain, temperature, and touch from the external ear; and (4) visceral sensory fibers, which function in the regulation of heart rate, blood pressure, and respiration by transmitting impulses from the stretch receptors in the heart, aorta, superior vena cava, and lungs. This component also receives sensory impulses from the abdominal viscera.

Cranial Nerve XI (Accessory).   The accessory nerve, the eleventh cranial nerve, is entirely motor in function. It leaves the cranial cavity through the jugular foramen and stimulates the trapezius and sternocleidomastoid muscles to contract.

Cranial Nerve XII (Hypoglossal).   The numerous roots of the twelfth cranial nerve emerge through the hypoglossal canal in the occipital bone. After passing through the canal, the roots unite to form the hypoglossal nerve. This nerve, which is motor in function, stimulates the muscles of the tongue to contract.

Summary of the Cranial Nerves.   The cranial nerves are summarized in Table 5-4. Most cranial nerves have both sensory and motor components. Three of the nerves (I, II, VIII) are associated with the special senses of smell, vision, hearing, and equilibrium and consist of sensory fibers only. Five other nerves (III, IV, VI, XI, XII) are primarily motor in function but have some sensory fibers for proprioception. The remaining four nerves (V, VII, IX, X) consist of significant amounts of both sensory and motor fibers.

QUICK CHECK

5.20   Which cranial nerve has the most extensive distribution?

5.21   Which cranial nerves pass through the cavernous sinus?

Orbital Cavity and Contents

Cavity Walls.   The orbital cavity is a pyramid-shaped structure with an apex, a base, and four triangular walls. The **optic foramen** is at the apex in the posterior part of the orbit. The base, which is the anterior part that opens onto the face, is formed by the zygomatic, maxillary, and frontal bones. The medial walls of the two orbits are nearly parallel and have portions of the ethmoid and sphenoid sinuses between them. Each medial wall is formed by the lacrimal bone and the fragile orbital plates of the ethmoid and palatine bones. The superior wall, or roof, of the cavity is formed by the orbital plate of the frontal bone. The maxilla and a small portion of the zygomatic bone make up the inferior wall, or floor. The lateral walls of the two orbits are positioned at right angles (90 degrees) to each other and, if extended, would intersect in the region of the pituitary gland. The sturdy lateral wall is formed by the zygomatic bone, or **zygoma,** and the greater wing of the sphenoid bone. A depression for the lacrimal gland is located in the superior portion of the lateral wall.

Bulbus Oculi.   The primary structure in the orbital cavity, of course, is the **bulbus oculi,** or **eyeball.** It is somewhat spherical, approximately 2 to 3 cm in diameter, and has an anterior bulge. The eyeball is surrounded by orbital fat within the orbital cavity.

The wall of the bulbus oculi is made up of three concentric coats, or tunics. The **external,** or **fibrous, tunic** is the supporting layer. It consists of the white, opaque **sclera,** which covers the posterior five sixths of the eyeball, and the transparent **cornea,** which covers the anterior one sixth.

The **middle vascular tunic** consists of the **choroid, ciliary body,** and **iris.** The **choroid** is a highly vascular, brown-pigmented layer that is located between the sclera and the retina. It is the largest part of the middle tunic, and it lines most of the sclera, although it is only loosely connected to the fibrous coat and can easily be stripped

TABLE 5-4   Summary of Cranial Nerves

Number	Name	Associated Foramen	Type	Function
I	Olfactory	Olfactory foramina in cribriform plate of ethmoid bone	Sensory	Sense of smell
II	Optic	Optic foramen of sphenoid bone	Sensory	Vision
III	Oculomotor	Superior orbital fissure of sphenoid bone	Motor	Movement of eye and eyelid
IV	Trochlear	Superior orbital fissure of sphenoid bone	Motor	Movement of the eye
V	Trigeminal		Mixed	
	Ophthalmic branch	Superior orbital fissure of sphenoid bone	Sensory	Cornea, skin of nose, forehead, scalp
	Maxillary branch	Foramen rotundum of sphenoid bone	Sensory	Cheek, nose, upper lip, and teeth
	Mandibular branch	Foramen ovale of sphenoid bone	Mixed	Skin over mandible, tongue, lower lip, and teeth; contraction of muscles of mastication
VI	Abducens	Superior orbital fissure of sphenoid bone	Motor	Eye movement
VII	Facial	Stylomastoid foramen of temporal bone	Mixed	Contraction of muscles of facial expression; lacrimal and submaxillary gland secretion; taste from anterior two thirds of tongue
VIII	Vestibulocochlear	Internal auditory meatus of temporal bone	Sensory	Hearing and equilibrium
IX	Glossopharyngeal	Jugular foramen of temporal bone	Mixed	Taste from posterior one third of tongue; contraction of muscles used in swallowing; parotid gland secretion
X	Vagus	Jugular foramen of temporal bone	Mixed	Contraction of muscles of pharynx and larynx; gastric motility; general visceral sensation; alters heart rate, respiration, blood pressure
XI	Accessory	Jugular foramen of temporal bone	Motor	Contraction of trapezius and sternocleidomastoid muscles
XII	Hypoglossal	Hypoglossal canal of occipital bone	Motor	Contraction of muscles of tongue

away. However, the choroid is firmly attached to the retina. Anteriorly, the choroid is continuous with the **ciliary body. Suspensory ligaments** connect the ciliary body to the lens of the eye. The ciliary body contains numerous, fingerlike ciliary processes that secrete the aqueous humor. Externally, the ciliary body contains ciliary muscle. When this muscle contracts, the suspensory ligaments relax and the lens bulges to allow focusing for close vision. The **iris** is the conspicuous, colored portion of the eye. It is a doughnut-shaped diaphragm with a central aperture, the **pupil.** The muscles of the iris are continually contracting and relaxing to change the size of the pupil, which regulates the amount of light entering the eye.

The **innermost nervous tunic** is the **retina,** which has several layers. The outer layer of the retina is deeply pigmented and firmly attached to the choroid. The rods and cones, which are the light receptor cells, are adjacent to the pigmented layer. Other layers consist of bipolar neurons and ganglion cells. The axons of the ganglion cells converge to form the optic nerve, which penetrates the tunics at the optic disc, then passes through the apex of the

orbital cavity to reach the brain. The slight depression in the retina is the fovea centralis.

A transparent, biconvex **lens** is located just posterior to the iris. The curvature of the lens surface changes by action of the ciliary muscles and suspensory ligaments to permit focusing on objects at different distances. The space anterior to the lens is the anterior cavity, which is filled with **aqueous humor.** The posterior cavity, between the lens and the retina, is filled with a colorless, transparent, gel-like **vitreous humor.** Unlike the aqueous humor, which is continually being replaced, the vitreous humor is formed during embryonic development and is not exchanged. Fig. 5-25 illustrates the structure of the bulbus oculi

Six extrinsic ocular muscles, which insert on the sclera, are associated with movements of the eye. These muscles are summarized in Table 5-5. They are illustrated in the axial MR image in Fig. 5-26 and the coronal MR image in Fig. 5-27.

Vascular Supply to the Orbital Contents.   Most of the vascular supply to the orbital contents is by way of the

FIG. 5-25. Structure of the bulbus oculi.

Lateral rectus muscle

Medial rectus muscle

Optic nerve

A

R◄─────►L

P

FIG. 5-26. Axial MR image showing the extrinsic muscles of the eye.

Superior rectus muscle

Optic nerve

Lateral rectus muscle

Medial rectus muscle

Inferior rectus mucle

FIG. 5-27. Coronal MR image showing the extrinsic muscles of the eye.

TABLE 5-5 Extrinsic Muscles Associated With Eye Movement

Muscle	Function	Innervation
Superior rectus	Rotates eye upward and laterally	Oculomotor (cranial nerve III)
Inferior rectus	Rotates eye downward and medially	Oculomotor (cranial nerve III)
Lateral rectus	Rotates eye laterally	Abducens (cranial nerve VI)
Medial rectus	Rotates eye medially	Oculomotor (cranial nerve III)
Superior oblique	Rotates eye downward and laterally	Trochlear (cranial nerve IV)
Inferior oblique	Rotates eye upward and laterally	Oculomotor (cranial nerve III)

ophthalmic artery, a branch of the internal carotid artery. Ciliary branches of the ophthalmic artery provide the blood supply to the sclera, choroid, ciliary body, and iris. One of the smallest but most important branches of the ophthalmic artery is the **central artery of the retina.** This vessel enters the bulbus oculi through the optic disc and then branches over the surface of the retina to provide the blood supply. If the central artery is blocked by a tumor, thrombus, or massive edema, the result is sudden blindness.

Venous drainage of the orbital cavity is furnished by the **superior** and **inferior ophthalmic veins,** which pass through the orbit to enter the cavernous sinus located adjacent to the pituitary gland. The **central vein of the retina** follows the pathway of the central artery along the optic nerve. The central vein drains into the cavernous sinus, along with the ophthalmic veins. Increased intracranial pressure restricts the blood flow in the central vein as it passes through the subarachnoid space. This restricted venous drainage results in edema at the optic disc, which is directly observable with an ophthalmoscope. Papilledema, or swelling at the optic disc, is one of the earliest indications of increased intracranial pressure.

Protective Features of the Eye.   The eyes are protected by the **eyelids,** or **palpebrae.** The upper eyelid consists of the **levator palpebrae superioris muscle,** which is covered by thin skin and lined by a highly vascular **conjunctiva.** The levator palpebrae superioris muscle elevates the upper eyelid to open the eye and is innervated by the oculomotor nerve.

The **lacrimal apparatus** is another protective structure associated with the eye. The **lacrimal gland,** located in the upper and lateral part of the orbit, produces the lacrimal fluid, or tears. The lacrimal fluid moistens the surface of the eye, lubricates the eyelids, and washes away foreign particles. It also contains an enzyme that destroys certain bacteria. After spreading across the surface of the eye, the fluid drains through the nasolacrimal duct into the inferior meatus of the nasal cavity.

QUICK CHECK

5.22   What opening is at the apex of the orbital cavity?
5.23   What small but important branch of the ophthalmic artery enters the bulbus oculi at the optic disc?
5.24   Where in the orbit is the lacrimal gland located?

Sectional Anatomy of the Head

Transverse Sections

Sections Through the Lateral Ventricles.   Sections superior to the lateral ventricles demonstrate the **cerebral gyri** and **sulci** with cortical gray matter and underlying white matter. The **longitudinal fissure** containing the **falx cerebri** and **superior sagittal sinus** is readily identifiable. In cadaveric specimens the **dura mater** and **arachnoid** may be seen; however, the subdural space is frequently exaggerated because of tissue shrinkage.

Sections taken a little more inferiorly, 6 to 7 cm from the top of the head, show the roof or upper portion of the **lateral ventricles** (Fig. 5-28). Just inferior to this, the lateral ventricles are separated by a thin partition, the **septum pellucidum.** The **genu** of the corpus callosum is between the anterior horns, and the **splenium** is between the posterior horns of the lateral ventricles. The body of the **caudate nucleus** is lateral to the lateral ventricles. Depending on the angle of the plane, the **inferior sagittal sinus** may be present. The axial MR image in Fig. 5-29 shows the lateral ventricles.

Section Through the Basal Ganglia.   Proceeding inferiorly from the upper portions of the lateral ventricles, numerous internal brain structures are noted (Fig. 5-30). This plane passes just above the tentorium cerebelli. The **genu** and the **splenium** of the **corpus callosum** are readily identified as bands of white fibers passing from one hemisphere to the other. Both the anterior and posterior horns of the **lateral ventricles** are present at this level. Just posterior and lateral to the anterior horns, in fact forming the floor of the anterior horns, are regions of gray matter, the head of the **caudate nucleus.** The **septum pellucidum** is seen as a thin midline partition between the two lateral ventricles. A slight enlargement of the septum pellucidum is the **fornix.** Posterior to the fornix, in a midline position, is a narrow slit representing the **third ventricle.** The **interventricular foramen,** sometimes called the *foramen of Monro,* is an opening between each of the lateral ventricles and the single midline third ventricle. Two regions of gray matter, the **thalami,** which make up a significant portion of the diencephalon, form the lateral walls of the third ventricle. The posterior horns of the lateral ventricles are posterior to the thalamic areas. **Choroid plexus,** a capillary network that produces cerebrospinal fluid, is evident in the wall of the ventricles. A small area of gray matter, the **tail of the caudate nucleus,** may be seen in the roof of the posterior horns. The posterior horns are separated by the splenium of the corpus callosum. The axial MR image in Fig. 5-31 shows horns of the lateral ventricles and the choroid plexus.

The **insula,** or island of Reil, which is buried deep within the lateral fissure, usually is evident at this level. Branches of the **middle cerebral artery** are within the lateral fissure and around the insula. Deep to the insula is a mass of gray matter, which is the **lentiform nucleus.** The lentiform nucleus is made up of two parts, an outer, darker segment, which is the **putamen,** and an inner, paler segment, which is the **globus pallidus.** The lentiform nucleus is separated from the caudate nucleus by a band of white fibers, which constitutes the **anterior limb of the internal capsule.** Between the thalamus and the lentiform nucleus, the internal capsule continues as the **posterior limb.** A thin strip of gray matter, the **claustrum,** is located between the insula and the putamen of the lentiform nucleus. A portion of the **frontal sinus** may be seen in some specimens at this level.

Section Through the Superior Cistern.   If the posterior portion of a section through the basal ganglia is at a slightly lower level, such as that obtained parallel to the

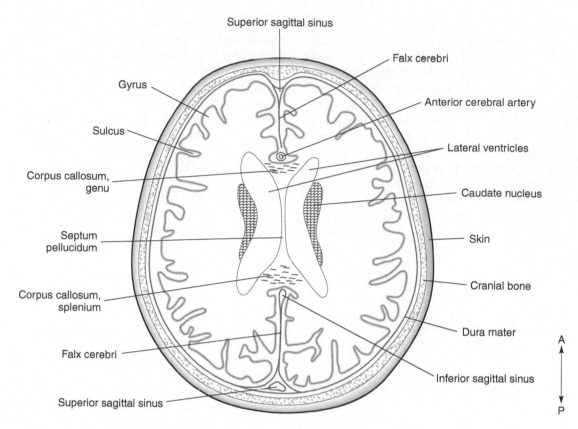

FIG. 5-28. Transverse section through the lateral ventricles.

FIG. 5-29. Axial MR image showing the lateral ventricles.

orbital-meatal line, some additional structures may be noted. The splenium of the corpus callosum may be absent, and the top portion of the **tentorium cerebelli** may be seen. Along with this will be the superior cistern, which is located between the splenium of the corpus callosum and the tentorium cerebelli (Fig. 5-32). The **great cerebral vein** and the **pineal gland** are located in the superior cistern, and the corpora quadrigemina project into this space. The **straight sinus,** which runs along the junc-

tion between the falx cerebri and the tentorium cerebelli, is present in sections showing the tentorium cerebelli. The straight sinus is continuous with the inferior sagittal sinus and also receives the great cerebral vein. The axial CT image in Fig. 5-33 shows the superior cistern.

QUICK CHECK

5.25 In transverse sections through the lateral ventricles, what portion of the basal ganglia is immediately lateral to the lateral ventricles?

5.26 In transverse sections through the basal ganglia, what is the midline space in the diencephalon?

5.27 In transverse sections through the superior cistern, what blood vessel is located in the same region as the pineal gland?

Section Through the Midbrain. The next few paragraphs deal with sections at the level of the midbrain. If the plane of section is parallel to the orbital-meatal line, sections at this level pass through the superior part of the orbit anteriorly and through the cerebellum posteriorly. If the plane of section is more oblique (e.g., a 15- to 20-degree angle to the orbital-meatal line), the anterior views are above the orbit, and more of the cerebellum is shown posteriorly.

Fig. 5-34 illustrates the area surrounding the **midbrain.** The two anteriorly projecting **cerebral peduncles** are

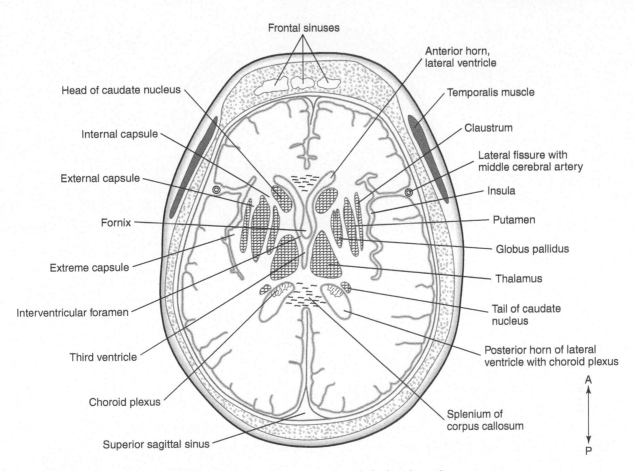

Frontal sinuses

Anterior horn,
lateral ventricle

Head of caudate nucleus

Temporalis muscle

Internal capsule

Claustrum

Lateral fissure with
middle cerebral artery

External capsule

Insula

Fornix

Putamen

Globus pallidus

Extreme capsule

Thalamus

Interventricular foramen

Tail of caudate
nucleus

Third ventricle

Posterior horn of lateral
ventricle with choroid plexus

Choroid plexus

Splenium of
corpus callosum

Superior sagittal sinus

FIG. 5-30. Transverse section through the basal ganglia.

Longitudinal fissure

Corpus callosum, genu

Lateral ventricle, anterior horn

Caudate nucleus

Septum pellucidum

Lateral ventricle, body

Third ventricle

Thalamus

Lateral ventricle, posterior horn, with choroid plexus

Corpus callosum, splenium

FIG. 5-31. Axial MR image showing the lateral ventricles.

particularly noticeable because of the presence of a very dark substance called **substantia nigra.** The **interpeduncular cistern** is between the two cerebral peduncles. Two **mammillary bodies,** which form a portion of the floor of the **third ventricle,** project into the interpeduncular cistern. The narrow space anterior to the mammillary bodies is the third ventricle. **Optic tracts** project posteriorly and laterally from the third ventricle. The aqueduct of Sylvius, or **cerebral aqueduct,** forms a small opening near the **superior colliculi of the corpora quadrigemina.** The space between the corpora quadrigemina and the cerebellum is the **superior cistern,** or cistern of the great cerebral vein. Compare the line drawing in Fig. 5-34 with the axial MR image in Fig. 5-35.

In sections that are nearly parallel to the orbital-meatal line, the frontal bone exhibits a large **frontal sinus.** The **orbits,** on either side, contain some **orbital fat,** or possibly some of the superior muscles, such as the **levator palpebrae superioris,** or superior rectus. Laterally, the **temporalis muscle** is superficial to the temporal bone. Posteriorly, the **cerebellum** is sectioned so that it shows the centrally located **vermis.** The **tentorium cerebelli** separates the cerebellum from the cerebrum. The **anterior cerebral arteries** are present in the longitudinal fissure, the **middle cerebral arteries** are in the lateral fissure, and the **posterior cerebral arteries** are in the superior cistern with the great cerebral vein.

In more oblique sections through the midbrain (e.g., at 15 or 20 degrees to the orbital-meatal line), the plane passes superior to the orbit and frontal sinus anteriorly and passes through the cerebellum at a more inferior level than

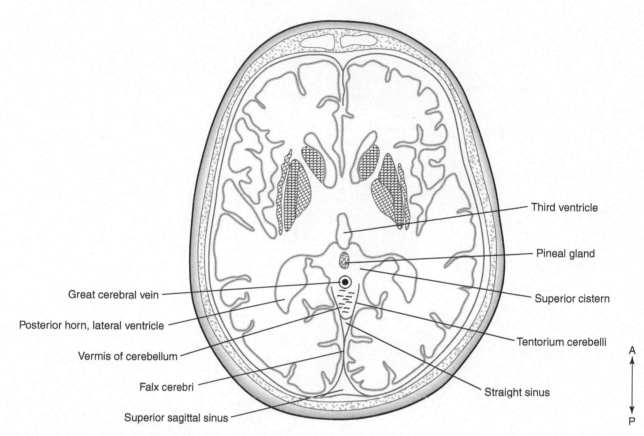

FIG. 5-32. Transverse section through the superior cistern.

Labels on figure: Third ventricle; Pineal gland; Superior cistern; Tentorium cerebelli; Straight sinus; Great cerebral vein; Posterior horn, lateral ventricle; Vermis of cerebellum; Falx cerebri; Superior sagittal sinus; A; P

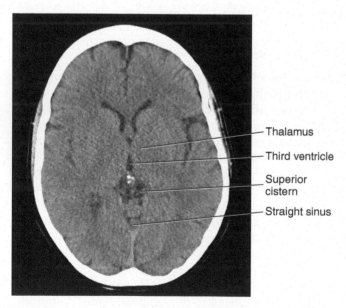

Labels on figure: Thalamus; Third ventricle; Superior cistern; Straight sinus

FIG. 5-33. Axial CT image through the superior cistern.

the section described previously. Either a **sigmoid sinus** or a **transverse sinus** probably will be present instead of the superior sagittal sinus.

Section Through the Pons. Transverse sections through the pons (Fig. 5-36) show the **pontine cistern** with the single **basilar artery.** The **fourth ventricle** is posterior to

the pons, with the **superior cerebellar peduncles** forming the walls of the ventricle. Large **middle cerebellar peduncles** are lateral to the superior cerebellar peduncles. Two **large trigeminal** nerves emerge laterally from the pons. In sections that are cut more or less parallel to the orbital-meatal line, the **pituitary gland** is just anterior to the pontine cistern. Some sections may also pass through the body of the **sphenoid bone,** with a cavernous sinus located on either side. The **internal carotid arteries** and some nerves are in the cavernous sinus (see Fig. 5-23). Sections at this level also show the **sphenoid sinuses** and **ethmoid air cells.** Compare the line drawing in Fig. 5-36 with the axial MR image in Fig. 5-37.

Fig. 5-36 also shows that the lateral walls of the orbit are perpendicular to each other, whereas the **medial walls** are parallel. The optic nerve is centrally located within each orbit, between the **lateral rectus muscle** and the **medial rectus muscle.** The axial CT image in Fig. 5-38 is at the level of the orbit and shows some of the features in this region.

In the posterior region, the dural venous sinuses are **transverse sinuses.** In the region of the pons, the **petrous portions of the temporal bone** project between the cerebellum and the temporal lobes of the cerebrum. The **sigmoid sinus** is present with the petrous portion of the temporal bone. The **temporalis muscle** is in the temporal fossa. In more oblique sections through the level of the pons, the anterior portion is cut above the level of the orbit and the nasal cavity and still shows the frontal lobes of the cerebrum.

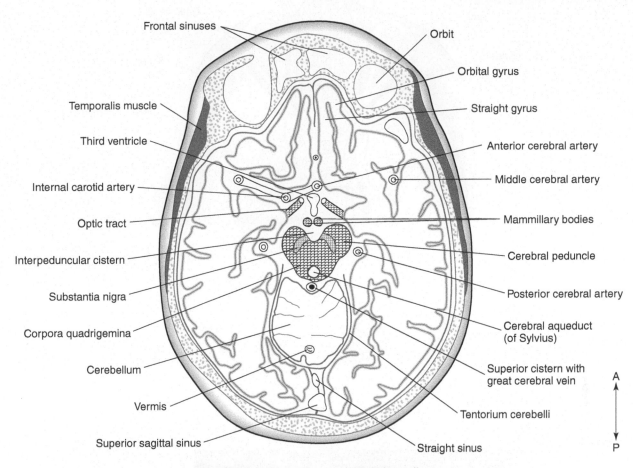

Frontal sinuses

Orbit

Orbital gyrus

Temporalis muscle

Straight gyrus

Third ventricle

Anterior cerebral artery

Internal carotid artery

Middle cerebral artery

Optic tract

Mammillary bodies

Interpeduncular cistern

Cerebral peduncle

Substantia nigra

Posterior cerebral artery

Corpora quadrigemina

Cerebral aqueduct (of Sylvius)

Cerebellum

Superior cistern with great cerebral vein

Vermis

Tentorium cerebelli

Superior sagittal sinus

Straight sinus

A

P

FIG. 5-34. Transverse section through the midbrain.

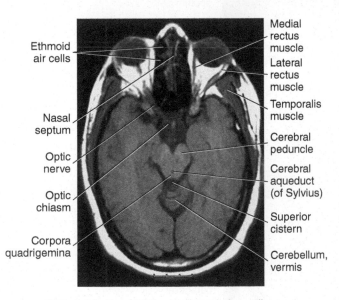

Ethmoid air cells

Medial rectus muscle

Lateral rectus muscle

Temporalis muscle

Nasal septum

Cerebral peduncle

Optic nerve

Cerebral aqueduct (of Sylvius)

Optic chiasm

Superior cistern

Corpora quadrigemina

Cerebellum, vermis

FIG. 5-35. Axial MR image through the midbrain.

Section Through the Medulla Oblongata. At the level of the medulla oblongata, the **right** and **left vertebral arteries** are present in the **cerebellomedullary cistern,** which is anterior to the medulla. The venous sinuses present in the **petrous portion of the temporal bone** are **sigmoid**

sinuses, which are continuations of the transverse sinuses. In some cases the **jugular foramen** is present at this level. The **internal carotid arteries** are lateral to the basilar portion of the occipital bone. In sections parallel to the orbital-meatal line (Fig. 5-39), the facial region shows the **nasal septum, middle nasal conchae,** and **maxillary sinuses.** The **zygomatic arch** is present in the cheek area, and the **temporalis muscle** is medial to the arch. This region is also illustrated by the axial MR image in Fig. 5-40.

The axial CT image in Fig. 5-41 is at a slightly lower level and passes through the ramus of the mandible and the mastoid process. Compare the features at this level with those at the level of the medulla oblongata.

QUICK CHECK

5.28   In transverse sections through the midbrain, what channel appears as a hole in the corpora quadrigemina?

5.29   What extension of dura mater is between the cerebrum and the cerebellum?

5.30   In transverse sections through the pons, what blood vessel is in the space anterior to the pons?

5.31   In transverse sections at the level of the medulla oblongata, is the internal carotid artery anterior or posterior to the internal jugular vein?

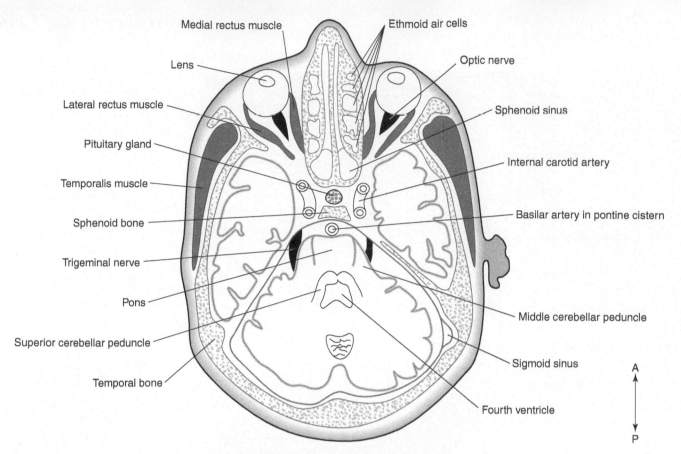

FIG. 5-36. Transverse section through the pons.

Medial rectus muscle

Ethmoid air cells

Lens

Optic nerve

Lateral rectus muscle

Sphenoid sinus

Pituitary gland

Internal carotid artery

Temporalis muscle

Sphenoid bone

Basilar artery in pontine cistern

Trigeminal nerve

Pons

Middle cerebellar peduncle

Superior cerebellar peduncle

Sigmoid sinus

Temporal bone

Fourth ventricle

A

P

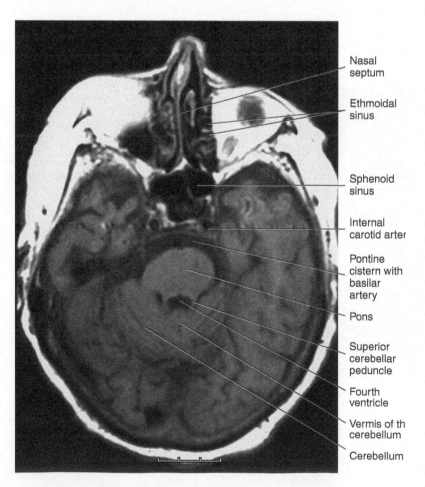

FIG. 5-37. Axial MR image through the pons.

Nasal septum

Ethmoidal sinus

Sphenoid sinus

Internal carotid arter

Pontine cistern with basilar artery

Pons

Superior cerebellar peduncle

Fourth ventricle

Vermis of th cerebellum

Cerebellum

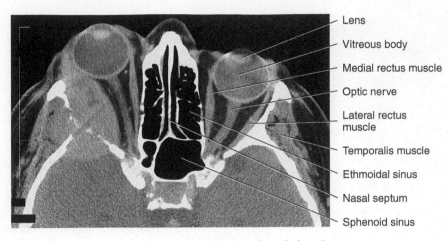

FIG. 5-38. Axial CT image through the orbit.

Lens
Vitreous body
Medial rectus muscle
Optic nerve
Lateral rectus muscle
Temporalis muscle
Ethmoidal sinus
Nasal septum
Sphenoid sinus

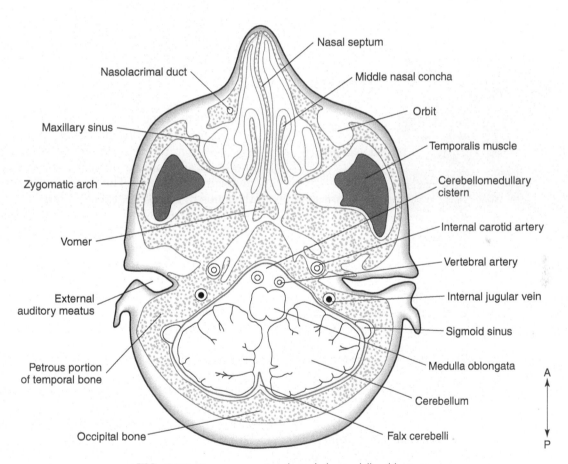

Nasal septum
Nasolacrimal duct
Middle nasal concha
Maxillary sinus
Orbit
Temporalis muscle
Zygomatic arch
Cerebellomedullary cistern
Internal carotid artery
Vomer
Vertebral artery
External auditory meatus
Internal jugular vein
Sigmoid sinus
Petrous portion of temporal bone
Medulla oblongata
Cerebellum
Occipital bone
Falx cerebelli

A
P

FIG. 5-39. Transverse section through the medulla oblongata.

Maxillary sinus
Inferior nasal concha
Nasal septum
Masseter muscle
Temporalis muscle
Pterygoid muscle
Nasopharynx
Internal jugular vein
Internal carotid arter
Medulla oblongata
Cerebellum

FIG. 5-40. Axial MR image through the base of the skull.

Nasal septum
Maxillary sinus
Nasopharynx
Masseter muscle
Ramus of mandible
Pterygoid muscle
Internal carotid artery
Internal jugular vein

FIG. 5-41. Axial CT image through the ramus of the mandible.

Sagittal Sections

Section Through the Temporomandibular Joint.
Fig. 5-42 illustrates a parasagittal section through the lateral surface of the head and neck, particularly through the **temporomandibular joint.** The **condyle of the mandible** articulates in the **mandibular fossa** of the temporal bone. Using the joint as a reference, the **zygomatic process** of the temporal bone projects anteriorly, the **external auditory meatus** is immediately posterior to the joint, and this is followed by the **mastoid process.** The superficial cheek muscle is the **masseter,** followed posteriorly by the **parotid gland** and the sternocleidomastoid muscle. The **sternocleidomastoid muscle,** a landmark muscle in the neck, courses obliquely along the neck to insert on the mastoid process. The **temporalis** muscle overlying the temporal

bone is superior to the masseter. Only the surface of the brain is visible inside the cranial cavity.

Section Through the Orbit.
Sagittal sections through the orbit (Fig. 5-43) are too lateral to show many details of the brain; however, numerous other structures of the head are illustrated. This plane passes through the **frontal, parietal, occipital,** and **temporal** lobes of the cerebrum. The **tentorium cerebelli,** with the **transverse sinus** in its posterior margin, forms a partition between the cerebrum and the cerebellum. Note that the tentorium cerebelli is anchored to the **petrous ridge** of the temporal bone, and the **sigmoid venous sinus** is along the posterior margin of the ridge.

The **frontal** and **maxillary** bones form the superior and inferior portions of the orbit. Within the orbit, fat surrounds the **bulbus oculi** and **extrinsic eye muscles.** The **mandible** is a recognizable structure in the face. The **buccinator muscle,** one of the muscles of mastication, is in the cheek superior to the mandible, and the **submandibular gland** is inferior to the mandible. The sublingual gland is not present, because it is nearer the midline. A portion of the **temporalis** and **pterygoid** muscles may be evident superior and posterior to the buccinator.

Midsagittal Section.
Fig. 5-44 illustrates a midsagittal section through the head. The midsagittal MR image in Fig. 5-45 is from the same region. Because many parts of the brain are midline or nearly so, they are evident on midsagittal sections. The **cerebrum** curves around the **thalamus** to enclose it, except inferiorly. The **lateral ventricle** is superior to the thalamus. Posteriorly, the **tentorium cerebelli** forms a partition between the cerebrum and the cerebellum. The brainstem, consisting of the **midbrain, pons,** and **medulla oblongata,** extends inferiorly from the thalamus. A large **middle cerebellar peduncle** connects the cerebellum with the pons. The **hypophysis,** or **pituitary gland,** is located in the sella turcica of the sphenoid bone, and the **sphenoid sinuses** are anterior to the sella turcica. Midsagittal sections show the **nasal septum,** made up of the vomer and the perpendicular plate of the ethmoid bone.

In the region of the mouth, the **maxilla** forms the upper jaw, the **mandible** forms the lower jaw, and the **hard** and **soft palates** form the roof of the mouth. The **uvula** is the terminal portion of the soft palate. The largest structure in the mouth is the **tongue.** Inferior to the tongue, between it and the mandible, the **sublingual gland** is visible as a midline structure.

QUICK CHECK
5.32 In parasagittal sections through the temporomandibular joint, what opening is between the mandibular condyle and the mastoid process?
5.33 In parasagittal sections through the orbit, what gland appears inferior to the mandible?
5.34 In midsagittal sections, what space is located posterior to the nasal cavity?

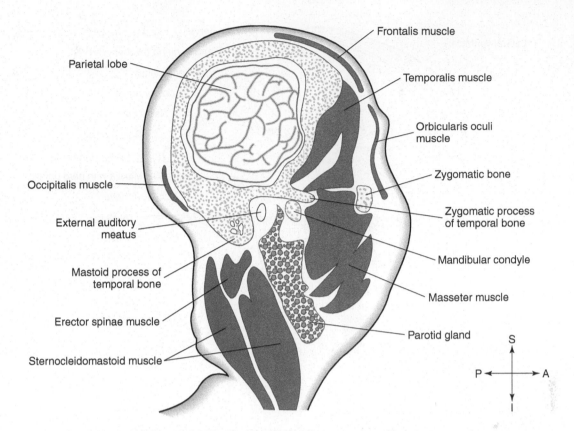

FIG. 5-42. Sagittal section through the temporomandibular joint.

FIG. 5-43. Sagittal section through the orbit.

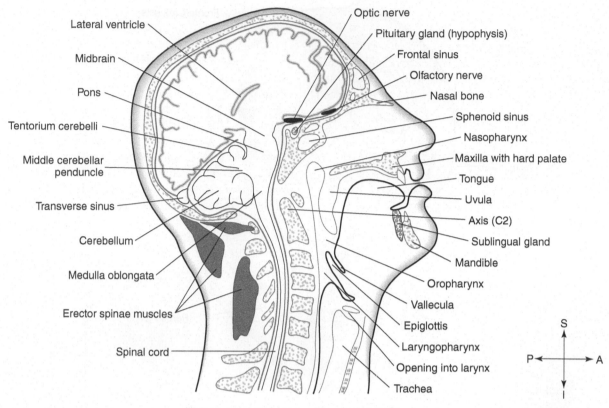

FIG. 5-44. Midsagittal section through the head.

Lateral ventricle
Midbrain
Pons
Tentorium cerebelli
Middle cerebellar peduncle
Transverse sinus
Cerebellum
Medulla oblongata
Erector spinae muscles
Spinal cord

Optic nerve
Pituitary gland (hypophysis)
Frontal sinus
Olfactory nerve
Nasal bone
Sphenoid sinus
Nasopharynx
Maxilla with hard palate
Tongue
Uvula
Axis (C2)
Sublingual gland
Mandible
Oropharynx
Vallecula
Epiglottis
Laryngopharynx
Opening into larynx
Trachea

FIG. 5-45. Midsagittal MR image of the brain.

Corpus callosum, body
Lateral ventricle
Corpus callosum, genu
Frontal lobe
Hypothalamus
Pituitary gland
Medulla oblongata

Parietal lobe
Thalamus
Corpus callosum, splenium
Occipital lobe
Pineal body
Superior cistern
Corpora quadrigemina
Cerebral aqueduct
Cerebral peduncle
Cerebellum
Fourth ventricle
Pons

Coronal Sections

Section Through the Third Ventricle and Brainstem. Fig. 5-46 illustrates a coronal section through the third ventricle and the brainstem. The two cerebral hemispheres are separated by the **longitudinal fissure,** which contains the **falx cerebri** and the **anterior cerebral arteries.** The **superior sagittal sinus** is in the superior margin of the falx cerebri. At the inferior margin of the falx cerebri, the **corpus callosum** forms a communicating band of white fibers between the two hemispheres. The two **lateral ventricles** are separated by a thin partition, the **septum pellucidum.** A region of gray matter, the **caudate nucleus,** forms the lateral portion of the floor of the lateral ventricle. Inferior to the lateral ventricles, in the midline, the **third ventricle** appears as a thin, slitlike opening, with the **thalamus** forming the wall on each side. Another region of gray matter, the **lentiform nucleus,** is lateral to the thalamus, between the thalamus and the **lateral sulcus.** The **cerebral peduncles** of the midbrain, easily identified by the small dark band of **substantia nigra,** extend inferiorly from the thalamus and third ventricle. The brainstem is completed by the **pons** and **medulla oblongata.** At the **foramen magnum,** between the occipital condyles, the medulla oblongata continues as the **spinal cord.** Large **middle cerebellar peduncles** form a connection between the cerebellar hemispheres and the pons. Fig. 5-46 shows the petrous and mastoid portions of the temporal bone. The **tentorium cerebelli** extends medially from the petrous ridge to form the dural partition between the cerebrum and the cerebellum. Sigmoid venous sinuses are associated with the petrous ridge. Fig. 5-47 is a coronal MR image slightly anterior to the illustration in Fig. 5-45 and shows lateral ventricles, the internal carotid artery, the optic chiasma, and other features in this region.

FIG. 5-46. Coronal section through the third ventricle and the brainstem.

FIG. 5-47. Coronal MR image through the ventricles.

Section Through the Orbit and Nasal Cavity. Fig. 5-48 illustrates a coronal section through the posterior portion of the orbit and the nasal cavity. This plane intersects the frontal lobes of the cerebral hemispheres, with the longitudinal fissure and the falx cerebri between them. Within the orbit, the **optic nerve** appears as a central structure with the extrinsic eye muscles and other nerves surrounding it. All are embedded in the orbital fat. The **bulbus oculi** is anterior to this plane and not visible. **Ethmoid sinuses** are medial to the orbits. Within the nasal cavity, the central structure is the thin **perpendicular plate of the ethmoid,** which forms the superior portion of the nasal septum. Three **nasal conchae** project medially from the lateral walls of the cavity. The superior and middle conchae are part of the ethmoid bone, but the inferior concha is a separate bone. A portion of the large **maxillary sinus** is lateral to the nasal cavity. The palate separates the nasal cavity from the oral cavity. Bones and muscle make up the framework of the sides of the face. Extending inferiorly from the temporal bone, the **temporalis muscle** inserts on the

medial side of the mandible. The **masseter muscle,** lateral to the mandible, originates on the zygomatic arch and maxilla and inserts on the mandible. The **submandibular gland** is near the inferior margin of the mandible. Fig. 5-49 is a coronal CT image through the nasal cavity. Compare this with the line drawing in Fig. 5-48.

QUICK CHECK
5.35   In coronal sections through the brainstem, what band of white fibers extends from the cerebellum to the pons?
5.36   In coronal sections through the third ventricle, what blood vessel appears in the lateral fissure?
5.37   In coronal sections through the orbit and nasal cavity, what is the muscle that appears lateral or external to the ramus of the mandible?
5.38   In coronal sections through the nasal cavity, what is the space between the middle nasal concha and the inferior nasal concha?

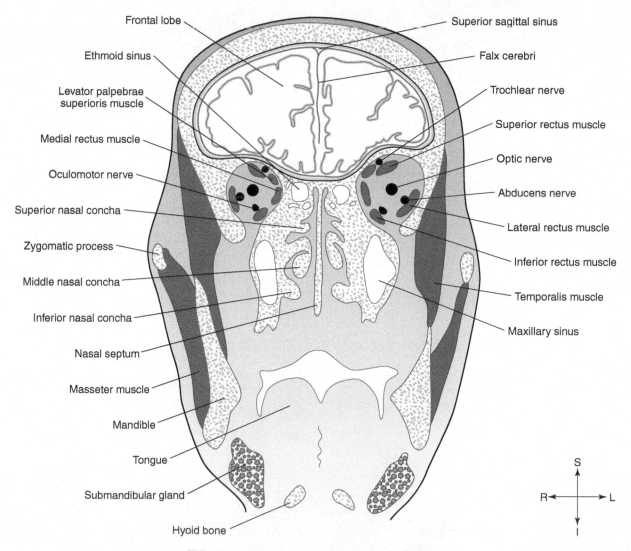

FIG. 5-48. Coronal section through the nasal cavity.

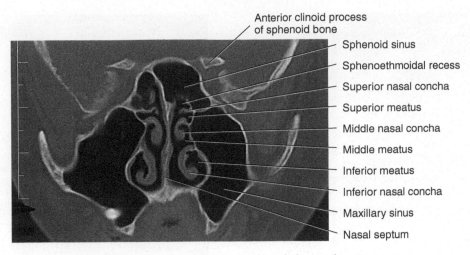

FIG. 5-49. Coronal CT image through the nasal cavity.

Working With Images of the Head

The axial CT image in Fig. 5-50 is through the superior portion of the cerebrum. It shows the two cerebral hemispheres separated by the falx cerebri. Gyri and sulci are clearly evident. The superior sagittal sinus is in the anterior and posterior margins of the falx cerebri.

The axial CT image in Fig. 5-51 is slightly inferior to the image in Fig. 5-50. It shows more of the cerebral hemispheres with gyri and sulci. Cerebrospinal fluid fills the sulci, because they are part of the subarachnoid space. The falx cerebri with the superior sagittal sinus in the margin separates the two hemispheres. The superior sagittal sinus is evident in the posterior margin of the falx cerebri.

The axial MR image in Fig. 5-52 shows the bodies of the two lateral ventricles. Anteriorly, the genu of the corpus callosum connects the two hemispheres. Two anterior cerebral arteries are present in the anterior por-

tion of the longitudinal fissure. The lateral sulcus with middle cerebral arteries is evident lateral to the insula on the left side. Posteriorly, the splenium of the corpus callosum connects the cerebral hemispheres. Some choroid plexus is evident in the ventricles.

The axial CT image in Fig. 5-53 is from a location similar to the MR image in Fig. 5-52. Notice how the two imaging modalities highlight different structures.

The axial MR image in Fig. 5-54 shows the third ventricle with the thalamus in its lateral walls. Anterior and posterior horns of the lateral ventricles are also present. The lateral fissure on each side delineates the insula. Anterior, middle, and posterior cerebral arteries are evident in the fissures.

The axial CT image in Fig. 5-55 shows the midline third ventricle and the diverging anterior horns of the lateral ventricles. The third ventricle is a narrow, midline slit with a thalamus on each side.

FIG. 5-50. Axial CT image through the superior portion of the cerebrum.

FIG. 5-51. Axial CT image through the cerebral hemispheres.

FIG. 5-52. Axial MR image through the lateral ventricles.

FIG. 5-54. Axial MR image through the third ventricle.

FIG. 5-53. Axial CT image through the lateral ventricles.

FIG. 5-55. Axial CT image through the third ventricle.

The axial MR image in Fig. 5-56 shows the midbrain in the center and the orbits of the eyes anteriorly. The midbrain includes the cerebral peduncles anteriorly and the corpora quadrigemina posteriorly. The cerebral aqueduct is a channel that passes through the midbrain as it proceeds from the third ventricle to the fourth ventricle. The interpeduncular cistern is between the two cerebral peduncles, and the corpora quadrigemina project into the superior cistern. Anteriorly, the orbits show the bulbus oculi, optic nerve, lateral and medial rectus muscles, and orbital fat. The temporalis muscle is lateral (superficial) to the temporal bone.

The axial MR image in Fig. 5-57 shows the pons with the basilar artery anterior to it, in the pontine cistern. The internal carotid arteries are present on either side of the sella turcica. A portion of the cerebellum is posterior to the pons and is separated from the cerebrum by the tentorium cerebelli. Anteriorly, ethmoid and sphenoid sinuses are present.

The axial CT image in Fig. 5-58 is similar to the MR image in Fig. 5-57, and many of the same structure are present. In this image, the fourth ventricle is a little larger, and the superior cerebellar peduncles are along the margin of the ventricle. The petrous ridge is on the left, with the sigmoid sinus along its wall.

FIG. 5-56. Axial MR image through the midbrain.

FIG. 5-58. Axial CT image through the pons.

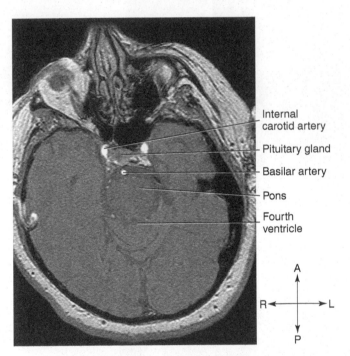

FIG. 5-57. Axial MR image through the pons.

FIG. 5-59. Axial CT image showing the circulus arteriosus cerebri (circle of Willis).

The axial CT image in Fig. 5-59 shows the contrast-enhanced vessels of the circulus arteriosus cerebri (circle of Willis). The arteries present that should be identified are the posterior cerebral, internal carotid, middle cerebral, anterior cerebral, and anterior communicating arteries.

The axial CT image in Fig. 5-60 shows the condyle of the mandible in the mandibular fossa of the temporal bone. The zygomatic arch is anterior to the joint, and the external auditory meatus is posterior to it. Mastoid air cells are posterior to the external auditory meatus. The portions of the brain that are present are the medulla oblongata and the cerebellum.

The temporalis muscle occupies the space medial to the zygomatic arch. Sphenoid, ethmoid, and maxillary sinuses are evident in the anterior portion of the image.

The axial CT image in Fig. 5-61 is at the C1 vertebral level. It shows the transverse foramina that are typical of cervical vertebrae. The odontoid process of C2 projects into C1. The ramus of the mandible is evident on both sides, with the masseter muscle lateral to the ramus and the temporalis muscle medial to it. The tiny styloid process is between the ramus and the atlas. The space in the center of the image is the nasopharynx. The nasal septum is in the center of the nasal cavity, with inferior nasal conchae on each side. Large maxillary sinuses are lateral to the nasal cavity.

The axial CT image in Fig. 5-62 shows the classic arrangement of the carotid and jugular vessels. The left internal carotid artery is anterior to the left internal jugular vein. The external carotid artery is lateral to the internal carotid artery. The external jugular vein is lateral to the

FIG. 5-60. Axial CT image through the temporomandibular joint.

- Maxillary sinus
- Mandibular condyle
- External auditory meatus

internal jugular vein, and the external carotid artery is anterior to the external jugular vein.

The axial CT image in Fig. 5-63 is near the same level as the image in Fig. 5-61, but this one has contrast to highlight the vasculature, and the muscles are more obvious. Pharyngeal constrictor muscles form the wall of the nasopharynx. Lateral and medial pterygoid muscles are evident lateral and medial to the pterygoid plate of the sphenoid bone. The masseter is lateral to the ramus of the mandible, and the temporalis inserts on the medial surface. Vertebral vessels are clearly evident in the transverse foramina of C1. Anterolateral to the vertebra, the internal carotid artery is anterior to the internal jugular vein, and the external vessels are lateral to the internal with the external carotid artery anterior to the external jugular vein. This is the same arrangement evident in Fig. 5-62.

The sagittal CT image in Fig. 5-64 clearly shows the anterior-to-posterior sequence of the temporomandibular joint, external auditory meatus, and mastoid. The ramus

FIG. 5-61. Axial CT image through the C1 vertebral level.

- Temporalis muscle
- Styloid process
- C1 vertebra

FIG. 5-63. Axial CT image through the C1 vertebral level with contrast to highlight the vasculature.

- Temporalis muscle
- Medial pterygoid muscle
- Pharyngeal constrictor muscle
- External carotid artery
- External jugular vein

FIG. 5-62. Axial CT image highlighting the relationships of the carotid arteries and jugular veins.

- External carotid artery
- Internal carotid artery
- External jugular vein
- Internal jugular vein

FIG. 5-64. Sagittal CT image through the temporomandibular joint.

- External auditory meatus
- Mastoid
- Mandibular condyle

FIG. 5-65. Coronal CT image through the nasal cavity.

and coronoid process of the mandible are evident, and a frontal sinus appears in the frontal bone.

The coronal CT image in Fig. 5-65 shows the nasal cavity and bulbus oculi. In the nasal cavity, the central structure is the perpendicular plate of the ethmoid, which forms the nasal septum. Three nasal conchae project medially from the lateral walls of the cavity. The superior and middle conchae are part of the ethmoid bone, but the inferior concha is a separate bone. The superior meatus is between the superior and middle conchae, the middle meatus is between the middle and inferior conchae, and the inferior meatus is below the inferior concha. The small space above the superior nasal concha is the sphenoethmoidal recess. A portion of the maxillary sinus is lateral to the nasal cavity. In the orbit, the optic nerve appears as a central structure with the superior, inferior, lateral, and medial rectus muscles surrounding it. All are embedded in the orbital fat. The temporalis muscle extends inferiorly from the temporal bone and inserts on the medial side of the mandible.

Important Anatomical Relationships in the Head

- The caudate nucleus basically follows the shape of the lateral ventricle. It is in the floor of the anterior horns and body of the lateral ventricle and in the roof of the inferior horns (see Figs. 5-10 and 5-28).
- The thalamus forms the lateral wall of the third ventricle (see Figs. 5-10 and 5-30).
- The third ventricle is a single, midline structure (see Figs. 5-10 and 5-30).
- The internal capsule is a band of white fibers that separates the caudate nucleus and thalamus medially from the lentiform nucleus laterally (see Figs. 5-10 and 5-30).
- The corpus callosum is a large band of white fibers that connects the two cerebral hemispheres (see Figs. 5-10, 5-13, and 5-29).
- The midbrain surrounds the cerebral aqueduct and consists of the cerebral peduncles anteriorly and the corpora quadrigemina posteriorly (see Figs. 5-34 and 5-35).
- The superior sagittal sinus is in the superior margin of the falx cerebri (see Figs. 5-15, 5-28, and 5-46).
- The inferior sagittal sinus is in the inferior margin of the falx cerebri (see Figs. 5-21 and 5-28).
- The tentorium cerebelli forms a partition between the cerebrum and cerebellum (see Figs. 5-34, 5-43, and 5-44).
- The straight sinus is in the junction between the tentorium cerebelli and the falx cerebri (see Figs. 5-12, 5-32, and 5-34).
- The corpora quadrigemina and pineal body project into the superior cistern (see Figs. 5-12, 5-32, and 5-35).
- The transverse sinus courses laterally along the internal surface of the occipital bone (see Figs. 5-21 and 5-44).
- The fourth ventricle is at the level of the pons and cerebellum (see Figs. 5-13, 5-14, and 5-36).
- Cerebellar peduncles connect the cerebellum with other parts of the central nervous system (see Figs. 5-36, 5-37, and 5-44).
- Sphenoid sinuses are anterior to the hypophysis (see Figs. 5-36, 5-37, and 5-44).
- The internal carotid arteries go through the cavernous sinus, which is lateral to the hypophysis (see Figs. 5-36 and 5-37).
- The basilar artery is in the pontine cistern anterior to the pons (see Figs. 5-36 and 5-37).
- The sigmoid sinus is related to the petrous ridge (see Figs. 5-39 and 5-43).
- The sigmoid sinus drains into the internal jugular vein (see Fig. 5-21).
- The internal carotid arteries are anterior and medial to the internal jugular veins in superior regions of the neck because the carotid canal is anterior to the jugular foramen (see Fig. 5-39 and 5-41).
- The masseter muscle is lateral to the ramus of the mandible, and the temporalis is medial to the ramus (see Figs. 5-40 and 5-41).
- The parotid gland is posterior to the ramus of the mandible, anterior to the mastoid, and lateral to the internal jugular vein and internal carotid artery (see Fig. 5-42).

Pathology

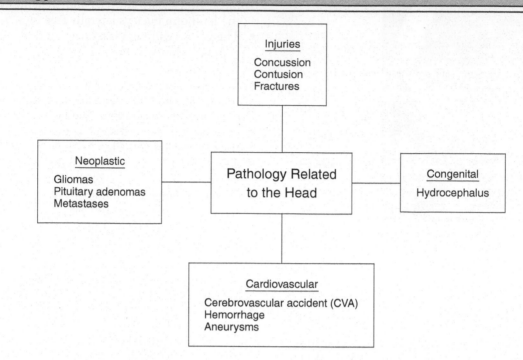

Concussion

A concussion results from a blow to the head that causes the brain to shift within the cranial vault and hit the cranial wall. Signs and symptoms include a short-term loss of consciousness following the injury, severe headache, nausea, and vertigo. This type of injury is common in automobile, motorcycle, and bicycle accidents, child abuse, and falls in the home.

Contusion

A contusion is injury to the brain tissue. It is a bruise of the brain, possibly accompanied by a collection of blood (hematoma) in the epidural or subdural space. This is more severe than a concussion and usually occurs as a result of direct impact by a blunt object, often in automobile accidents and violent acts.

Fractures

Fractures of the bones of the skull are often accompanied by damage to brain tissue, such as concussion or contusion. Skull fractures are of additional concern when they cross an artery because the vessel may tear, resulting in an epidural hematoma. Because bleeding from an artery is usually rapid, intracranial pressure increases quickly. If the fracture enters the mastoid air cells or a sinus, there is the danger that an infection from these areas may potentially spread throughout the cranial vault and possibly result in encephalitis or meningitis.

Hydrocephalus

Hydrocephalus is excessive accumulation of cerebrospinal fluid (CSF) in the ventricles of the brain (internal hydrocephalus), in the subarachnoid space (external hydrocephalus), or in both locations. Noncommunicating hydrocephalus is caused by an obstruction in the channels between the ventricles. Communicating hydrocephalus results when there is diminished resorption of cerebrospinal fluid by the arachnoid villi. The accumulation of cerebrospinal fluid leads to ventricular enlargement, compression of brain tissue, and increased intracranial pressure.

Cerebrovascular Accident (CVA or Stroke)

A cerebrovascular accident is sudden interruption of cerebral circulation. The loss of cerebral circulation results in a diminished supply of oxygen (ischemia) and leads to an area of necrosis in brain tissue. This area is referred to as an infarct. There are two major causes of a cerebrovascular accident. The most common is the blockage of a blood vessel, either by a thrombus (more common) or an embolus. The second, more serious cause, is cerebral hemorrhage. The precipitating cause is usually chronic hypertension or an aneurysm that weakens the vessel wall. Symptoms depend on the arteries involved. The internal carotid, anterior cerebral, middle cerebral, vertebral, and basilar arteries are most commonly affected.

Hemorrhage

Hemorrhage is the escape of blood from a ruptured vessel. A ruptured or torn artery bleeds faster than a vein because of the higher pressure in the arterial system. There are four primary types of hemorrhage. **Epidural** hemorrhage is external to the dura mater and usually is in the temporal region as a result of rupture of the middle meningeal artery. **Subdural** hemorrhage is between the dura mater and arachnoid and usually is the result of slow venous leakage. **Subarachnoid** hemorrhage occurs between the arachnoid and pia mater, often as the result of a ruptured berry aneurysm. The intersections, or junctions, along the circle of Willis are vulnerable locations for berry aneurysms. **Intracerebral** hemorrhage occurs within the brain, often with the bleeding originating from a hemangioma that develops as a result of chronic hypertension. With all types of hemorrhage, the surrounding brain tissue is usually swollen and edematous.

Pathology—cont'd

Aneurysm

An aneurysm is a sac formed by a localized dilation of a vessel wall, usually an artery. It is caused by a weakness in the vessel wall. Most aneurysms enlarge with time and become increasingly susceptible to rupture with subsequent hemorrhage. Cerebral aneurysms are most often associated with the circle of Willis.

Glioma

A glioma is a primary tumor of the brain that is composed of neuroglia. Approximately one half of all primary brain tumors are gliomas of some type, such as glioblastomas (most common), astrocytomas, oligodendrogliomas, and ependymomas. Often the location of the tumor is just as important as the malignancy of the tumor. Any tumor, whether benign or malignant, primary or metastatic, usually causes an increase in intracranial

pressure resulting in headaches, vomiting, and blurred vision. Seizures may occur as a result of the presence of a tumor.

Pituitary Adenoma

Pituitary adenomas are tumors of the pituitary gland. These tumors grow out of the sella turcica and usually are benign, slow growing, and well encapsulated. These features contribute to a high rate of cure with surgery and irradiation. Symptoms of pituitary adenomas include headaches and, if the tumor compresses the optic chiasm, visual disturbances.

Metastatic Tumors

Metastases of tumors from other sites may invade any intracranial structure. Usually the metastases arise from lung carcinoma, adenocarcinoma of the breast, or malignant melanoma.

Summary

- The 8 bones of the cranium are the frontal (1), parietal (2), temporal (2), occipital (1), ethmoid (1), and zygomatic (1).
- The 14 bones of the face are the maxillae (2), palatine (2), zygomatic (2), nasal (2), lacrimal (2), vomer (1), inferior nasal conchae (2), and mandible (1).
- The four types of paranasal sinuses are the frontal, maxillary, sphenoidal, and ethmoidal sinuses.
- All muscles of facial expression are innervated by the facial nerve (VII) and insert on the skin of the face. These muscles include the frontalis, orbicularis oculi, orbicularis oris, buccinator, and platysma.
- The muscles of mastication are innervated by the mandibular division of the trigeminal nerve (V) and insert on the mandible. These muscles are the masseter, temporalis, lateral pterygoid, and medial pterygoid.
- The parotid gland is the largest salivary gland. It is wedged between the ramus of the mandible and the mastoid portion of the temporal bone.
- The submandibular gland is located medial to the body and the angle of the mandible.
- The sublingual gland is the smallest salivary gland and is located in the floor of the mouth adjacent to the lingual frenulum.
- Each cerebral hemisphere is divided into five lobes: frontal, parietal, occipital, temporal, and insula.
- Basal ganglia are regions of gray matter scattered throughout the cerebral white matter. The basal ganglia include the caudate nucleus, lentiform nucleus, and claustrum.
- The diencephalon is centrally located and surrounded by the cerebral hemispheres. It consists of the epithalamus, thalamus, and hypothalamus.
- The brainstem is subdivided into the midbrain, pons, and medulla oblongata. The midbrain is further divided into the cerebral peduncles and corpora quadrigemina.

- The cerebellum is located posterior to the brainstem. It has two hemispheres, which are connected by the vermis. Gray matter surrounds the branching white matter, called *arbor vitae*.
- Cerebrospinal fluid (CSF) is produced by the choroid plexus in the ventricles. From the lateral ventricles, the CSF flows through the short interventricular foramen into the third ventricle, then through the cerebral aqueduct into the fourth ventricle. From the fourth ventricle, the CSF enters the subarachnoid space through median and lateral apertures.
- Dura mater is the tough outer layer of meninges. The middle layer is the thin, delicate arachnoid. The innermost layer, which is intimately adherent to the cerebral cortex, is the thin, highly vascular pia mater.
- Six subarachnoid cisterns are the cerebellomedullary, pontine, interpeduncular, and chiasmatic cisterns, the cistern of the lateral sulcus, and the cisterna ambiens.
- The cerebellomedullary cistern is between the medulla oblongata and the cerebellum. It receives CSF from the fourth ventricle through the foramen of Magendie.
- The pontine cistern is ventral to the pons and contains the basilar artery. The cistern of the lateral sulcus contains the middle cerebral artery. The circle of Willis is in the interpeduncular cistern, the optic chiasma is in the chiasmatic cistern, and the great cerebral vein is in the cisterna ambiens.
- Arterial blood supply to the brain is from the two internal carotid arteries and the two vertebral arteries.
- Venous sinuses that return blood to the internal jugular vein are the superior sagittal sinus, inferior sagittal sinus, straight sinus, transverse sinus, and sigmoid sinus.
- Cranial nerves are designated by name and Roman numerals: olfactory (I), optic (II), oculomotor (III), trochlear (IV), trigeminal (V), abducens (VI), facial (VII),

vestibulocochlear (VIII), glossopharyngeal (IX), vagus (X), accessory (XI), and hypoglossal (XII).

- The bulbus oculi is made up of three tunics. The sclera and cornea form the outer fibrous tunic. In the middle, the choroid, ciliary body, and iris form the vascular tunic. The innermost layer is the retina, or nervous tunic; this layer contains the photoreceptors for vision.

- Six extrinsic muscles are associated with eye movements: the superior oblique, inferior oblique, superior rectus, inferior rectus, lateral rectus, and medial rectus muscles.
- Most of the vascular supply to the orbit is from the ophthalmic artery.
- Protective features of the eye include the eyelids and the lacrimal apparatus, which produces tears.

• REVIEW QUESTIONS •

1. Indicate whether each of the following is a bone of the face or a bone of the cranium:
   a. Maxilla
   b. Frontal
   c. Ethmoid
   d. Temporal
   e. Zygomatic
2. What nerve innervates the muscles of facial expression?
3. On what bone do all of the muscles of mastication insert?
4. What salivary glands are medial to the angle of the mandible?
5. Where are the basal ganglia located?
6. What is the largest portion of the diencephalon?
7. Name the three parts of the brainstem.
8. Where are the ventricles located:
   a. Lateral ventricles
   b. Third ventricle
   c. Fourth ventricle
9. Between which layers of meninges are the subarachnoid cisterns located?
10. Name six subarachnoid cisterns.
11. What are the two pairs of arteries that supply blood to the brain?
12. What venous structures collect blood and cerebrospinal fluid from the brain and return it to the internal jugular vein?
13. Name the three cranial nerves that are primarily sensory in function.
14. Name the three tunics, or coats, in the wall of the bulbus oculi.
15. What is contained in the anterior and posterior cavities of the eye, and what separates the two cavities?

• CHAPTER QUIZ •

Name the Following:

1. The largest of the paranasal sinuses
2. The bone that has a mastoid process, spinous process, and external auditory meatus
3. The muscle of mastication that is superficial to the ramus of the mandible
4. The salivary gland between the ramus of the mandible and the mastoid process
5. The component of the basal ganglia that is closely associated with the lateral ventricles
6. The portion of the diencephalon that forms the lateral walls of the third ventricle
7. The passageway between the third and fourth ventricles
8. The largest of the subarachnoid cisterns
9. The venous sinus that empties into the internal jugular vein
10. The anterior portion of the fibrous tunic of the eye

True/False:

1. The sphenoid bone is a facial bone.
2. The falx cerebri is an extension of the arachnoid that is found in the longitudinal fissure.
3. The tentorium cerebelli is between the cerebrum and the cerebellum.
4. The internal capsule is a band of white matter between the globus pallidus and the putamen.
5. The cerebrospinal fluid is located in the subarachnoid space between the arachnoid and the dura mater.
6. The two vertebral arteries join to form the basilar artery, which passes over the midbrain.
7. The longitudinal sulcus (fissure) separates the frontal lobe from the parietal lobe.
8. The cavernous sinus contains the internal jugular vein.
9. The venous sinus that follows along the tentorium cerebelli from the inferior sagittal sinus to the confluence of sinuses is the straight sinus.
10. The lacrimal gland for the production of tears is located in the superior and medial margin of the orbit.

Answers to the Review Questions and Chapter Quiz questions can be found at http://evolve.elsevier.com/Applegate/SAlearning/

The Vertebral Column, Spinal Cord, and Neck

6

OBJECTIVES

Upon completion of this chapter, the student should be able to do the following:
- Describe the general structure of vertebrae and identify the structural components on a diagram.
- State the characteristics that distinguish cervical vertebrae from other types.
- Distinguish the first two cervical vertebrae from other cervical vertebrae and state their specific names.
- Identify the characteristic features that distinguish thoracic vertebrae from other vertebrae.
- Identify the characteristic features that distinguish lumbar vertebrae from other vertebrae.
- Describe the structural features of the sacrum and coccyx.
- Discuss the composition and purpose of intervertebral discs.
- Identify the curvatures of the vertebral column and state the direction of the curvatures.
- Identify three types of abnormal curvatures of the vertebral column.
- Describe and state the location of the following ligaments associated with the vertebral column: anterior and posterior longitudinal ligaments, ligamenta flava, interspinous ligaments, supraspinous ligaments, ligamentum nuchae, and intertransverse ligaments.
- Identify the muscles in the superficial, intermediate, and deep layers of the intrinsic back muscles.
- Describe the meninges of the spinal cord.
- Identify the structural features of the spinal cord in longitudinal and cross-sectional views.
- Name the five groups of spinal nerves and state the number of nerves in each group.
- Distinguish between dorsal and ventral nerve roots and state the components of each.
- Describe the location, components, and functions of the four major nerve plexuses and name the principal nerves that emerge from each plexus.
- Describe the vasculature of the spinal cord.
- Identify the margins of the anterior and posterior triangles of the neck and name the principal components in each triangle.
- Identify the regions of the pharynx by describing the location and features of each region.
- Describe the features of the larynx.
- Discuss the relationships of the esophagus and trachea as they descend through the neck.
- Describe the location of the thyroid and parathyroid glands relative to the trachea.

- Discuss the relationships of the internal jugular vein to other vessels and anatomical structures as it descends from the jugular foramen to the brachiocephalic vein.
- Describe the pathways and relationships of the common carotid, external carotid, and internal carotid arteries.
- State the origin and pathway of the vertebral arteries.
- Explain what is meant by the term *sympathetic trunk* and describe its location.
- Name one cranial nerve located in the neck.
- Identify the nerve plexus located in the neck and name one nerve that emerges from this plexus.
- Describe the composition and location of the brachial plexus and name the region innervated by the nerves that emerge from this plexus.
- Identify the features of the neck, including vertebrae, muscles, viscera, and blood vessels, in transverse and midsagittal sections.

Key Terms, Structures, and Features to Be Identified and/or Described

Anterior and posterior longitudinal ligaments
Anterior scalene muscle
Anterior triangle
Anulus fibrosus
Atlas
Axis
Brachial plexus
Carotid sheath
Carotid sinus
Cauda equina
Central canal
Centrum
Cervical curvature
Cervical enlargement
Cervical nerves
Cervical plexus
Cervical vertebrae
Coccygeal nerve
Coccyx
Columns of white matter in spinal cord
Common carotid artery
Conus medullaris
Costal facets
Cricoid cartilage
Dens
Dorsal (posterior) median sulcus
Dorsal root
Dorsal root ganglion
Epiglottis
Erector spinae muscles
Esophagus
External carotid artery
External jugular vein
Filum terminale
Gray commissure

Horns of gray matter in spinal cord
Hypopharynx
Internal carotid artery
Internal jugular vein
Intervertebral discs
Intervertebral foramina
Lamina
Larynx
Levator costarum muscle
Levator scapulae muscle
Ligamenta flava
Ligamentum nuchae
Lumbar curvature
Lumbar nerves
Lumbar plexus
Lumbar vertebrae
Lumbosacral enlargement
Mandible
Masseter muscle
Meninges
Middle scalene muscle
Nasopharynx
Nerve plexus
Nerve tracts
Nucleus pulposus
Odontoid process
Oropharynx
Parathyroid glands
Parotid gland
Pedicle
Pharyngeal constrictor muscle
Pharynx
Posterior scalene muscle
Posterior triangle
Prevertebral muscles
Pterygoid muscle

Retropharyngeal space
Rima glottidis
Sacral curvature
Sacral foramina
Sacral hiatus
Sacral nerves
Sacral plexus
Sacral promontory
Sacroiliac joints
Sacrum
Scapula
Spinal arteries
Spinal nerves
Spinous process
Sternocleidomastoid muscle
Sublingual gland
Submandibular gland
Superior and inferior articular processes
Thoracic curvature
Thoracic nerves
Thoracic vertebrae
Thyroid cartilage
Thyroid gland
Tonsils
Trachea
Transverse foramina
Transverse processes
Trapezius muscle
Uvula
Vagus nerve
Ventral (anterior) median fissure
Ventral root
Vertebral arch
R & L vertebral arteries
Vertebral foramen
Vertebral notch

Anatomical Review of the Vertebral Column

The vertebral column is a bony structure composed of individual vertebrae and the fibrocartilaginous pads, called *intervertebral discs*, that are between the vertebrae. The column supports the body weight, helps to maintain posture, and protects the spinal cord.

Structure of the Vertebrae

General Structure. All vertebrae have a common structural pattern (Fig. 6-1), although variations exist between them. The thick, anterior, weight-bearing portion of a vertebra is the **body,** or **centrum.** The posterior, curved portion is the **vertebral arch.** Together, the body and vertebral arch surround a central opening, the **vertebral foramen.** When the vertebrae are stacked together, the vertebral foramina make a vertebral canal, which contains and protects the spinal cord. The vertebral arch is formed by the transverse processes, the spinous process, the pedicles, the laminae, and the superior and inferior articular processes. **Transverse processes** project laterally from the vertebral arch, and the **spinous process** is in the posterior midline. These processes are places for muscle attachment. The spinous processes can be felt as bony projections along the midline of the back. The portion of the vertebral arch adjacent to the body, between the body and the transverse process, is the **pedicle.** A concave surface on the upper and lower margins of the pedicles is called the **vertebral notch.** When the superior and inferior vertebral notches of adjacent vertebrae meet, they form **intervertebral foramina,** which transmit **spinal nerves** and blood vessels. The portion between the transverse process and the spinous process is the **lamina. Superior** and **inferior articular processes** project superiorly and inferiorly, respectively, from the vertebral arch. The superior articular process of one vertebra articulates with the inferior articular process of the preceding vertebra in the column. Fig. 6-2 is a radiograph of cervical vertebrae that demonstrates some of these features.

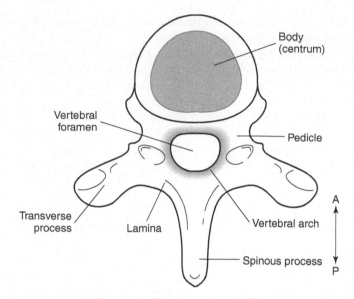

FIG. 6-1. General features of vertebrae.

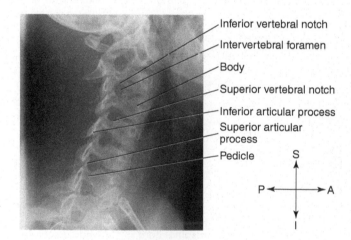

FIG. 6-2. Radiograph of cervical vertebrae.

FIG. 6-3. Cervical vertebra.

QUICK CHECK

6.1   Together the centrum and the vertebral arch surround an opening. What is the name of this opening?

6.2   What opening is formed by the superior and inferior notches of adjacent vertebrae?

Cervical Vertebrae. The seven **cervical vertebrae** are designated C1 through C7. In general, the cervical vertebrae (Figs. 6-3 and 6-4) can be distinguished from other vertebrae because the cervicals have **transverse foramina** in the transverse processes. The foramina allow passage of the vertebral arteries as they ascend through the neck to the brain. Also, the spinous processes of cervical vertebrae are forked, or bifid. The exception to this is the seventh

cervical vertebra (C7), which has a long spinous process that typically is not bifid. The C7 spinous process is easily palpable at the base of the neck.

The first two cervical vertebrae are modified and have no disc between them. The **atlas** (C1), shown in Figs. 6-5 and 6-6, has no body and no spinous process, and it has

FIG. 6-4. Transverse CT image of a cervical vertebra.

FIG. 6-5. Atlas (C1).

FIG. 6-7. Axis (C2).

short transverse processes. It is a ring that consists of an anterior arch, a posterior arch, and two large lateral masses that have large articular facets. The superior facets articulate with the occipital condyles on the occipital bone, and the inferior facets articulate with the vertebra below. The **axis** (C2), shown in Figs. 6-7 to 6-9, has a **dens,** or **odontoid process,** that projects upward from the vertebral body like a tooth. The odontoid process acts as a pivot for rotation of the atlas.

Thoracic Vertebrae. The 12 **thoracic vertebrae** are designated T1 through T12. These can be distinguished from other vertebrae by the **costal facets,** located on the

bodies and transverse processes, for articulation with the ribs. The head of the rib articulates with the vertebral body, and the tubercle of the rib articulates with the transverse process. They also have long, pointed spinous processes. These features are illustrated in Fig. 6-10. The axial CT image in Fig. 6-11 shows the articulations of a thoracic vertebra with ribs. The sagittal CT image in Fig. 6-12 shows the long, pointed spinous processes that are typical of thoracic vertebrae.

Lumbar Vertebrae. The five **lumbar vertebrae,** designated L1 through L5, make up the part of the vertebral column in the small of the back. The lumbar vertebrae (Figs. 6-13 and 6-14) have large, heavy bodies because they support most of the body weight and have many back muscles attached to them. They also have short, blunt spinous processes. The sagittal MR image in Fig. 6-15 shows the thick, heavy bodies of the lumbar vertebrae and the intervertebral discs between the vertebrae.

Sacrum and Coccyx. The sacral region of the vertebral column (Fig. 6-16) consists of five vertebrae that fuse to form the **sacrum.** The transverse processes of the

FIG. 6-6. Transverse CT image of C1 with odontoid process of C2.

Odontoid process
of C2

C1

C2

S

R←——→L

I

FIG. 6-8. Coronal CT image of C2.

Odontoid process
of C2

Anterior arch
of C1

S

A←——→P

I

FIG. 6-9. Sagittal CT image of C2.

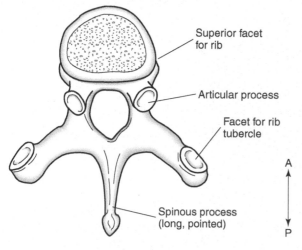

Superior facet
for rib

Articular process

Facet for rib
tubercle

Spinous process
(long, pointed)

A

P

FIG. 6-10. Thoracic vertebra.

Body of vertebra

Rib

Transverse
process

Spinal
cord

Spinous
process

A

R←——→L

P

FIG. 6-11. Axial CT image of a thoracic vertebra showing articulations with ribs.

FIG. 6-12. Sagittal CT image of thoracic vertebrae showing their long, pointed spinous processes.

FIG. 6-15. Sagittal MR image of the lumbar vertebrae. (Modified from Weir J, Abrahams PH: *Imaging atlas of human anatomy,* ed 3, St Louis, 2003, Elsevier/Mosby.)

FIG. 6-13. Lumbar vertebra.

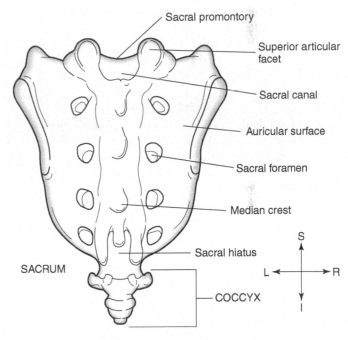

FIG. 6-16. Sacrum and coccyx.

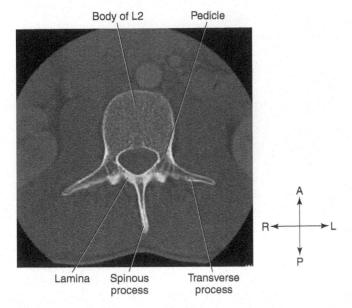

FIG. 6-14. Axial CT image of lumbar vertebra. (From Kelley LL, Petersen CM: *Sectional anatomy for imaging professionals,* ed 2, St Louis, 2007, Elsevier/Mosby.)

vertebrae fuse to form the **lateral masses (alae),** which articulate with the pelvic girdle laterally at the **sacroiliac joints.** Within the lateral masses, **sacral foramina** allow for passage of nerves. The first sacral segment has a prominent ridge, called the **sacral promontory,** on the visceral surface. The region inferior to this landmark is the true pelvic cavity. The spinous process of the S5 segment is absent, leaving an opening called the **sacral hiatus.** The coronal CT image in Fig. 6-17 shows these features.

FIG. 6-17. Coronal CT image of the sacrum and coccyx. (From Kelley LL, Petersen CM: *Sectional anatomy for imaging professionals,* ed 2, St Louis, 2007, Elsevier/Mosby.)

The **coccyx,** or tailbone, is the most inferior region of the vertebral column. The child has four separate small bones (the number can vary from three to five), which fuse to form a single bone in the adult. Several muscles have some point of attachment on the coccyx. The CT reconstruction in Fig. 6-18 shows features of the sacrum and coccyx.

QUICK CHECK

6.3 What feature distinguishes cervical vertebrae from all other types of vertebrae?

6.4 What is the primary distinguishing feature of thoracic vertebrae?

6.5 Where do the fused transverse processes of the sacral vertebrae articulate with the appendicular skeleton?

Intervertebral Discs

The **intervertebral discs,** located between the vertebral bodies, are fibrocartilaginous pads classified as symphysis joints; they are designed for strength. In addition to the discs, the vertebral bodies are joined by ligaments. Each disc consists of a soft central core, called the **nucleus pulposus,** and a firm outer ring, called the **anulus fibrosus.** Fig. 6-19 illustrates an intervertebral disc. The sagittal MR image in Fig. 6-20 shows lumbar vertebrae with intervertebral discs. The nucleus pulposus acts as a shock absorber and as a ball bearing during flexion, extension, and lateral bending of the vertebral column. The anulus fibrosus is composed of rings of fibrocartilage that run obliquely from one vertebra to another to form strong bonds between the vertebrae. The intervertebral discs are thickest in the cervical and lumbar regions, which provides greater flexibility in these regions. As people get older, the nucleus pulposus may become thinner. This

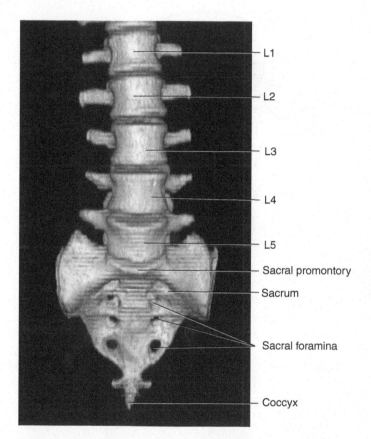

FIG. 6-18. CT reconstruction of the lumbar spine. (From Kelley LL, Petersen CM: *Sectional anatomy for imaging professionals,* ed 2, St Louis, 2007, Elsevier/Mosby.)

accounts for some of the loss of height that occurs as a result of aging. Changes also may occur in the anulus fibrosus that permit the nucleus pulposus to protrude through the outer ring; this is called a *herniated disc* (Fig. 6-21). The protrusion may compress an adjacent spinal nerve and cause pain in the lower back and/or leg.

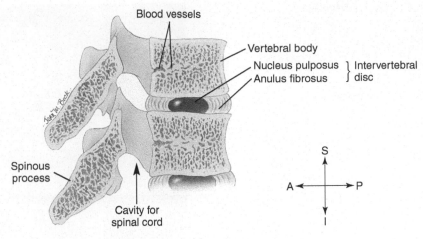

FIG. 6-19. Intervertebral disc. (Modified from Thibodeau GA, Patton KT: *Anatomy & physiology,* ed 6, St Louis, 2007, Elsevier/Mosby.)

FIG. 6-20. Sagittal MR image of intervertebral discs. (Modified from Weir J, Abrahams PH: *Imaging atlas of human anatomy,* ed 3, St Louis, 2003, Elsevier/Mosby.)

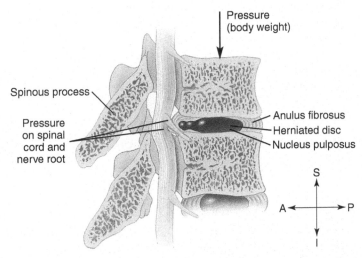

FIG. 6-21. Herniated disc. (Modified from Thibodeau GA, Patton KT: *Anatomy & physiology,* ed 6, St Louis, 2007, Elsevier/Mosby.)

Curvatures of the Vertebral Column

Normally, when viewed from the side (Fig. 6-22), the vertebral column has four curvatures. These curvatures increase the strength, resilience, and flexibility of the vertebral column. The **thoracic curvature** and the **sacral curvature** are concave anteriorly (convex posteriorly) and are present at birth. The cervical and lumbar curvatures are convex anteriorly (concave posteriorly). The **cervical curvature** develops when the baby holds its head erect, and the **lumbar curvature** develops when the child begins to stand. Fig. 6-23 is a radiograph of the lumbar spine that shows the anteriorly convex curvature. Several types of abnormal variations occur in the curvatures of the vertebral column. Some of these are congenital, whereas others may be due to poor posture, disease, or unequal muscle pull on the column. **Scoliosis** is an abnormal lateral curvature that most commonly occurs in the thoracic region. If left untreated, it may become severe and result in breathing difficulties. **Kyphosis** is an exaggerated dorsal curvature in the thoracic region. It is frequently seen in older individuals as a result of osteoporosis. It also may be due to a bone deformity known as rickets. **Lordosis** is an exaggerated lumbar curvature. This may occur temporarily in pregnant women when they throw back their shoulders and accentuate the lumbar curvature in an attempt to maintain their center of gravity. Fig. 6-24 illustrates abnormal spinal curvatures.

QUICK CHECK

6.6 What is the central core of an intervertebral disc called?

6.7 In what regions of the vertebral column are the intervertebral discs the thickest?

6.8 What two curvatures of the vertebral column are normally present at birth?

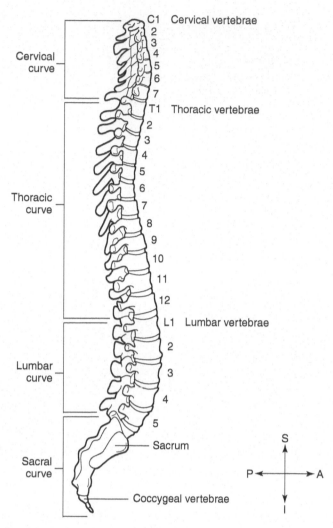

FIG. 6-22. Curvatures of the vertebral column.

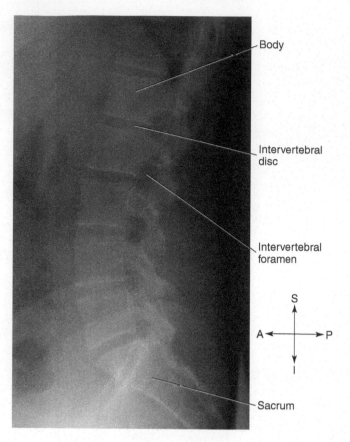

FIG. 6-23. Radiograph of the lumbar curvature.

Ligaments of the Vertebral Column

The vertebral column is held in place by straplike ligaments. The major supporting ligaments are the **anterior** and **posterior longitudinal ligaments.** The anterior longitudinal ligament begins at C1 and extends downward along the entire anterior surface of the vertebral bodies to the sacrum. It is strongly attached to the bony vertebral bodies and to the discs to maintain stability of the joints and to prevent hyperextension (bending too far backward). The posterior longitudinal ligament is a narrow ligamentous band that runs inside the vertebral canal, along the posterior surface of the vertebral bodies, for the entire length of the vertebral column. It is somewhat weaker than the anterior longitudinal ligament. The ligament is attached to the intervertebral discs and the posterior edges of the vertebral bodies. The posterior longitudinal ligament tends to prevent hyperflexion (bending too far forward) of the vertebral column. **Ligamenta flava** are short bands of yellow elastic fibers on each side of the spinous process. These ligaments connect the laminae of adjacent vertebrae and help to maintain the normal curvature of the vertebral column. The margins of adjacent spinous processes from C7 to the sacrum are joined by **interspinous ligaments. Supraspinous ligaments** join the tips of the spinous processes in the same region. From C7 upward to the occipital bone, the interspinous and supraspinous ligaments are represented by the **ligamentum nuchae. Intertransverse ligaments** connect adjacent transverse processes. These consist of a few scattered ligamentous fibers, except in the lumbar region, where they are membranous. The ligaments associated with the vertebral column are summarized in Table 6-1. Fig. 6-25 illustrates some of the ligaments.

Muscles Associated With the Vertebral Column

The muscles associated with the back are arranged in three layers. The superficial and intermediate layers are extrinsic muscles and are concerned with respiration and movement of the limbs. These muscles, described in other portions of this book, include the trapezius, the latissimus dorsi, the levator scapulae, the rhomboids, and the serratus posterior. The deep muscle layer includes the true back muscles; these are the intrinsic muscles, which are concerned with the maintenance of posture and

FIG. 6-24. Abnormal spinal curvatures. **A,** Lordosis. **B,** Kyphosis. **C,** Scoliosis. **D,** Radiographic appearance of scoliosis. (Modified from Thibodeau GA, Patton KT: *Anatomy & physiology,* ed 6, St Louis, 2007, Elsevier/Mosby.)

FIG. 6-25. A, Coronal oblique view of spinal ligaments. **B,** Midsagittal view of spinal ligaments. (From Kelley LL, Petersen CM: *Sectional anatomy for imaging professionals,* ed 2, St Louis, 2007, Elsevier/Mosby.)

TABLE 6-1   Ligaments of the Vertebral Column

Ligament	Description and Location
Anterior longitudinal ligament	Extends from C1 to sacrum; attached to anterior surface of vertebral bodies and discs; prevents hyperextension
Posterior longitudinal ligament	Extends from C1 to sacrum; narrow band that is attached to posterior edges of vertebral bodies and discs; located within vertebral canal; prevents hyperflexion
Ligamenta flava	Short bands that connect laminae of adjacent vertebrae on each side of spinous process; help maintain normal curvature of column
Interspinous ligaments	Short bands that connect the margins of adjacent spinous processes in thoracic and lumbar regions
Supraspinous ligaments	Short bands that connect the tips of adjacent spinous processes in thoracic and lumbar regions
Intertransverse ligaments	Short bands that connect adjacent transverse processes; poorly developed except in lumbar region
Ligamentum nuchae	Combination of interspinous and supraspinous ligaments in the cervical region

movements of the vertebral column. The intrinsic muscles are summarized in Table 6-2.

The deep layer of muscles associated with the vertebral column, which are the intrinsic back muscles, is further subdivided into superficial, intermediate, and deep layers. The superficial layer includes the **splenius capitis** and the **splenius cervicis.** The fibers of these muscles run superolaterally, with their origin on the ligamentum nuchae and spinous processes of vertebrae C7 to T6. The insertion of the splenius capitis is on the mastoid process of the temporal bone and the adjacent portion of the occipital bone, whereas the splenius cervicis fibers insert on the transverse processes of C2 to C4. As a group, these muscles pull the head posteriorly (extend the head). If the muscles on one side act alone, they bend or rotate the neck to turn the face to the same side.

The largest muscle mass associated with the vertebral column is in the intermediate layer of intrinsic muscles. As a group, these muscles are the **erector spinae muscles;** with both sides working together, they extend the vertebral column to maintain posture. The erector spinae are arranged in three longitudinal columns with their fibers parallel to the long axis of the body. The most lateral column is the **iliocostalis,** the intermediate column is the **longissimus,** and the most medial column is the **spinalis.** Fig. 6-26 illustrates the erector spinae muscles.

When the mass of erector spinae muscles is removed, the deep layer, consisting of several small muscles, is visible in the space between the spinous processes and the transverse processes. Collectively these muscles are called **transversospinal muscles,** and their fibers run obliquely in a superomedial direction from transverse processes to spinous processes above. The transversospinal muscles include the **semispinalis,** the **multifidus,** and the **rotatores.** They act synergistically with other intrinsic muscles. In addition to the transversospinal muscles,

small, rather insignificant muscle fibers run between the spinous processes of adjacent vertebrae (**interspinales**) and between the transverse processes of adjacent vertebrae (**intertransversarius**). These are usually well developed only in the cervical region.

QUICK CHECK

6.9   What are the major supporting ligaments of the vertebral column?

6.10   What term is given to the combination of interspinous and supraspinous ligaments from C7 to the occipital bone?

6.11   What term denotes the three columns of muscles in the intermediate layer of intrinsic back muscles?

Iliocostalis muscle

Spinalis muscle

Longissimus muscle (cut)

Iliocostalis muscle (cut)

Longissimus muscle (cut)

FIG. 6-26. Erector spinae muscles. (From Larsen WJ: *Anatomy: development, function, clinical correlations,* St Louis, 2002, Elsevier/ Saunders.)

TABLE 6-2 Intrinsic Muscles Associated With the Vertebral Column

Muscle	Origin	Insertion	Function	Description
Superficial Layer				
Splenius capitis	Ligamentum nuchae and spinous processes of C7 to T6	Mastoid process of temporal bone and adjacent occipital bone	Extend the head; rotate neck if one side contracts	Superficial intrinsic muscle in the neck
Splenius cervicis	Ligamentum nuchae and spinous processes of C7 to T6	Transverse processes of C2 to C4	Extend the head; rotate neck if one side contracts	Superficial intrinsic muscle in the neck
Intermediate Layer				
Iliocostalis	Iliac crests and ribs	Angles of ribs and transverse processes of C4 to C6	Extend vertebral column to maintain posture; if one side contracts, column bends to that side	Most lateral column of the erector spinae muscle group
Longissimus	Transverse processes of lumbar through cervical vertebrae	Transverse processes of thoracic and cervical vertebrae, ribs superior to origin, and mastoid process of temporal bone	Extend vertebral column; if one side contracts, column bends to that side	Intermediate column of erector spinae muscle group
Spinalis	Spinous processes of upper lumbar and lower thoracic vertebrae	Spinous processes of upper thoracic and cervical vertebrae	Extend vertebral column	Most medial column of erector spinae muscle group
Deep Layer				
Semispinalis	Transverse processes of C7 to T12	Occipital bone, spinous processes of cervical and thoracic vertebrae	Extend vertebral column	Composite muscle of deep layer; extends from thoracic region to head; part of the transversospinal group
Multifidus	Transverse processes of vertebrae	Spinous processes of preceding vertebrae	Stabilize vertebral column and rotate to opposite side	Short muscle bundles that pass superiorly over two to five vertebrae and then insert; part of the transversospinal group
Rotatores	Transverse processes of vertebrae	Spinous process of vertebra immediately superior to origin	Extend, rotate, and stabilize the vertebral column	Shortest muscles in the transversospinal group
Interspinales	Spinous processes of vertebrae	Spinous process of vertebra immediately superior to origin	Extend vertebral column	Insignificant muscle; well developed only in cervical region
Intertransversarius	Transverse processes of vertebrae	Transverse process of vertebra immediately superior to origin	Laterally bends vertebral column	Insignificant muscle; well developed only in cervical region

Anatomical Review of the Spinal Cord

The spinal cord is part of the central nervous system. It is located within the vertebral canal of the vertebral column. Like the brain, it is protected by bone, cerebrospinal fluid, and meninges. The spinal cord has two main functions. It is a conduction pathway for impulses going to and from the brain, and it serves as a reflex center.

Meninges

The three layers of **meninges** that surround the spinal cord are the same as those that surround the brain: the dura mater, the arachnoid, and the pia mater. These were described in Chapter 5. Unlike the dura mater around the brain, the dura mater of the spinal cord consists of a single layer and is separated from the vertebral bones by an epidural space, which is filled with loose connective tissue and adipose tissue (Fig. 6-27). The spinal cord terminates at vertebral level L1, but the meninges extend beyond the end of the cord, down to the upper part of the sacrum. From there, a fibrous cord of pia mater, the **filum terminale,** extends down to the coccyx, where it is anchored. Cerebrospinal fluid circulates in the subarachnoid space between the arachnoid and the pia mater. The subarachnoid space beyond the end of the spinal cord, between the end of the cord and the termination of the dura mater and arachnoid at the sacrum, provides a region for withdrawing cerebrospinal fluid with little danger of damage to the spinal cord.

Structure of the Spinal Cord

The spinal cord (Fig. 6-28) begins as a continuation of the medulla oblongata, the inferior portion of the brainstem, at the level of the foramen magnum and continues downward for about 43 to 46 cm until it terminates at the level of the first lumbar vertebra. Distally, at L1, the spinal cord terminates in a triangular or cone-shaped region called the **conus medullaris.** The spinal cord is divided into 31 segments, and each segment gives rise to a pair of spinal nerves. The spinal cord has eight cervical segments (C1 through C8), 12 thoracic segments (T1 through T12), five lumbar segments (L1 through L5), five sacral segments (S1 through S5), and one coccygeal segment. These segments do not correspond directly with the vertebral levels (Fig. 6-29). At the distal end of the cord, many spinal nerves extend beyond the conus medullaris to form a collection that resembles a horse's tail. This is the **cauda equina.** The cord has two enlarged sections, one in the cervical region and one in the lumbar region. The **cervical enlargement** includes the C4 to T1 segments of the cord and extends from approximately the C3 to the C7 vertebral bodies. It gives rise to the nerves that supply the upper extremity. The **lumbosacral enlargement** includes the L2 to S3 segments of the cord and extends from approximately the T11 to the L1 vertebral bodies. Nerves from this enlargement supply the lower extremity.

In cross section (Fig. 6-30), the spinal cord appears oval in shape. A narrow, deep **dorsal (posterior) median sulcus** and a shallower but wider **ventral (anterior) median fissure** partially divide the cord into right and left halves. Peripheral white matter surrounds a core of gray matter that resembles a butterfly or the letter H. Each side of the gray matter is divided into **dorsal, lateral,** and **ventral** horns. These contain the terminal portions of sensory neuron axons, entire interneurons, and the dendrites and cell bodies of motor neurons. The central connecting bar between the two large areas of gray matter is the **gray commissure.** This surrounds the **central canal,** which contains cerebrospinal fluid. The gray matter divides the surrounding white matter into three regions on each side. These regions are the **dorsal, lateral,** and **ventral funiculi,** or **columns.** The white matter contains longitudinal bundles of myelinated nerve fibers, called **nerve tracts.**

> ### QUICK CHECK
> 6.12 What is the difference in structure between the dura mater around the brain and the dura mater around the spinal cord?
> 6.13 What is the distal triangular terminal portion of the spinal cord?
> 6.14 In what two regions is the spinal cord enlarged?

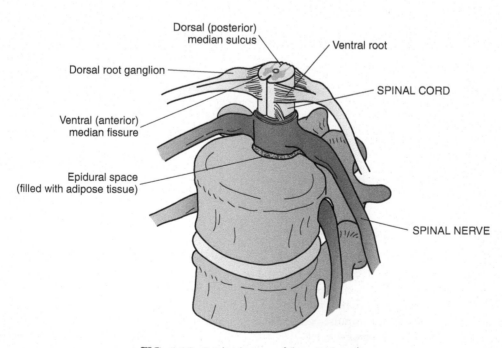

FIG. 6-27. Epidural space of the spinal cord.

Cervical nerves

Thoracic nerves

Lumbar nerves

Sacral nerves

Coccygeal nerve

Dura mater

Cervical plexus

Brachial plexus

Lumbar enlargement

Conus medullaris

Cauda equina

Lumbosacral plexus

Filum terminale

FIG. 6-28. Gross anatomy of the spinal cord.

Spinal Nerves

Thirty-one pairs of spinal nerves emerge laterally from the spinal cord. Each pair of nerves corresponds to a segment of the cord, and they are named accordingly: there are eight **cervical nerves** (C1 through C8), 12 **thoracic nerves** (T1 through T12), five **lumbar nerves** (L1 through L5), five **sacral nerves** (S1 through S5), and one **coccygeal nerve** (Co).

Spinal Nerve Roots.   Each spinal nerve is connected to the spinal cord by a **dorsal root** and a **ventral root** (see Figs. 6-27 and 6-30). The dorsal root can be recognized by an enlargement, the **dorsal root ganglion,** which contains the cell bodies of afferent (sensory) neurons that transmit impulses from the periphery of the body to the central nervous system. The cell bodies of efferent (motor) neurons are in the ventral horns of the gray matter. The dorsal root has only sensory fibers, and the ventral root has only motor fibers. The two roots join to form the spinal nerve just before the nerve leaves the vertebral column through the corresponding intervertebral foramen. Because all spinal

nerves have both afferent (sensory) and efferent (motor) components, they are all mixed nerves.

Nerve Plexuses.   Immediately after leaving the vertebral column, each spinal nerve divides into **dorsal** and **ventral rami.** Each ramus contains both sensory and motor fibers. The dorsal rami supply the skin and muscles of the posterior portion of the body trunk. In the thoracic region, the ventral rami of nerves T2 through T12 go directly to the thoracic wall, where they are called **intercostal nerves.** In other regions, the ventral rami form complex networks, called **plexuses,** which supply the skin and muscles of the extremities. In the plexus, the fibers are sorted and recombined so that the fibers associated with a particular body part are together, even though they may originate from different regions of the cord. The four major nerve plexuses are the **cervical, brachial, lumbar,** and **sacral plexuses,** which are summarized in Table 6-3.

The **cervical plexus,** located deep in the neck and under the sternocleidomastoid muscle, arises from the ventral rami of spinal nerves C1 through C4. It supplies the skin

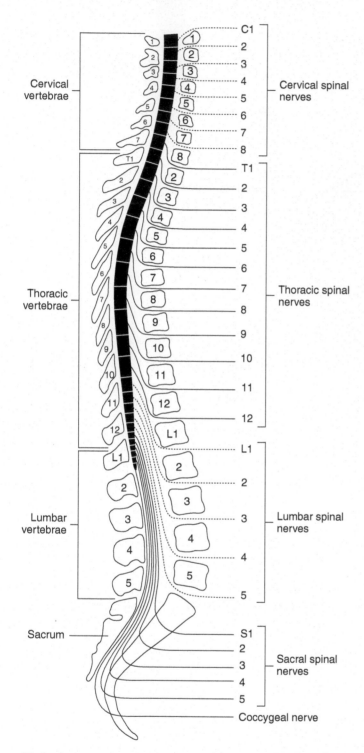

FIG. 6-29. Relationship of spinal cord segments to vertebral bodies.

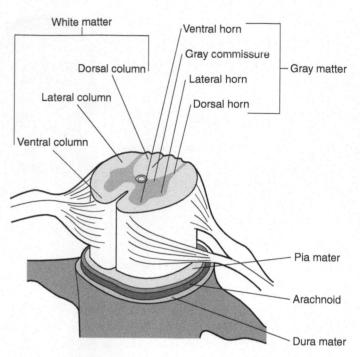

FIG. 6-30. Cross section of the spinal cord.

C5 through C8 and T1 form this plexus. Five major nerves and several smaller nerves emerge from the brachial plexus to supply the skin and muscles of the upper extremity. The larger nerves are the **musculocutaneous, ulnar, median, radial,** and **axillary nerves.**

The **lumbar plexus** is formed within the psoas major muscle by the ventral rami of the first four lumbar nerves. In about 50% of people, the ventral ramus of T12 also contributes. The nerves from the lumbar plexus innervate the skin and muscles of the lower abdominopelvic region, the buttocks, and the anterior thighs. The largest and most important branches that emerge from the lumbar plexus are the **femoral** and the **obturator nerves.**

The **sacral plexus** is located in the true pelvis, where it is closely associated with the anterior surface of the piriformis muscle. Branches from this plexus innervate the pelvic diaphragm, the external genitalia, the posterior thigh, and the leg and foot. Important nerves that emerge from the sacral plexus are the **pudendal nerve** and the **sciatic nerve,** which is the largest nerve in the body. The sacral plexus is formed by the ventral rami of spinal nerves L4 and L5 and by the ventral rami of S1 through S4. Note that L4 contributes to both the lumbar plexus and the sacral plexus. The lumbar and sacral plexuses are closely related and are sometimes collectively referred to as the **lumbosacral plexus.**

Vasculature of the Spinal Cord

The arterial blood supply for the spinal cord comes from three longitudinal vessels, a single **anterior spinal artery** and two **posterior spinal arteries.** The anterior spinal artery runs

and muscles of the neck and shoulder. One of the important nerves that emerges from the plexus is the **phrenic nerve,** which supplies the diaphragm. Trauma in the cervical region may damage the phrenic nerve and result in paralysis of the diaphragm.

The **brachial plexus** is located deep to the clavicle, between the neck and axilla. It runs between the anterior and middle scalene muscles. Ventral rami of spinal nerves

TABLE 6-3 Spinal Nerve Plexuses

Plexus	Location	Spinal Nerves Involved	Region Supplied	Major Nerves Leaving Plexus
Cervical	Deep in the neck; under the sternocleidomastoid muscle	C1 through C4	Skin and muscles of the neck and shoulder; diaphragm	Phrenic
Brachial	Deep to the clavicle, between neck and axilla; between anterior and middle scalene muscles	C5 through C8 and T1	Skin and muscles of the upper extremity	Musculocutaneous Ulnar Median Radial Axillary
Lumbar	Within psoas major muscle	T12 and L1 through L4	Skin and muscles of lower abdominopelvic region, buttocks, and anterior thighs	Femoral Obturator
Sacral	Within the true pelvis where it is associated with the anterior surface of the piriformis muscle	L4, L5, and S1 through S4	Pelvic diaphragm, external genitalia, posterior thigh, leg, and foot	Sciatic Pudendal

the entire length of the cord in the ventral (anterior) median fissure. It is formed by two small branches of the vertebral arteries, and it supplies the anterior two thirds of the spinal cord. The posterior spinal arteries also arise as branches of the vertebral arteries and are adjacent to the dorsal roots of spinal nerves. These arteries anastomose freely with each other and supply the posterior one third of the spinal cord. The blood from the vertebral arteries that enters the anterior and posterior spinal arteries is sufficient only for the cervical segments of the cord. Blood for the remaining segments comes from the numerous **radicular arteries** that contribute blood to the anterior and posterior spinal arteries. Radicular arteries arise as branches of the **segmental arteries,** which are formed by the parietal branches of the thoracic and abdominal aorta, particularly the intercostal and lumbar arteries. The radicular arteries enter the vertebral canal through the intervertebral foramina and provide the blood supply for the vertebrae and meninges in addition to contributing blood to the spinal arteries.

Spinal veins have a distribution similar to that of the spinal arteries. The veins are arranged longitudinally and anastomose freely with each other. In the vertebral canal is a plexus of veins that surrounds the spinal dura. The vertebral venous plexus and the anterior and posterior spinal veins drain into intervertebral veins, which then empty into the vertebral veins, the ascending lumbar veins, and the azygous venous system. The arteries and veins of the spinal cord are difficult to visualize in cross sectional images because of their small size.

QUICK CHECK

6.15 How many spinal nerves arise from the spinal cord?

6.16 What vitally important nerve emerges from the cervical plexus?

6.17 From which nerve plexus does the sciatic nerve arise?

Anatomical Review of the Neck

The principal bony structures in the neck are the cervical vertebrae. These bones and the muscles in the neck provide support for the head, yet they permit some degree of movement. The digestive and respiratory systems begin with openings in the head and continue as passageways in the neck. The thyroid and parathyroid glands, which are important endocrine organs, are located in the neck region. The neck also serves as a passageway for the spinal cord, blood vessels, and nerves. As you can see, many important structures are located in the limited region of the neck, and an understanding of the relationships of these structures is important for the imaging professional.

Osseous Components

The bony skeleton of the neck consists of seven cervical vertebrae (see Fig. 6-3 to review the features of the cervical vertebrae). These vertebrae are distinguished from other types of vertebrae by their transverse foramina for the passage of the vertebral arteries. Another unique feature is the bifid spinous processes on the first six cervical vertebrae. The spinous process of the seventh cervical vertebra may not be bifid and is usually long and pointed, which makes it easily palpable. This is a good reference point for counting the vertebrae.

The first two cervical vertebrae are modified and have special names. The first cervical vertebra, C1, is called the *atlas*. The second cervical vertebra, C2, is called the *axis* (see Figs. 6-5 to 6-7 to review the features of C1 and C2).

Muscular Components

Numerous muscles are located in the neck; however, many of them are small and difficult to separate from adjacent muscles. They may be even more difficult to isolate by imaging techniques. These muscles have functional significance, because they deal with deglutition and with movements of the head, neck, and shoulder. The muscles of the neck are often described as being located within one of two triangles, which are separated by the sternocleidomastoid muscle. Fig. 6-31 illustrates the boundaries of the anterior and posterior triangles of the neck. Only the larger and more significant muscles are presented in this discussion.

Anterior Triangle of the Neck.   The **anterior triangle** extends from the midline of the neck to the anterior margin of the sternocleidomastoid muscle. The lower border of the mandible forms the base, and the manubrium of the sternum forms the apex of the triangle.

The muscles of the anterior triangle, which are generally considered throat muscles, also help to form the floor of the oral cavity, and all are attached to the hyoid bone. They are involved with movements of the tongue and aid in swallowing. These muscles, summarized in Table 6-4, may be divided into two groups, the **suprahyoid muscles** and

the **infrahyoid muscles.** As a group, the suprahyoid muscles are superior to the hyoid bone and raise the hyoid bone during swallowing, or open the jaw when the hyoid bone is fixed. These muscles are the digastric, stylohyoid, mylohyoid, and geniohyoid. The infrahyoid muscles are inferior to the hyoid bone and pull down on the larynx and hyoid to return them to their normal positions after swallowing. These muscles are the sternohyoid, sternothyroid, thyrohyoid, and omohyoid.

In addition to the muscles, a significant structure located in the anterior triangle is the **carotid sheath,** which is a tubular arrangement of fascia that extends from the base of the skull to the inferior portion of the neck. The sheath encloses the common carotid artery, internal jugular vein, and vagus nerve (Fig. 6-32). Superior to the bifurcation of the common carotid artery, the internal carotid artery is in the position previously occupied by the common carotid artery. Branches of the external carotid artery are within the anterior triangle but are not enclosed by the carotid sheath.

Other components in the anterior triangle include the carotid sinus, carotid body, lymph nodes, and submandibular salivary gland. The carotid sinus and carotid body are closely related to the common carotid artery near its point of bifurcation. The carotid sinus, which reacts to changes in arterial blood pressure, is an enlargement of the internal carotid artery as it branches from the common carotid artery. The carotid body, a small ovoid mass of tissue in the region of the carotid sinus, responds to changes in the chemical composition of the blood.

Posterior Triangle of the Neck.   The **posterior triangle** of the neck extends from the posterior margin of the sternocleidomastoid muscle to the trapezius, with the apex of the triangle at the junction of these two muscles. The base is formed by the clavicle. The muscular floor of the triangle is formed by the splenius capitis, the levator scapulae, and the middle and posterior scalene muscles. These muscles are summarized in Table 6-5. The external jugular vein, the phrenic and accessory nerves, and

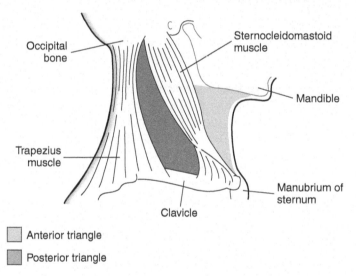

Anterior triangle

Posterior triangle

FIG. 6-31. Boundaries of the anterior and posterior triangles in the neck.

TABLE 6-4   Muscles Associated With the Anterior Triangle of the Neck

Muscle	Origin	Insertion	Action	Innervation
Sternocleidomastoid	Sternum and clavicle	Mastoid of temporal	Turn head side to side; flex neck	Spinal accessory (XI)
Suprahyoid Muscles				
Digastric	Mandible	Hyoid	Elevate hyoid; open mouth	Trigeminal (V)
Stylohyoid	Temporal	Hyoid	Elevate hyoid; retract tongue	Facial (VII)
Mylohyoid	Mandible	Hyoid	Elevate hyoid and floor of mouth	Trigeminal (V)
Geniohyoid	Mandible	Hyoid	Protracts hyoid	Hypoglossal (XII)
Infrahyoid Muscles				
Sternohyoid	Sternum	Hyoid	Depress hyoid	Hypoglossal (XII)
Sternothyroid	Sternum	Thyroid cartilage and hyoid	Depress thyroid cartilage and hyoid	Hypoglossal (XII)
Thyrohyoid	Thyroid cartilage	Hyoid	Depress hyoid	Hypoglossal (XII)
Omohyoid	Scapula	Hyoid and clavicle	Depress hyoid	Hypoglossal (XII)

FIG. 6-32. Contents and location of the carotid sheath.

portions of the brachial plexus are located within the posterior triangle.

QUICK CHECK

6.18 What bones form the skeleton of the neck?
6.19 What muscle divides the neck into anterior and posterior triangles?
6.20 What are the three main structures within the carotid sheath?

Viscera of the Neck

The neck region represents the connection between the head and the trunk of the body. Although the term *viscera* usually refers to the organs of the thoracic and abdominopelvic cavities, it is used here as a collective term for the miscellaneous structures of the neck that cannot be classified as nerves, muscles, or blood vessels. This includes the pharynx, larynx, trachea, and esophagus, which represent passageways for food and air, and the thyroid and parathyroid glands, which are important endocrine glands in the neck. The MR image in Fig. 6-33 shows some of the viscera in the neck.

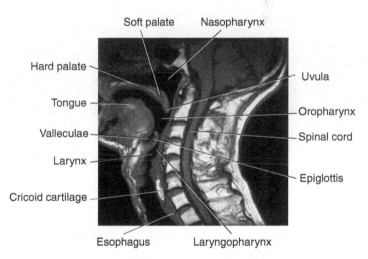

FIG. 6-33. Midsagittal MR image of the neck (T1 weighted). (From Kelley LL, Petersen CM: *Sectional anatomy for imaging professionals,* ed 2, St Louis, 2007, Elsevier/Mosby.)

TABLE 6-5   Muscles Associated With the Posterior Triangle of the Neck

Muscle	Origin	Insertion	Action	Innervation
Trapezius	Occipital bone and vertebral spines	Scapula	Elevates scapula	Spinal accessory (XI)
Splenius capitis	Cervical and thoracic vertebrae	Occipital bone	Extends head	Cervical nerves
Levator scapulae	Cervical vertebrae	Vertebral border of scapula	Elevates scapula	Dorsal scapular
Middle scalene	Cervical vertebrae	First rib	Elevates rib	Cervical plexus
Posterior scalene	Cervical vertebrae	Second rib	Elevates rib	Cervical plexus

Pharynx.   The **pharynx** is a muscular tube about 12 cm long that extends from the base of the skull to the level of the sixth cervical vertebra and cricoid cartilage, where it becomes the esophagus. The wall of the pharynx consists of overlapping pharyngeal constrictor muscles lined with mucous membrane. For descriptive purposes, it is divided into the nasal, oral, and laryngeal portions.

The **nasopharynx,** which is the region posterior to the nose, extends from the base of the skull to the soft palate. The anterior wall of the pharynx is somewhat lacking in structural elements but presents open space where the nasal cavity communicates with the pharynx through the **choanae,** or internal nares. The **eustachian,** or auditory, **tubes** open into the lateral walls of the nasopharynx. The openings are recognized by the **torus tubarius,** a rounded protuberance of cartilage that outlines the posterior wall of the opening. Posterior to the torus tubarius, the walls of the nasopharynx extend laterally to form the **pharyngeal recess.** Aggregations of lymphoid tissue, the **pharyngeal tonsils,** are found in the mucosa of the posterior wall of the nasopharynx. When enlarged, these **tonsils** are commonly called "adenoids."

The **oropharynx,** which is posterior to the oral cavity, extends from the soft palate to the tip of the epiglottis. The opening from the oral cavity into the pharynx is called the **fauces.** Collections of lymphoid tissue, the **palatine tonsils,** are in the wall of the oropharynx; these are commonly referred to as "the tonsils." The base of the tongue, with the associated lymphoid tissue called **lingual tonsils,** forms part of the anterior wall of the oropharynx. Between the tongue and the epiglottis are two valleys, called **valleculae,** which present a potential hazard, because foreign objects may become lodged there.

The laryngeal portion of the pharynx, called the **laryngopharynx,** or **hypopharynx,** extends from the superior border of the epiglottis to the cricoid cartilage, which is located at the junction between the larynx and trachea at the level of the sixth cervical vertebra. The walls extend laterally around the opening of the larynx to form the **piriform recesses.** Foreign objects that enter the pharynx may become lodged in the recesses. Inferiorly the laryngopharynx is continuous with the esophagus.

The **retropharyngeal space** is a potential space between the fascia that surrounds the pharynx and the fascia that surrounds the vertebral column and its associated **prevertebral muscles.** The space contains loose connective tissue and permits the movement of the pharynx, larynx, trachea, and esophagus during swallowing. The retropharyngeal space is closed off by the skull superiorly, but it opens into the mediastinum of the thorax inferiorly. Laterally, the carotid sheath forms a barrier to the space. Infections in the region of the fascial layers may penetrate the fascia and enter the retropharyngeal space. Pus from infections may form abscesses that bulge into the pharynx and cause difficulty with speaking or swallowing. Once an infection enters the retropharyngeal space, it has a direct pathway into the mediastinum.

Larynx.   Although the **larynx** is an essential part of the air passageway, it is especially modified for voice production. The larynx is anterior to the laryngeal portion of the pharynx, the laryngopharynx or hypopharynx. In the male, the larynx typically extends from the epiglottis at the level of the third cervical vertebra (C3) to the cricoid cartilage at the level of the sixth cervical vertebra (C6). The cricoid cartilage, which is the most inferior portion of the larynx, rests on the first tracheal cartilage. It is usually somewhat higher than this in females and children. The skeleton of the larynx is formed by nine cartilages joined by ligaments. The major cartilages are the single **thyroid cartilage, cricoid cartilage,** and **epiglottic cartilage** and the paired **arytenoids.** In addition there are small **corniculate** and **cuneiform cartilages,** which are paired. The thyroid and cricoid cartilages and the arytenoids are hyaline cartilage. With age, the hyaline cartilage may calcify, making these cartilages visible on radiographs. The other cartilages (the epiglottic, corniculate, and cuneiform cartilages) are elastic cartilage. The corniculate cartilages are attached to the tips of the arytenoids and are covered by a fold of tissue called the *aryepiglottic fold.* The cuneiform cartilages are enclosed within the aryepiglottic fold lateral to the arytenoids.

The interior of the larynx is subdivided into three portions by folds of tissue that project from the lateral laryngeal wall. The upper folds are the **vestibular folds.** These form the inferior margin of the **vestibule,** which is the most superior chamber of the larynx. The opening between the two vestibular folds is called the **rima vestibuli.** Because the vestibular folds are frequently mistaken for the vocal cords, they are sometimes referred to as the *false vocal cords,* even though they play little or no part in voice production. The lower projections are the **vocal folds,** or true vocal cords, and the slit or opening between them is the **rima glottidis.** This aperture changes shape according to the position of the folds during breathing and phonation. The space between the vestibular folds and the vocal folds is the **ventricle** of the larynx. Sometimes the ventricle is called the *laryngeal sinus.* This is the smallest and middle of the three regions. The remainder of the laryngeal cavity is the **infraglottic portion,** which extends from the vocal folds to the trachea. The term *glottis* refers to the true vocal folds and the rima glottidis collectively. Fig. 6-34 illustrates the structure of the larynx.

If a foreign particle, such as a bit of food, enters the larynx, the musculature goes into a spasm and creates tension on the vocal folds, which closes the rima glottidis. This prevents air from reaching the trachea and lower air passageways, and the individual is in danger of asphyxiation.

QUICK CHECK

6.21   The eustachian tube opens into which region of the pharynx?

6.22   In which region of the pharynx are the palatine tonsils located?

6.23   What is the opening or slit between the vocal folds called?

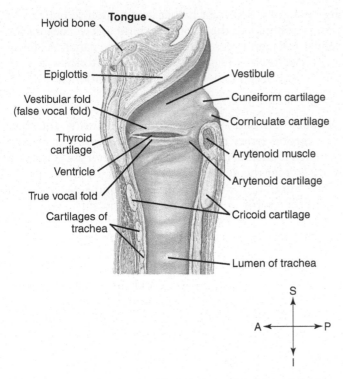

Hyoid bone
Tongue
Epiglottis
Vestibular fold (false vocal fold)
Thyroid cartilage
Ventricle
True vocal fold
Cartilages of trachea

Vestibule
Cuneiform cartilage
Corniculate cartilage
Arytenoid muscle
Arytenoid cartilage
Cricoid cartilage
Lumen of trachea

S
A ← → P
I

FIG. 6-34. Midsagittal view of the larynx. (Modified from Thibodeau GA, Patton KT: *Anatomy & physiology*, ed 6, St Louis, 2007, Elsevier/ Mosby.)

Trachea. The **trachea** begins as a continuation of the larynx in the neck at vertebral level C6. It descends through the thorax, anterior to the esophagus, and enters the **superior mediastinum** of the thorax a little to the right of midline. It extends to vertebral level T5, where it bifurcates into the right and left **bronchi.** The walls of the trachea are supported by 16 to 20 incomplete rings of hyaline cartilage. The rings are deficient on the posterior side, where they are related to the esophagus; therefore the posterior margin of the trachea is flattened. The tracheal airway is kept open by the rings of cartilage; the soft tissue filling the posterior gap, between the tips of the rings, allows for expansion of the esophagus during swallowing. The common carotid arteries and the lobes of the **thyroid gland** are lateral to the trachea in the neck (see Fig. 6-32). At lower levels, near the aortic arch, the **brachiocephalic artery** (trunk) is anterior and to the right of the trachea.

Esophagus. The **esophagus** is a thick, distensible, muscular tube that extends from the pharynx at the level of the cricoid cartilage (C6) in the neck to the stomach in the abdomen. As it descends through the neck, it is near the midline between the trachea and the vertebral bodies. At the root of the neck, on the right side, the esophagus is related to the **parietal pleura** of the apex of the lung. On the left, the **thoracic duct** and **subclavian artery** are between the esophagus and the pleura. These relationships are illustrated in Fig. 6-35.

Thyroid and Parathyroid Glands. The **thyroid,** an important endocrine gland, consists of right and left lobes

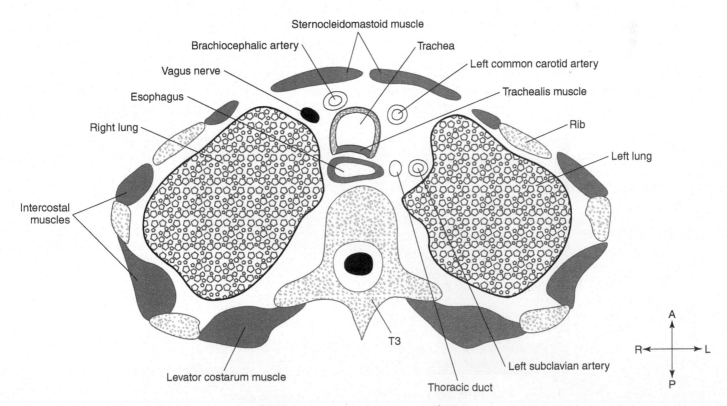

Sternocleidomastoid muscle
Brachiocephalic artery
Vagus nerve
Esophagus
Right lung
Intercostal muscles
Trachea
Left common carotid artery
Trachealis muscle
Rib
Left lung
Levator costarum muscle
T3
Thoracic duct
Left subclavian artery

A
R ← → L
P

FIG. 6-35. Relationships of the esophagus.

that usually are connected by an **isthmus.** The lobes are lateral to the lower portion of the larynx and the upper part of the trachea, and they may extend posteriorly enough to be related to the esophagus. The isthmus connecting the lobes passes over the second and third tracheal rings, and the lobes may extend inferiorly to the sixth tracheal ring. Four small **parathyroid glands** are usually embedded along the posterior margin of the thyroid, but these are difficult to visualize. The sonogram in Fig. 6-36 shows the right lobe of the thyroid gland with a portion of the isthmus. The right internal jugular vein and right common carotid artery are lateral to the gland.

QUICK CHECK

6.24   What structure is immediately posterior to the trachea in the neck?

6.25   What glands are embedded along the posterior margin of the thyroid gland?

6.26   What is between the trachea the carotid sheath in the neck?

Vascular Components

Internal Jugular Veins.
The **internal jugular vein** begins as a continuation of the **sigmoid sinus** at the jugular foramen in the posterior cranial fossa. It is usually the largest vein in the neck, and it is generally larger on the right side than on the left. As the internal jugular vein descends toward the heart, it passes deep to the **sternocleidomastoid muscle,** then courses anteriorly to unite with the **subclavian vein.** Posterior to the sternal end of the clavicle, the internal jugular vein joins with the subclavian vein to form the **brachiocephalic vein.** The internal jugular vein is located within the carotid sheath with the common carotid artery (or internal carotid artery at higher levels) and vagus nerve. Within the sheath, the internal jugular vein is lateral to the common carotid artery, and the vagus nerve is between the two vessels and slightly posterior to them (see

Figs. 6-32 and 6-36). At higher levels the internal jugular vein is posterior to the internal carotid artery, because the jugular foramen is posterior to the carotid canal. At lower levels the internal jugular vein is anterior to the common carotid artery because of the anteriorly positioned brachiocephalic veins.

Common Carotid Arteries.
On the right side, the **common carotid artery** begins posterior to the sternoclavicular joint as a branch of the **brachiocephalic artery.** On the left, it arises from the **aortic arch.** It ascends the neck, medial to the internal jugular vein in the carotid sheath, to the level of the superior border of the thyroid cartilage, where it divides into the **external** and **internal carotid arteries.** This is at the level of the disc between the third and fourth cervical vertebrae. At the bifurcation, the common carotid artery and the continuing internal carotid artery dilate to form the **carotid sinus.** The carotid sinus contains receptors for the regulation of blood pressure.

The angiogram in Fig. 6-37, A, and the sonogram in Fig. 6-37, B, show the bifurcation of the common carotid artery into the internal and external carotid arteries.

Internal Carotid Arteries.
Arising as a direct continuation of the common carotid artery, the **internal carotid artery** ascends almost vertically within the carotid sheath to enter the carotid canal in the petrous portion of the temporal bone. The right and left internal carotid arteries are two of the four major vessels supplying blood to the brain. Branches also supply the pituitary gland and orbit. The internal jugular vein is lateral to the internal carotid artery, and the vagus nerve is posterolateral (see Fig. 6-32).

External Carotid Arteries.
The **external carotid artery** arises at the bifurcation of the common carotid artery. As the name implies, the external carotid artery and its numerous branches supply structures external to the skull. At low levels, near the bifurcation of the common

FIG. 6-36. Sonogram of the right lobe of the thyroid gland.

FIG. 6-37. Angiogram **(A)** and sonogram **(B)** showing the bifurcation of the common carotid artery.

carotid artery, the external carotid artery is anterior and medial to the internal carotid artery. At higher levels the external carotid artery becomes more superficial, such that it is anterior and lateral to the internal carotid artery.

Vertebral Arteries. The **right** and **left vertebral arteries** begin as branches of the right and left **subclavian arteries.** The arteries ascend through the transverse foramina of cervical vertebrae C6 through C1. The vessels then course along the superior portion of the atlas and enter the **foramen magnum.** As they pass through the foramen magnum, the arteries pierce the dura mater and arachnoid to enter the subarachnoid space of the **cerebellomedullary cistern.** Within the skull, at the base of the pons, the right and left vertebral arteries join to form a single basilar artery. The vertebral arteries are two of the four major arteries that supply the brain. The other two arteries are the right and left internal carotid arteries.

QUICK CHECK
6.27   Within the carotid sheath, what is the position of the internal jugular vein relative to the common carotid artery?
6.28   Where is the carotid sinus located?
6.29   Where are the vertebral arteries located as they ascend through the neck?

Major Nerves of the Neck

Sympathetic Trunks. The **sympathetic trunks** are strands of nerve fibers and ganglia that lie lateral to the vertebral column. They extend from the base of the skull to the coccyx. In the cervical region, the trunks are posterior to the carotid sheath and are immediately anterior to the transverse processes of the vertebrae. Three ganglia are present in the cervical region of the sympathetic trunk. The **superior cervical ganglion** is located at the level of the axis, and because it is large, it serves as a good landmark for locating the trunk. The **middle cervical ganglion** is small and is located just anterior to the vertebral artery at the level of the transverse process of the sixth cervical vertebra. The **inferior cervical ganglion** is usually found posterior to the vertebral artery at the level of the superior border of the neck of the first rib.

Vagus Nerve. Cranial nerve X is called the **vagus nerve** because of its wide distribution. The vagus nerve leaves the skull through the jugular foramen with the internal jugular vein. It descends in the anterior triangle of the neck in the carotid sheath, and it is slightly posterior to and between the internal jugular vein and the carotid artery, either common or internal depending on the level (see Fig. 6-32).

Cervical Plexus. The **cervical plexus** is a network of nerve fibers that are derived from the first four cervical nerves. It is located within the posterior triangle of the neck, lateral to the first four cervical vertebrae and deep to the internal jugular vein and sternocleidomastoid muscle. Branches from this plexus innervate the skin and muscles of the neck and portions of the head and shoulders. The **phrenic nerve,** an important branch of the cervical plexus, is the only nerve that supplies motor impulses to stimulate contraction of the diaphragm. It descends the neck along the anterior surface of the anterior scalene muscle. At the root of the neck, it enters the thorax between the subclavian artery and subclavian vein.

Brachial Plexus. The **brachial plexus** is a network of nerve fibers that are derived from the last four cervical nerves and the first thoracic nerve. Nerves from the brachial plexus innervate the upper extremity. The **supraclavicular portion** of this plexus is in the anterior and inferior portion of the posterior triangle of the neck, lying between the anterior and middle scalene muscles. The **infraclavicular portion** of the brachial plexus is located in the axilla. This plexus is discussed further with the thorax in Chapter 2.

QUICK CHECK

6.30   What nerve is associated with the internal jugular vein and common carotid artery in the neck?

6.31   What nerve plexus innervates the skin and muscles of the neck?

Sectional Anatomy of the Vertebral Column, Spinal Cord, and Neck

Transverse Sections of the Neck

Tranverse Section Through the Neck at the Level of C1. Sections through the neck at the level of the first cervical vertebra (Figs. 6-38 and 6-39) typically pass through the **hard** and **soft palate.** The **pharyngeal constrictor muscle** forms the wall of the **oropharynx** at the posterior edge of the soft palate. The dens, or odontoid process, of C2 projects upward, posterior to the anterior arch of C1. The **ramus of the mandible** appears as a thin slice of bone, with the **masseter muscle** lateral to it and the **pterygoid muscle** medial to it. Another significant structure at this level is the **parotid gland.** The **sternocleidomastoid muscle** is posterior to the parotid gland, and the masseter muscle, the medial pterygoid muscle, and the ramus of the mandible are anterior to the gland. Medially, the parotid gland is related to the **styloid process** of the temporal bone and the **internal jugular vein.** The tissue of the parotid gland may surround the **external jugular vein.**

Tranverse Section Through the Neck at the Level of C3. Sections through the third cervical vertebrae (Figs. 6-40 and 6-41) will likely pass through the **mandible** and the **muscles of the tongue.** The **submandibular gland** is medial to the mandible, and a small portion of the **parotid gland** may still be present at this level. The arrangement of the vessels

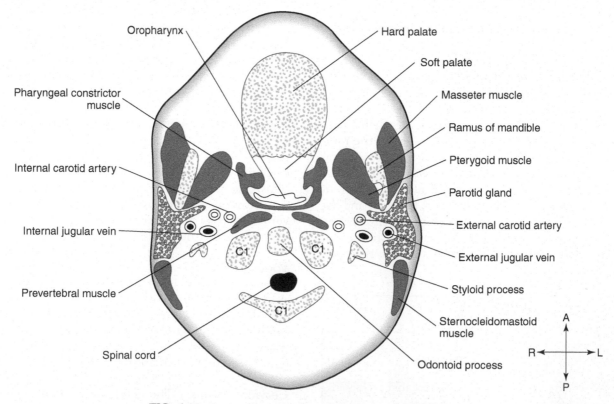

FIG. 6-38. Transverse section through the neck at the level of C1.

Masseter muscle
Ramus of mandible
Parotid gland
Styloid process
Transverse foramen
C1
Spinal cord

Pterygoid muscle
Oropharynx
Pharyngeal constrictor muscle
Prevertebral muscle
Odontoid process of C2

A
R←→L
P

FIG. 6-39. Transverse CT image through the neck at the level of C1.

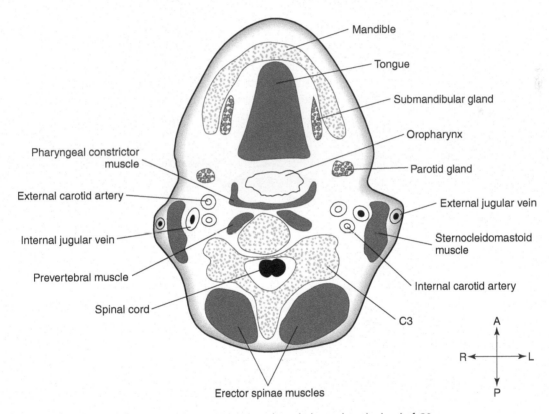

Mandible
Tongue
Submandibular gland
Oropharynx
Parotid gland
External jugular vein
Sternocleidomastoid muscle
Internal carotid artery
C3

Pharyngeal constrictor muscle
External carotid artery
Internal jugular vein
Prevertebral muscle
Spinal cord

Erector spinae muscles

A
R←→L
P

FIG. 6-40. Transverse section through the neck at the level of C3.

in the region is particularly significant. The **external** and **internal carotid arteries** are close together, which indicates that this is near their junction point. The external carotid artery is anterior to the internal carotid artery, and the **internal jugular vein** is lateral to both of these. The **external jugular vein** is lateral to the sternocleidomastoid muscle.

Tranverse Section Through the Neck at the Larynx. A representative transverse section through the larynx is

illustrated in Figs. 6-42 and 6-43. The laminae of the laryngeal **thyroid cartilage** are usually evident at vertebral level C3 or C4. Near the upper margin of the thyroid laminae, the **common carotid arteries** bifurcate into the **external** and **internal carotid arteries.** At this junction, the common carotid artery and the internal carotid artery that continues from it dilate to form the **carotid sinus,** which contains baroreceptors to monitor blood pressure. The pharynx continues through this region as the

Tongue
Masseter muscle
Ramus of mandible
Submandibular gland
Internal carotid artery
Sternocleido-mastoid muscle
Internal jugular vein
C3
Spinal cord
Parotid gland
Oropharynx

FIG. 6-41. Transverse CT image through the neck at the level of C3.

laryngopharynx. Muscles forming the floor of the posterior triangle of the neck are lateral to the transverse processes of the vertebrae.

Section Through the Neck at the Thoracic Inlet. Sections through the thoracic inlet, or superior thoracic aperture, are inferior to the larynx and show the structures that pass through the root of the neck into the thorax. Figs. 6-44

and 6-45 illustrate this region. At this level the **trachea** is present, with a lobe of the **thyroid gland** on each side. In some cases the isthmus of the thyroid will be present anterior to the trachea. The posterior soft tissue of the trachea, namely the **trachealis muscle,** allows for expansion of the **esophagus,** which is posterior to the trachea, during swallowing. At this level the **sternocleidomastoid muscles** are more anteriorly positioned than they are at higher levels. The **common carotid arteries** and **internal jugular veins** are lateral to the thyroid gland, with the artery medial to the vein.

Some of the components of the posterior triangle are evident in transverse sections at this level. The **anterior scalene, middle scalene,** and **levator scapulae muscles** are present, and the **brachial plexus** is visible between the anterior and middle scalene muscles. Sections at this level also show the shoulder region with the pectoral girdle and the upper extremity. The details of these regions are discussed in Chapters 2 and 7.

Midsagittal Section Through the Neck

Figs. 6-46 and 6-47 illustrate a midsagittal section through the neck. These illustrations show features of the brain and oral cavity, but this discussion focuses on the neck region.

Thyroid cartilage
Pharyngeal constrictor muscle
Vagus nerve
Internal jugular vein
Prevertebral muscle
Vertebral artery
Trapezius muscle
Vestibular fold of larynx
Arytenoid cartilage
Laryngopharynx
Sternocleidomastoid muscle
Common carotid artery
External jugular vein
Levator scapulae muscle
Erector spinae muscle
C6

FIG. 6-42. Transverse section through the larynx.

FIG. 6-43. Transverse CT image through the larynx. (From Kelley LL, Petersen CM: *Sectional anatomy for imaging professionals*, ed 2, St Louis, 2007, Elsevier/Mosby.)

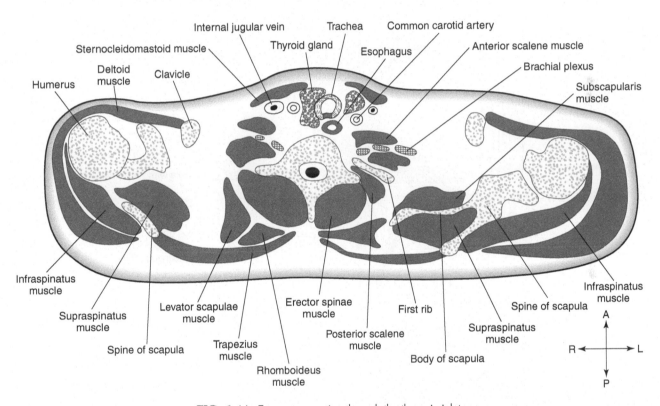

FIG. 6-44. Transverse section through the thoracic inlet.

The leaf-shaped **epiglottis,** one of the laryngeal cartilages, is quite obvious. The trachea, with its cartilaginous rings, is inferior to the larynx.

The pharynx is immediately anterior to the vertebral column. The nasopharynx, which is located posterior to the nasal cavity, extends from the superior pharyngeal margin to the **uvula.** At the uvula, the nasopharynx becomes the oropharynx, which continues inferiorly to the epiglottis. The laryngopharynx continues inferiorly from the epiglottis, posterior to the larynx. At the level of the first tracheal cartilage, the laryngopharynx becomes the esophagus. Midsagittal sections provide nice views of the vertebral bodies, the intervertebral discs, and the spinal cord.

QUICK CHECK

6.32 In transverse sections through the neck, what muscle is lateral to the ramus of the mandible?

6.33 In transverse sections through the neck at the level of C3, what are the relative positions of the internal and external jugular veins to the sternocleidomastoid muscle?

6.34 In transverse sections through the thoracic inlet, what group of nerves is between the anterior and middle scalene muscles?

6.35 In a midsagittal section, what is the space posterior to the nasal cavity?

FIG. 6-45. Transverse CT image through the thoracic inlet.

Thyroid gland

Internal jugular vein

Internal carotid artery

Trachea

Sternocleido-mastoid muscle

Esophagus

Brachial plexus

Spinal cord

Levator scapulae muscle

FIG. 6-46. Midsagittal section through the neck.

Atlas (C1)

Erector spinae muscles

Spinal cord

Nasopharynx

Uvula

Maxilla with hard palate

Tongue

Axis (C2)

Sublingual gland

Mandible

Oropharynx

Vallecula

Epiglottis

Laryngopharynx

Opening into larynx

Trachea

Esophagus

Working With Images of the Vertebral Column, Spinal Cord, and Neck

The radiograph in Fig. 6-48 shows the cervical vertebrae, with the superior and inferior vertebral notches forming the intervertebral foramina. The bodies of the vertebrae are separated by intervertebral discs.

The transverse CT image in Fig. 6-49 shows the hyoid bone anterior to the oropharynx and posterior to the tongue. The hyoid bone is located in the neck just superior to the larynx. The hyoid is unique because it does not articulate directly with any other bone; instead, it is suspended by ligaments. Throat muscles, which are located in the anterior triangle of the neck, help form the floor of the oral cavity, and all are attached to the hyoid bone. The image shows the parotid gland lateral to the hyoid and the sternocleidomastoid muscle posterior to the

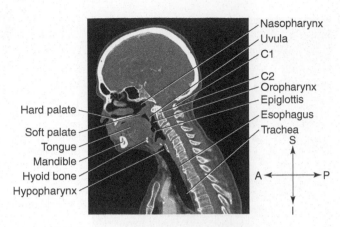

FIG. 6-47. Midsagittal CT image through the neck.

Nasopharynx
Uvula
C1
C2
Oropharynx
Epiglottis
Esophagus
Trachea

Hard palate
Soft palate
Tongue
Mandible
Hyoid bone
Hypopharynx

parotid gland. A typical cervical vertebra with transverse foramina containing vertebral vessels is present. The internal and external jugular veins are separated by the sternocleidomastoid muscle, and the external carotid artery is anterior to the internal carotid artery.

The transverse CT image in Fig. 6-50 is similar to the one in Fig. 6-49 but is from a different individual. It shows many of the same structures seen in Fig. 6-49. Of particular note is the base of the epiglottis and vallecula. The levator scapulae muscles are lateral to the cervical vertebra. Note the bifid spinous process on the vertebra.

The transverse CT image in Fig. 6-51 shows the thyroid and cricoid cartilages of the larynx. Vestibular folds project into the lumen, creating a narrow slit called the *rima vestibuli.* The larger space is the vestibule of the larynx. Because this section is inferior to the bifurcation of the common carotid artery, that is the only artery present. The vagus nerve, though difficult to see, is slightly posterior to and between the common carotid artery and the internal jugular vein.

The transverse CT image in Fig. 6-52 is near the junction of the cricoid cartilage and the first tracheal cartilage. The opening, or space, is the most interior cavity of the larynx, the infraglottic region. The lobes of the thyroid gland are adjacent to the cartilage and medial to the internal jugular vein. The esophagus is posterior the tracheal cartilage.

The transverse CT image in Fig. 6-53 is slightly inferior to the one in Fig. 6-52 and shows the typical shape and

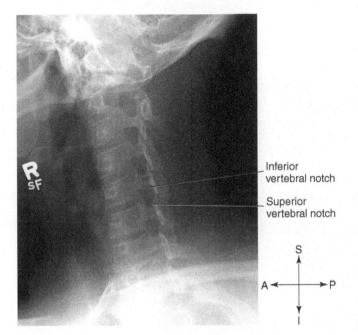

FIG. 6-48. Radiograph of the cervical vertebrae.

Inferior vertebral notch

Superior vertebral notch

Tongue
Hyoid bone
Pharyngeal constrictor muscle
Retropharyngeal space
Internal jugular vein

FIG. 6-49. Transverse CT image through the hyoid bone.

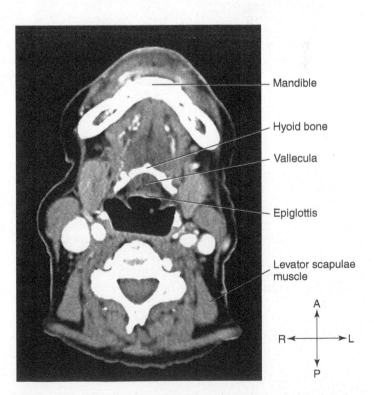

Mandible
Hyoid bone
Vallecula
Epiglottis
Levator scapulae muscle

FIG. 6-50. Transverse CT image of the neck at the level of the hyoid bone and the attachment of the epiglottis.

Rima vestibuli
Vestibular fold
Thyroid cartilage
Cricoid cartilage
Vagus nerve

FIG. 6-51. Transverse CT image through the larynx.

Trachea
Esophagus
Rib
Spinal cord

FIG. 6-53. Transverse CT image through the trachea and esophagus.

Sternocleidomastoid muscle
Thyroid gland
Internal jugular vein

FIG. 6-52. Transverse CT image through the neck at the level of the trachea.

relationships of the trachea. This image shows ribs articulating with the thoracic vertebra.

The sonogram in Fig. 6-54 shows both lobes of the thyroid gland connected by the isthmus that is located anterior to the trachea. The internal jugular veins are lateral to the thyroid gland.

The midsagittal CT image in Fig. 6-55 offers a review of some of the structures in the head and shows the upper region of the neck. In the brain it shows the tentorium cerebelli with the straight sinus, the cerebral aqueduct,

and the fourth ventricle. The great cerebral vein is visible in the superior cistern with the calcified pineal gland. The midbrain, pons, and medulla oblongata form the brainstem, and the basilar artery is in the pontine cistern. The sphenoidal sinus and pituitary gland are in the sphenoid bone. Frontal sinuses are in the frontal bone. The hard palate separates the nasal cavity from the oral cavity. The nasopharynx is posterior to the nasal cavity and continues as the oropharynx in the region of the oral cavity. Cervical vertebrae form the skeletal structure of the neck.

FIG. 6-54. Bilateral sonogram of the thyroid gland.

FIG. 6-55. Midsagittal CT image of the head and upper neck.

Important Anatomical Relationships in the Vertebral Column, Spinal Cord, and Neck

- Cervical and lumbar curvatures are convex anteriorly (see Fig. 6-22).
- Thoracic and sacral curvatures are concave anteriorly (see Fig. 6-22).
- Superior and inferior vertebral notches of adjacent vertebrae form intervertebral foramina, which transmit spinal nerves and blood vessels (see Figs. 6-2, 6-12, and 6-23).
- The dura mater of the spinal cord consists of a single layer and is separated from vertebral bones by an epidural space, which is filled with loose connective tissue and adipose tissue (see Fig. 6-27).
- In the spinal cord, gray matter is in the central region and is surrounded by white matter (see Fig. 6-30).
- The spinal cord is shorter than the vertebral column, therefore spinal cord segments do not correspond directly with vertebral levels. In most regions, spinal nerves descend before passing through the corresponding intervertebral foramen (see Fig. 6-29).

- Each spinal nerve has a dorsal root with a ganglion and a ventral root; these join to form the spinal nerve (see Fig. 6-27).
- The sternocleidomastoid muscle separates the neck into an anterior triangle and a posterior triangle (see Fig. 6-31).
- The submandibular gland is anterior to the parotid gland and medial to the angle of the mandible (see Fig. 6-40).
- The oropharynx is posterior to the oral cavity (see Figs. 6-33 and 6-38).
- The laryngopharynx (hypopharynx) is posterior to the larynx (see Fig. 6-33).
- The internal carotid arteries are anterior and medial to the internal jugular veins in superior regions of the neck, because the carotid canal is anterior to the jugular foramen (see Fig. 6-38).
- The masseter muscle is lateral to the ramus of the mandible, and the temporalis is medial to the ramus (see Figs. 6-38 and 6-39).
- In the carotid sheath, the internal jugular vein is anterior and lateral to the common carotid artery (see Figs. 6-32 and 6-36).
- In the neck, the vagus nerve is within the carotid sheath and is between the internal jugular vein and the common carotid artery (see Fig. 6-32).
- The parotid gland is posterior to the ramus of the mandible, anterior to the mastoid, and lateral to the internal jugular vein and internal carotid artery (see Figs. 6-38, 6-39, and 6-41).
- The external jugular vein is lateral to the internal jugular vein and is separated from the internal jugular vein by the parotid gland or the sternocleidomastoid muscle (see Figs. 6-38 and 6-40).
- At higher levels, the external carotid artery is lateral to the internal carotid artery, but at lower levels, near the bifurcation of the common carotid artery, the external carotid artery may be medial to the internal carotid artery. The external carotid artery typically is anterior to the internal carotid artery (see Figs. 6-38 and 6-40).

- The lobes of the thyroid gland are lateral to the trachea. The isthmus of the thyroid, which connects the two lobes, is anterior to the trachea (see Figs. 6-32 and 6-36).
- The esophagus is posterior to the trachea (see Figs. 6-32 and 6-35).
- The internal jugular vein is anterior to the common carotid artery in inferior regions of the neck, because the internal jugular veins drain into the anteriorly positioned brachiocephalic veins (see Figs. 6-32 and 6-36).
- The brachial plexus is posterior to the clavicle and is between the anterior scalene and middle scalene muscles (see Fig. 6-44).

Summary

- Typical vertebrae have a centrum, vertebral arch, transverse processes, spinous process, laminae, pedicles, vertebral notch, and articular processes.
- Cervical vertebrae have a transverse foramen in each transverse process and bifid spinous processes.
- The atlas is C1; it has no body and no spinous process, and it has short transverse processes. The axis is C2, which has an odontoid process.
- Thoracic vertebrae have costal facets and long spinous processes.
- Lumbar vertebrae have a large, heavy body and a short, blunt spinous process.
- The sacrum consists of five vertebrae that fuse to form one piece. The coccyx consists of three to five bones that fuse into one.
- Intervertebral discs have a central core, called the *nucleus pulposus*, and an outer ring, called the *anulus fibrosus*. The discs are designed for strength, act as shock absorbers, and lend flexibility to the vertebral column.
- The cervical and lumbar curvatures are convex anteriorly. The thoracic and sacral curves are concave anteriorly. Curvatures increase the strength, resilience, and flexibility of the vertebral column.
- Scoliosis is an abnormal lateral curvature; kyphosis is an exaggerated thoracic curvature; and lordosis is an exaggerated lumbar curvature.
- Anterior longitudinal ligaments extend along the anterior surface of the vertebral bodies; posterior longitudinal ligaments extend along the posterior surface of the vertebral bodies, inside the vertebral canal; ligamenta flava are short bands that connect the laminae of adjacent vertebrae; interspinous ligaments extend between adjacent spinous processes; supraspinous ligaments join the tips of adjacent spinous processes; ligamentum nuchae are the interspinous and supraspinous ligaments from C7 upward to the occipital bone; intertransverse ligaments connect adjacent transverse processes.
- The superficial layer of intrinsic back muscles includes the splenius capitis and splenius cervicis; the intermediate layer is composed of the erector spinae muscles; and the deep layer is the transversospinal muscles.

- The meninges of the spinal cord are the dura mater, arachnoid, and pia mater. The pia mater extends beyond the cord to form the filum terminale, which attaches to the coccyx.
- The spinal cord extends from the foramen magnum to L1, where it terminates in a cone-shaped conus medullaris. Each of the 31 segments gives rise to a pair of spinal nerves. There is a cervical enlargement and a lumbosacral enlargement.
- In the spinal cord, white matter surrounds the gray matter. White matter is divided into columns, and gray matter is divided into horns. The gray commissure surrounds the central canal and connects the two sides of gray matter.
- There are 8 cervical nerves, 12 thoracic nerves, 5 lumbar nerves, 5 sacral nerves, and 1 coccygeal nerve.
- Dorsal nerve roots contain only sensory nerve fibers and are distinguished by dorsal root ganglia. Ventral roots contain only motor fibers.
- The cervical plexus arises from the ventral rami of nerves C1 to C4; the phrenic nerve is an important nerve that emerges from the plexus.
- The brachial plexus is between the anterior and middle scalene muscles. It arises from C5 to T1 and supplies the muscles and skin of the upper extremity through the musculocutaneous, ulnae, median, radial, and axillary nerves.
- Important nerves from the sacral plexus (L4, L5, and S1 to S4) are the pudendal and sciatic nerves.
- Arterial supply to the spinal cord is from a single anterior spinal artery and two posterior spinal arteries. Veins follow a pattern similar to arteries, but they anastomose freely.
- The anterior triangle of the neck extends from the midline to the anterior margin of the sternocleidomastoid muscle. The base is the mandible, and the apex is the manubrium of the sternum.
- The posterior triangle of the neck extends from the posterior margin of the sternocleidomastoid muscle to the trapezius muscle. The apex is the junction of the two muscles, and the base is the clavicle.
- The pharynx is divided into the nasopharynx, oropharynx, and hypopharynx.
- The skeleton of the larynx is formed by nine cartilages. The three largest cartilages are the unpaired thyroid, cricoid, and epiglottic cartilages. The smaller cartilages are paired and are the arytenoids, corniculate, and cuneiform cartilages.
- The trachea descends the neck anterior to the esophagus. The common carotid arteries are lateral to the trachea.
- Lobes of the thyroid gland are lateral to the trachea. Parathyroid glands are embedded on the posterior surface of the thyroid gland.
- The internal jugular vein begins as a continuation of the sigmoid sinus at the jugular foramen. It descends deep to the sternocleidomastoid muscle and then courses anteriorly to unite with the subclavian vein. It is associated with the common carotid artery and vagus nerve in the carotid sheath.

- The common carotid artery ascends the neck medial to the internal jugular vein and then divides into external and internal carotid arteries at the level of the thyroid cartilage. The internal carotid artery continues through the carotid canal to supply the brain. The external carotid artery, with its numerous branches, supplies the structures external to the skull.
- Vertebral arteries arise as branches of the subclavian arteries and ascend the neck in the transverse foramina of the cervical vertebrae. After passing through the foramen magnum, they join at the level of the pons to form the basilar artery.
- A sympathetic trunk is a band of nerve fibers and ganglia that extends from the base of the skull to the coccyx. There are two trunks, one on each side of the vertebral column.
- The vagus nerve leaves the skull through the jugular foramen with the internal jugular vein. It descends in the carotid sheath in the posterior triangle of the neck.
- The cervical plexus is located in the posterior triangle of the neck lateral to the first four cervical vertebrae. The phrenic nerve, which supplies the diaphragm, arises from the cervical plexus.
- The brachial plexus is derived from C5 to T1 and is located in the posterior triangle of the neck. Nerves from this plexus innervate the upper extremity.

• REVIEW QUESTIONS •

1. What are the unique features that distinguish each type of vertebra from all the other types?
2. What special names are given to C1 and C2?
3. What is the most inferior region of the vertebral column?
4. In what two regions of the vertebral column are the intervertebral discs the thickest?
5. What are the two parts of an intervertebral disc and which is the inner portion?
6. What is the purpose or advantage of the curvatures in the vertebral column?
7. What are the three columns of erector spinae muscles and what is their sequence from lateral to medial?
8. Inferior to the termination of the spinal cord, what is present in the vertebral canal?
9. What is in the epidural space around the spinal cord?
10. Where are the two enlargements of the spinal cord located?
11. What type of tissue is in the horns of the spinal cord?
12. How many segments are in the spinal cord?
13. How many nerves are in each of the five groups, or categories, of spinal nerves?
14. Name four nerve plexuses and at least one nerve that emerges from each plexus?

15. Name the longitudinal vessels that provide the arterial blood supply for the spinal cord and state where each one is located.
16. What muscle forms the dividing line between the anterior and posterior triangles of the neck?
17. In which triangle, anterior or posterior, is the carotid sheath located?
18. What are the three components located within the carotid sheath?
19. What three structures form the boundaries of the posterior triangle?
20. What are the three regions of the pharynx and where are they located?
21. What are the three largest and unpaired cartilages of the larynx?
22. What two structures are immediately lateral to the trachea in the neck?
23. What distensible tube is between the trachea and the vertebral bodies in the neck?
24. What vein descends in the neck to join with the subclavian vein?
25. What is the cervical plexus and at what vertebral level is it located?

• CHAPTER QUIZ •

Name the Following:

1. The portion of a vertebra that is between the transverse process and the spinous process
2. The superiorly projecting process on C2
3. The outer ring of an intervertebral disc
4. The strongest major supporting ligament of the vertebral column
5. The triangular terminal portion of the spinal cord
6. The spinal cord enlargement that gives rise to nerves that supply impulses to the upper extremity
7. The bone that forms the base of the anterior triangle of the neck
8. The most lateral component in the carotid sheath
9. The glandular structure immediately lateral to the trachea
10. The structure in the neck that contains receptors for the regulation of blood pressure

True/False:

1. Cervical vertebrae are unique because they are the only ones that have laminae and pedicles.
2. With a herniated disc, the anulus fibrosus protrudes through the nucleus pulposus.
3. The filum terminale is a fibrous cord of pia mater that anchors the spinal cord to the coccyx.
4. The anterior spinal artery is located in the ventral median fissure.
5. In the spinal cord, the gray matter is peripherally located and the white matter is more central.
6. The phrenic nerve that innervates the diaphragm originates from the brachial plexus.
7. The epiglottis is one of the unpaired laryngeal cartilages.
8. On the right side, the esophagus is related to the pleura, and on the left side, it is related to the thoracic duct and subclavian artery.
9. In the carotid sheath, the internal jugular vein is lateral to the common carotid artery and anterior to the vagus nerve.
10. The vertebral arteries ascend the neck in the transverse foramina of the cervical vertebrae and enter the skull through the foramen magnum.

Answers to the Review Questions and Chapter Quiz questions can be found at http://evolve.elsevier.com/Applegate/SAlearning/

CHAPTER SEVEN

The Upper Extremity

OBJECTIVES

Upon completion of this chapter, the student should be able to do the following:
- Identify the bones that make up the pectoral girdle.
- Describe the location and functions of three groups of muscles associated with the attachment of the pectoral girdle and the upper extremity to the trunk of the body.
- Describe the boundaries and contents of the axilla.
- Identify the skeletal, muscular, vascular, and neural components of the arm.
- Describe the boundaries and contents of the cubital fossa and identify its components in a transverse section.
- Identify the skeletal, muscular, vascular, and neural components of the forearm.
- Name and locate the eight bones in the wrist and discuss the structure and significance of the carpal tunnel.
- Identify the structural components of the arm in transverse sections through the proximal and distal regions.
- Identify the structural components of the forearm in transverse sections through the proximal and distal regions.
- Describe the structure of the shoulder joint and discuss the anatomical relationships of its components.
- Identify structural components of the shoulder joint in transverse sections through the humeral head and the glenoid fossa, and in a coronal section.
- Describe the structure of the elbow joint and discuss the anatomical relationships of its components, including the humeroulnar, humeroradial, and radioulnar articulations.
- Identify the structural components of the elbow joint in sagittal sections through the humerus and the ulna, through the humerus and the radius, and in a transverse section through the radius and the ulna.

Key Terms, Structures, and Features to Be Identified and/or Described

Acromion process of the scapula
Annular ligament
Axilla
Axillary nerve
Basilic vein
Biceps brachii muscle
Brachial artery and vein
Brachial plexus
Brachialis muscle
Brachioradialis muscle
Bursae
Capitate bone

Capitulum of the humerus
Cephalic vein
Clavicle
Coracobrachialis muscle
Coracoid process of the scapula
Coronoid fossa of the humerus
Coronoid process of the ulna
Cubital fossa
Deltoid muscle
Flexor retinaculum
Glenoid fossa
Glenoid labrum

Hamate bone
Humerus
Infraspinatus muscle
Interosseous membranes
Lunate bone
Median cubital vein
Median nerve
Musculocutaneous nerve
Olecranon fossa of the humerus
Olecranon process of the ulna
Pectoral girdle
Pectoralis minor muscle

Pectoralis major muscle
Pisiform bone
Pronator teres muscle
Radial artery
Radial nerve
Radius
Rotator cuff muscles
Scaphoid bone

Scapula
Spine of the scapula
Subscapularis muscle
Supraspinatus muscle
Teres major muscle
Teres minor muscle
Trapezium bone
Trapezoid

Triceps brachii muscle
Triquetral
Trochlea of the humerus
Ulna
Ulnar artery
Ulnar nerve

Anatomical Review of the Upper Extremity

The upper extremity (limb) consists of the arm, forearm, wrist, hand, and fingers. It is attached to the trunk at the shoulder by the pectoral girdle. The arm is the region between the shoulder and the elbow. A single bone, the **humerus,** makes up the framework of the arm. The forearm extends from the elbow to the wrist. Two bones, the radius on the lateral side and the ulna on the medial side, form the framework of the forearm. The wrist, or carpus, consists of eight small bones, collectively called *carpals*. The hand has five bones, which are known as the *metacarpals*, and distal to these are 14 phalanges that form the fingers. These bones are covered with muscle, fascia, and skin. Note that in common use, the terms "upper extremity" and "arm" often are used synonymously. Anatomically, however, this is not correct. "Arm" refers only to the portion of the upper extremity between the shoulder and the elbow.

Attachment of the Upper Extremity to the Trunk

The scapula and the **clavicle** make up the **pectoral girdle,** which provides the connection between the upper extremity and the axial skeleton. The bones of the pectoral girdle are shown in Fig. 7-1. Muscles anchor the upper extremity and the pectoral girdle to the trunk of the body. These muscles can be divided into three groups.

One group of muscles extends from the trunk to the scapula. In appropriate combinations, the muscles in this group can move the scapula upward, downward, forward, backward, clockwise, or counterclockwise. These actions assist in movement of the shoulder.

A second group of muscles extends between the scapula and the humerus. These muscles move the arm at the glenohumeral (shoulder) joint. The muscles and tendons that extend over the shoulder strengthen and stabilize the joint.

A third group extends from the trunk to the humerus. This group, which includes the pectoralis major and the latissimus dorsi, adducts the arm. Table 7-1 summarizes the muscles associated with the trunk, the scapula, and the humerus.

QUICK CHECK

7.1   How many bones are in each upper extremity?
7.2   What is the function of the muscle group that extends from the trunk to the scapula?
7.3   Muscles that adduct and abduct the arm insert on what bone?

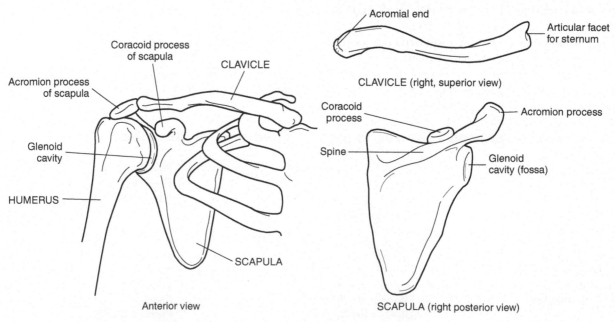

FIG. 7-1. Components of the pectoral girdle.

TABLE 7-1   Muscles Associated with Trunk, Scapula, and Humerus

Muscle	Origin	Insertion	Action	Innervation
Extend from Trunk to Scapula				
Trapezius	Thoracic vertebrae	Spine of scapula	Adduct scapula	Accessory (XI)
Rhomboids	Cervical and thoracic vertebrae	Medial border and spine of scapula	Adduct scapula	Dorsal scapular
Levator scapulae	Cervical vertebrae	Medial border of scapula	Elevate scapula	Dorsal scapular
Pectoralis minor	Third to fifth ribs	Coracoid process of scapula	Pull scapula inferiorly	Medial pectoral
Serratus anterior	First eight ribs	Medial border of scapula	Rotate scapula	Long thoracic nerve
Extend from Scapula to Humerus				
Deltoid	Acromion and spine of scapula; clavicle	Deltoid tuberosity of humerus	Abduct arm	Axillary
Supraspinatus	Supraspinous fossa	Greater tubercle of humerus	Abduct arm	Suprascapular
Subscapularis	Subscapular fossa	Lesser tubercle of humerus	Medial rotation of arm	Subscapular
Infraspinatus	Infraspinous fossa	Greater tubercle of humerus	Lateral rotation of arm	Suprascapular
Teres minor	Lateral margin of scapula	Greater tubercle of humerus	Lateral rotation of arm	Axillary
Teres major	Superior lateral margin of scapula	Intertubercular groove of humerus	Adduct arm	Subscapular
Coracobrachialis	Coracoid process of scapula	Shaft of humerus	Adduct arm	Musculocutaneous
Extend from Trunk to Humerus				
Pectoralis major	Clavicle, sternum, costal cartilages	Intertubercular groove of humerus	Adduct and medially rotate humerus	Medial and lateral pectoral
Latissimus dorsi	Thoracic and lumbar vertebrae; crest of ilium	Intertubercular groove of humerus	Adduct and medially rotate humerus	Thoracodorsal

Axilla

The space at the junction of the arm and the thorax, between the upper limb and the chest wall, is called the **axilla.** The anterior wall of the axilla is formed by the **pectoralis major muscle** and the **pectoralis minor muscle.** Predominant structures in the posterior wall are the **scapula** and the **subscapularis muscle.** Medially, the axilla is delineated by the ribs, the intercostal muscles, and the serratus anterior muscle. The narrow lateral wall is formed by the head of the humerus; specifically, it is formed by the intertubercular (bicipital) groove, where the anterior and posterior walls converge. The long head of the biceps brachii muscle is located in the intertubercular groove. The short head of the biceps brachii muscle and the **coracobrachialis muscle** are closely associated in this same region. The boundaries of the axilla are illustrated in Fig. 7-2.

The axilla functions as a passageway for vessels and nerves that pass between the root of the neck and the arm. The vessels in this region include the axillary artery and vein, together with their branches. The nerves that pass through the axilla are branches of the **brachial plexus** and innervate the upper extremity. The axilla also contains numerous lymph nodes, which are drained by axillary lymph vessels that pass through this region. The axillary lymph nodes are of particular significance because a large

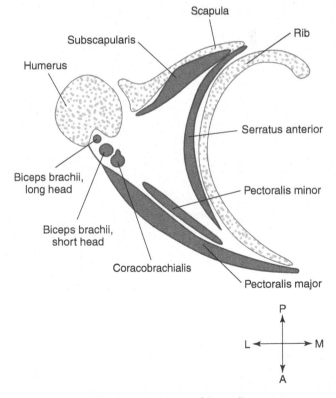

FIG. 7-2. Boundaries of the axilla.

portion of the lymphatic drainage from the breast filters through these nodes, and they are frequently involved with breast cancer.

General Anatomy of the Arm

Osseous Components.   The region from the shoulder to the elbow is the arm, or brachium. The only bone in this region is the humerus, which is the longest bone in the upper extremity. The features of the humerus are shown in Fig. 7-3.

Muscular Components.   The muscles of the arm, or brachium, are arranged in anterior and posterior compartments, which are separated by an intermuscular septum of fascia (Fig. 7-4). The muscles of the arm are summarized in Table 7-2.

The anterior muscle compartment consists of three muscles that act as flexors and are innervated by the musculocutaneous branch of the brachial plexus. The largest of the muscles is the **biceps brachii muscle.** As the name implies, the biceps brachii has two heads of origin. The short head originates on the **coracoid process of the scapula,** and the long head originates from a tubercle just above the glenoid cavity (supraglenoid tubercle). The two heads merge to form a single muscle belly that inserts on the radial tuberosity and on the ulna by way of an aponeurosis. In addition to being a flexor of the forearm at the elbow, the biceps brachii is a supinator of the forearm. The muscle originates superior to the shoulder and passes over the joint; it therefore helps stabilize and strengthen the shoulder joint. The biceps brachii muscle also acts as a flexor of the arm at the shoulder.

The coracobrachialis is a short muscle on the medial surface of the superior part of the arm. It has a common origin with the short head of the biceps brachii on the coracoid process of the scapula, and it inserts on the medial side of the humerus near the midpoint of the shaft. The coracobrachialis, along with the biceps brachii, acts as a weak flexor and adductor of the shoulder. This muscle is visible only in sections through the upper part of the arm. The coracobrachialis is the only muscle that, although predominantly located in the arm, acts on the shoulder joint.

The third muscle of the anterior compartment is the **brachialis muscle.** This is a deep muscle, underlying the biceps brachii. It has an extensive origin along the anterior surface of the distal half of the humerus, and it terminates on the coronoid process of the ulna. The brachialis is a strong flexor of the forearm at the elbow joint. It is seen only in sections through the lower part of the arm.

The posterior compartment of the arm is occupied by a single, large muscle, the triceps brachii. As the name implies, this muscle has three heads of origin. The long head originates via a tendon from the infraglenoid tubercle. The lateral head attaches to the posterior surface of the proximal shaft of the humerus. The medial head is deep to both the long and the lateral heads. Its origin is on the posterior surface of the shaft of the humerus, distal to the origin of the lateral head. All three heads merge to form a single muscle belly that inserts on the olecranon process of the ulna via a single tendon. An olecranon bursa is located between the tendon and the olecranon process. The **triceps brachii muscle** is a powerful extensor of the elbow. The long head spans the shoulder joint; consequently, it also helps stabilize that joint. The **radial nerve** innervates the triceps brachii.

Vascular Components.   The primary arterial blood supply to the arm is the brachial artery and its branches. The brachial artery begins at the inferior border of the **teres major muscle,** as a continuation of the axillary artery, and ends in the cubital fossa, where it divides into the radial and ulnar arteries. The vessel is superficial throughout its length, and it runs its course in the fascia of the medial intermuscular septum, which divides the muscles into the anterior and posterior compartments. In the septum, it is associated with the **basilic vein,** the **median nerve,** and the **ulnar nerve.** Numerous branches supply the muscles of the arm.

One, or possibly two, brachial veins accompany the **brachial artery.** These deep veins ascend through the arm

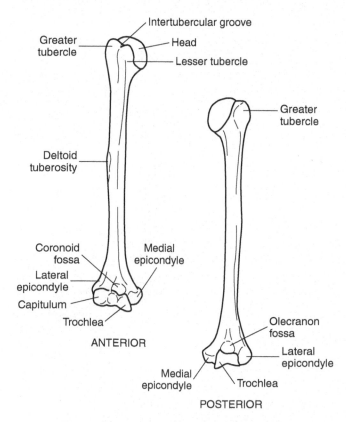

Greater tubercle
Intertubercular groove
Head
Lesser tubercle
Greater tubercle
Deltoid tuberosity
Coronoid fossa
Medial epicondyle
Lateral epicondyle
Capitulum
Trochlea
ANTERIOR
Olecranon fossa
Lateral epicondyle
Medial epicondyle
Trochlea
POSTERIOR

FIG. 7-3. Features of the humerus.

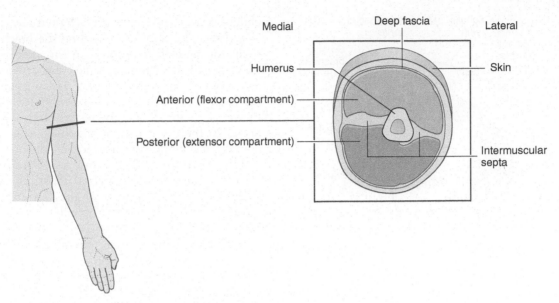

FIG. 7-4. Muscle compartments of the arm. (Modified from Drake R, Vogl W, Mitchell AW: *Gray's anatomy for students*, London, 2005, Elsevier/Churchill Livingstone.)

TABLE 7-2 Muscles Located in the Arm

Muscle	Origin	Insertion	Action	Innervation
Anterior Compartment				
Biceps brachii	Long head: supraglenoid tubercle	Radius and ulna	Flex and supinate forearm	Musculocutaneous
	Short head: coracoid process			
Coracobrachialis	Coracoid process	Medial humerus	Flex and adduct shoulder	Musculocutaneous
Brachialis	Distal humerus	Ulna	Flex forearm	Musculocutaneous
Posterior Compartment				
Triceps brachii	Long head: infraglenoid tubercle	Olecranon process of ulna	Extend arm at elbow and stabilize shoulder	Radial
	Lateral head: proximal shaft of humerus			
	Medial head: distal shaft of humerus			

to continue as the axillary vein. In addition to the deep **brachial vein,** two important superficial veins are in the arm. The **cephalic vein** is in the superficial fascia, anterolateral to the biceps brachii muscle. As it courses superiorly, it passes between the deltoid and the pectoralis major muscles to empty into the axillary vein. The basilic vein is in the superficial fascia on the medial side of the arm. About one third of the way up the arm from the elbow, the basilic vein passes deep to the superficial fascia and continues upward to merge with the brachial vein to form the axillary vein. Both the superficial cephalic and basilic veins are frequently visible through the skin. Fig. 7-5 shows some of the vascular relationships in the arm.

Nerves in the Arm.   The major nerves traversing the arm are the musculocutaneous, median, ulnar, and radial nerves. A fifth nerve, the axillary nerve, supplies the skin over the upper part of the arm. The nerves are all terminal branches of the brachial plexus. Both the median and ulnar nerves descend the arm without giving off branches. They supply the elbow joint and the forearm. In the uppermost part of the arm, the median nerve may be either lateral or anterior to the brachial artery. About midway down the arm, the nerve crosses over the vessel to the medial side. The ulnar nerve is situated near the brachial artery in the upper half of the arm. It then penetrates the intermuscular septum and descends through the arm just anterior to the medial

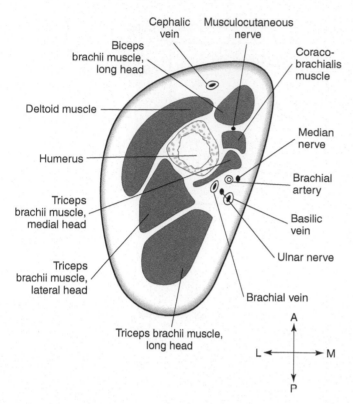

Cephalic vein
Musculocutaneous nerve
Biceps brachii muscle, long head
Coraco-brachialis muscle
Deltoid muscle
Median nerve
Humerus
Brachial artery
Triceps brachii muscle, medial head
Basilic vein
Triceps brachii muscle, lateral head
Ulnar nerve
Brachial vein
Triceps brachii muscle, long head

A
L ← → M
P

FIG. 7-5. Relationships of vessels associated with the humerus.

head of the triceps brachii. The musculocutaneous and radial nerves give off branches to supply the muscles of the arm. The **musculocutaneous nerve** descends between the biceps brachii and the brachialis muscles. As it descends, its branches innervate those two muscles and the coracobrachialis muscle. The radial nerve enters the arm on the medial side of the humerus, then curves around the bone, in the radial groove, to descend in the intermuscular septum on the lateral side.

QUICK CHECK

7.6   What is the primary function of the muscles in the posterior compartment of the arm?

7.7   What is the largest muscle in the anterior compartment of the arm?

7.8   What two nerves are associated with the brachial artery in the medial intermuscular septum of the arm?

Cubital Fossa

The **cubital fossa,** a triangular area on the anterior side of the elbow joint, contains vessels and nerves that pass from the arm to the forearm. The base of the triangular area is an imaginary line between the lateral and medial epicondyles of the humerus. The two sides are formed by the **brachioradialis muscle** laterally and the **pronator teres muscle** medially. Both of these muscles follow a somewhat

oblique course, and they meet to form the apex of a triangle (Fig. 7-6). The floor is formed by the brachialis and the supinator muscles. The roof consists of deep fascia and a triangular sheet of tendon called the *bicipital aponeurosis*. The contents of the fossa, from medial to lateral, include the median nerve, the brachial artery with its accompanying veins, the tendon of the biceps brachii, and the radial nerve. In the distal part of the fossa, near the apex, the brachial artery branches into the radial and ulnar arteries, and the radial nerve divides into the superficial radial and posterior interosseous branches. All these structures are embedded in fatty connective tissue within the fossa. The superficial fascia, overlying the cubital fossa, contains superficial blood vessels and nerves. One of the most significant of these is the **median cubital vein,** which connects the basilic and cephalic veins and frequently is used for venipuncture. A transverse section through the cubital fossa is shown in Fig. 7-7.

QUICK CHECK

7.9   Where is the cubital fossa located?

7.10 What is the most lateral structure within the cubital fossa?

7.11 What significant vein is located in the superficial fascia that overlies the cubital fossa?

General Anatomy of the Forearm

Osseous Components.   The forearm, or antebrachium, extends from the elbow to the wrist. The skeleton of the forearm consists of two bones, the **radius** and the **ulna.** In anatomical position, the bones are parallel, with the radius on the lateral side and the ulna on the medial side. An interosseous membrane connects the two bones and also

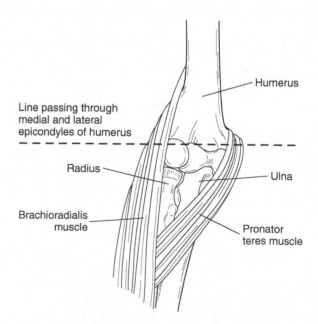

Humerus

Line passing through medial and lateral epicondyles of humerus

Radius

Ulna

Brachioradialis muscle

Pronator teres muscle

FIG. 7-6. Diagram of the boundaries of the cubital fossa.

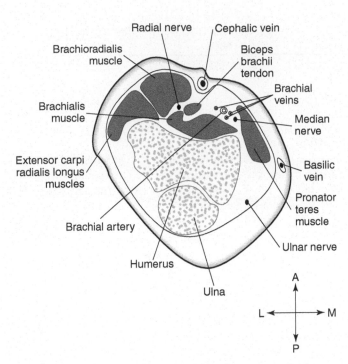

FIG. 7-7. Transverse section through the cubital fossa showing the boundaries and contents of the fossa.

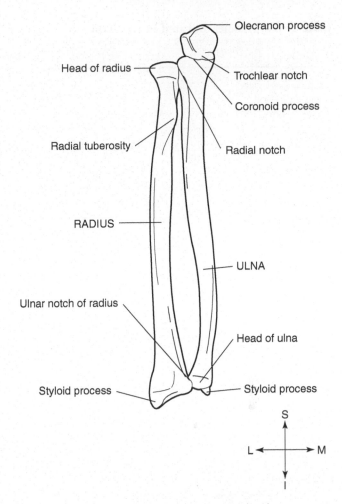

FIG. 7-8. Features of the radius and the ulna.

separates the muscles of the forearm into the anterior flexor compartment and the posterior extensor compartment. Rotation of the proximal and distal radioulnar joints allows the hand to function in either the pronated or supinated position. Some of the features of the radius and the ulna are shown in Fig. 7-8.

Muscular Components, In general, the muscles of the forearm act on the wrist, the hand, and the digits (Table 7-3). Exceptions to this include the brachioradialis, which flexes the elbow joint, and the pronator and supinator muscles. The radius, ulna, interosseous membrane, and an intermuscular septum divide the muscles of the forearm into anterior and posterior compartments (Fig. 7-9).

The anterior muscle compartment contains the flexor/pronator group of muscles. Superficial muscles in this group arise from the medial epicondyle of the humerus by a common flexor origin. These muscles cross the elbow joint and are anterior to it; consequently, they act as weak flexors of the elbow in addition to their function with the wrist or hand. All of the superficial muscles, except the flexor carpi ulnaris, are innervated by the median nerve. The flexor carpi ulnaris is innervated by the ulnar nerve.

The deep muscles of the anterior compartment, which include two flexor muscles and a pronator, originate from the anterior surfaces of the radius and the ulna. These are innervated by the anterior interosseous branch of the median nerve. A portion of the flexor digitorum profundus is supplied by the ulnar nerve.

The posterior muscle compartment contains the extensor/supinator group of muscles. In addition, the brachioradialis muscle is considered part of this compartment. Four of the superficial extensors arise from a common origin on the lateral epicondyle of the humerus.

The brachioradialis and the extensor carpi radialis longus arise from the lateral supracondylar ridge of the humerus rather than from the common extensor origin with the other superficial muscles. The brachioradialis is a lateral muscle that inserts on the styloid process of the radius, and it flexes the elbow joint rather than acting on the wrist or hand. Four of the five deep muscles are extensors. The fifth muscle, the supinator, acts on the forearm, rather than on the hand and digits. The radial nerve and its branches innervate all the muscles of the posterior compartment.

QUICK CHECK

7.12   In the forearm, what separates the muscles into anterior and posterior compartments?

7.13   In general, the muscles in the anterior compartment have what function?

TABLE 7-3   Muscles Located in the Arm

Muscle	Origin	Insertion	Action	Innervation
Anterior Compartment				
Superficial Muscles				
Flexor carpi radialis	Medial epicondyle	Metacarpals, second and third	Flex hand	Median
Flexor carpi ulnaris	Medial epicondyle	Carpals: pisiform and hamate	Flex hand	Ulnar
Palmaris longus	Medial epicondyle	Flexor retinaculum	Flex hand	Median
Pronator teres	Medial epicondyle	Radius, lateral surface	Pronate hand	Median
Flexor digitorum superficialis	Medial epicondyle	Middle phalanges of fingers	Flex fingers	Median
Deep Muscles				
Flexor digitorum profundus	Ulna	Distal phalanges of fingers	Flex fingers	Median and ulnar
Flexor pollicis longus	Radius	Distal phalanx of thumb	Flex thumb	Median
Pronator quadratus	Distal ulna	Distal radius	Pronate hand	Median
Posterior Compartment				
Superficial Muscles				
Extensor carpi ulnaris	Lateral epicondyle	Fifth metacarpal	Extend hand	Radial
Extensor carpi radialis brevis	Lateral epicondyle	Third metacarpal	Extend hand	Radial
Extensor digiti minimi	Lateral epicondyle	Proximal phalanx of fifth finger	Extend fifth finger	Radial
Extensor digitorum	Lateral epicondyle	Phalanges	Extend fingers	Radial
Extensor carpi radialis longus	Lateral supracondylar ridge	Second metacarpal	Extend hand	Radial
Brachioradialis	Lateral supracondylar ridge	Styloid of radius	Flex forearm	Radial
Deep Muscles				
Extensor pollicis brevis	Radius	Proximal phalanx of thumb	Extend thumb	Radial
Extensor pollicis longus	Ulna	Distal phalanx of thumb	Extend thumb	Radial
Extensor indicis	Ulna	Phalanx of index finger	Extend index finger	Radial
Abductor pollicis longus	Radius and ulna	First metacarpal	Abduct thumb	Radial
Supinator	Lateral epicondyle	Proximal radius	Supinate hand	Radial

Vascular Components. The brachial artery, which is located in the arm, divides into the radial and ulnar arteries in the cubital fossa. The **radial artery,** which is the smaller of the two vessels, courses distally, deep to the brachioradialis muscle. Near the wrist it becomes more superficial and can be palpated against the anterior surface of the radius. The radial artery enters the palm and terminates in the deep palmar arch. Along its course, the radial artery gives off branches to nearby muscles.

The **ulnar artery** continues distally from the cubital fossa, between the superficial and deep muscle layers on the medial side of the anterior compartment. Near its origin in the cubital fossa, the ulnar artery gives off a common interosseous branch. This branch immediately divides into the anterior and posterior interosseous arteries. The anterior branch courses distally along the anterior surface of the interosseous membrane. The posterior interosseous artery enters the posterior compartment and supplies the muscles in that region. The ulnar artery terminates in superficial and deep palmar arches. Veins accompany most of the arteries.

Nerves in the Forearm. The largest nerve in the forearm is the median nerve. It begins in the axilla as a branch of the brachial plexus and descends through the arm without dividing into branches. In the cubital region, the median nerve passes over the ulnar artery and then descends through the forearm, lateral to the ulnar artery, between the superficial and deep muscle layers in the anterior compartment. Near the wrist, the nerve becomes superficial. The median nerve supplies all the superficial

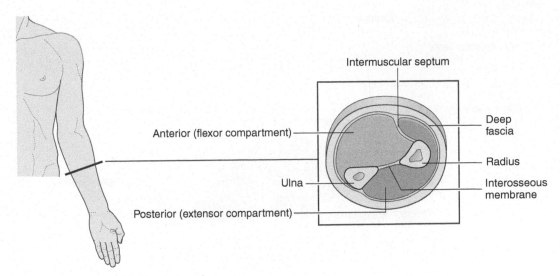

FIG. 7-9. Muscle compartments of the forearm. (Modified from Drake R, Vogl W, Mitchell AW: *Gray's anatomy for students,* London, 2005, Elsevier/Churchill Livingstone.)

muscles in the anterior compartment except the flexor carpi ulnaris. The anterior interosseous branch of the median nerve supplies most of the deep muscles of the anterior compartment.

The **ulnar nerve** is on the medial side of the anterior compartment. It supplies the flexor carpi ulnaris muscle. The radial nerve descends along the lateral side of the arm and supplies muscles of the posterior compartment. In the region of the elbow, the radial nerve divides into the superficial and deep branches. The superficial branch continues distally under the brachioradialis muscle and innervates the brachioradialis and flexor carpi radialis muscles. The deep branch becomes the posterior interosseous nerve, which descends along the posterior surface of the interosseous membrane. This nerve supplies all the muscles of the posterior compartment except for two muscles that are supplied by the superficial branch of the radial nerve. Fig. 7-10 shows some of the vessels and nerves in the forearm.

> ### QUICK CHECK
> **7.14** What are the two major arteries in the forearm?
> **7.15** What is the largest nerve in the forearm?

Wrist and Carpal Tunnel

The wrist, or carpus, consists of eight bones arranged in two irregular rows of four bones each (Fig. 7-11). The proximal row, from lateral to medial, contains the scaphoid, lunate, **triquetral,** and pisiform. The distal row, from lateral to medial, contains the trapezium, trapezoid, capitate, and hamate. Fig. 7-12 shows a radiograph of the carpal bones.

The eight carpal bones in the wrist are tightly bound together by ligaments in such a way that they form an anterior depression, or concavity, called the *carpal groove.*

A fibrous connective tissue sheet, called the **flexor retinaculum,** bridges over the carpal groove, making it into a carpal tunnel. On the medial side, the flexor retinaculum is anchored to the hook of the **hamate bone.** On the lateral side, it attaches to the **trapezium bone.**

The carpal tunnel (Fig. 7-13) is completely filled with the flexor tendons that pass from the forearm to the hand and digits. In addition to the tendons, the median nerve is just beneath the flexor retinaculum on the lateral side. At times the tendons may compress the nerve, leading to "carpal tunnel syndrome." The ulnar artery and ulnar nerve are more medially located and are superficial to the retinaculum.

> ### QUICK CHECK
> **7.16** What fibrous connective tissue sheet forms a bridge over the carpal groove?
> **7.17** What nerve is on the lateral side of the carpal tunnel?

Sectional Anatomy of the Upper Extremity

Sectional Anatomy of the Brachium (Upper Arm)

Transverse Section Through the Proximal Humerus.   Fig. 7-14 shows a transverse section through the upper region of the arm. The **deltoid muscle** is superficial on the lateral side of the humerus, and the long head of the biceps brachii is anterior. The cephalic vein is in the superficial fascia, anterior to these two muscles. At upper levels (Fig. 7-14), the coracobrachialis muscle is adjacent to the long head of the biceps brachii. The coracobrachialis has a common origin with the short head of the biceps, and at this level the two may be indistinguishable. The musculocutaneous nerve enters the arm by penetrating the coracobrachialis

Cephalic vein

Pronator teres
muscle

Flexor muscles

Radial artery

Ulnar nerve

Brachioradialis
muscle

Basilic vein

Radial nerve

Ulnar artery

Radius

Ulna

Radial nerve (deep)

Median nerve

Extensor muscles

Interosseus membrane

Supinator muscle

A

L ◄───► M

P

FIG. 7-10. Major vessels and nerves in the forearm.

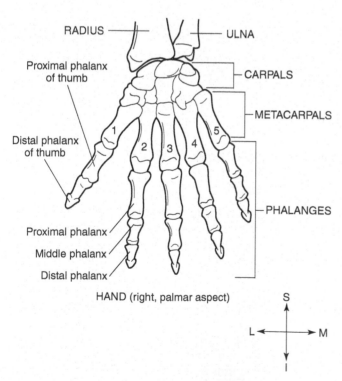

RADIUS

ULNA

Proximal phalanx
of thumb

CARPALS

METACARPALS

Distal phalanx
of thumb

1

5

2   3   4

PHALANGES

Proximal phalanx

Middle phalanx

Distal phalanx

HAND (right, palmar aspect)

S

L ◄───► M

I

FIG. 7-11. Bones of the wrist (carpus).

muscle; in Fig. 7-14, this nerve is apparent between the coracobrachialis and the biceps brachii muscles. The posterior compartment contains the lateral head and the long head of the triceps brachii. A small portion of the medial head is evident on the posterior surface of the humerus. Several vessels and nerves are apparent in the fascia of the medial intermuscular septum. The artery of note is the brachial artery, with the median nerve anterior to it and the ulnar nerve posterior to it. The deep vein is the brachial vein; the basilic vein is more superficial.

Transverse Section Through the Distal Humerus. In the distal half of the arm (Fig. 7-15), the anterior muscle compartment includes the biceps brachii and the brachialis muscles. The brachialis is lateral and deep to the biceps brachii. The coracobrachialis muscle, seen in the proximal arm, is not evident in the lower sections, because this short muscle inserts near the middle of the humeral shaft. The posterior compartment continues to contain the triceps brachii. The radial nerve is now lateral to the shaft of the humerus, between the triceps brachii and the brachialis muscles. At this level the median nerve is medial to the brachial artery. The ulnar nerve is closely associated with the triceps brachii on the medial side.

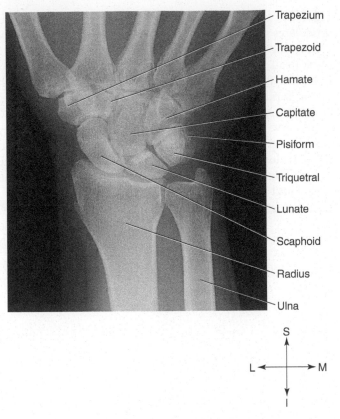

FIG. 7-12. Radiograph of the wrist.

Labels (top to bottom):
- Trapezium
- Trapezoid
- Hamate
- Capitate
- Pisiform
- Triquetral
- Lunate
- Scaphoid
- Radius
- Ulna

S / L — M / I

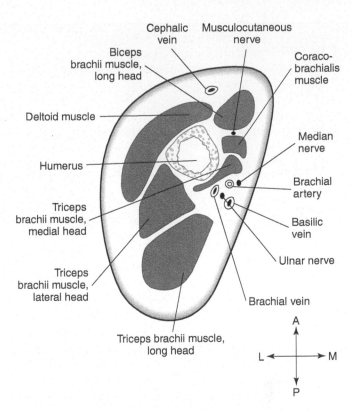

FIG. 7-14. Transverse section through the proximal portion of the humerus.

Labels:
- Cephalic vein
- Musculocutaneous nerve
- Biceps brachii muscle, long head
- Coraco-brachialis muscle
- Deltoid muscle
- Median nerve
- Humerus
- Brachial artery
- Triceps brachii muscle, medial head
- Basilic vein
- Triceps brachii muscle, lateral head
- Ulnar nerve
- Brachial vein
- Triceps brachii muscle, long head

A / L — M / P

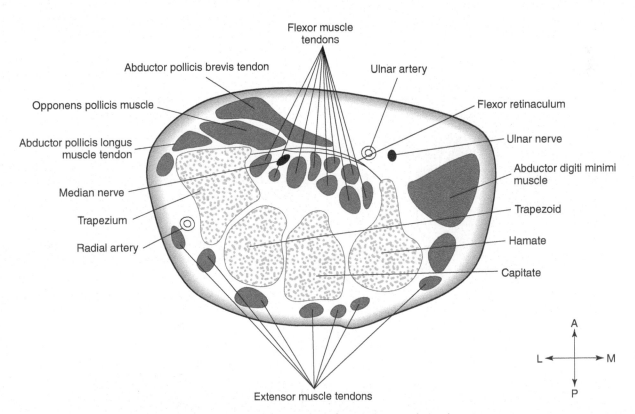

FIG. 7-13. Transverse section through the carpal tunnel.

Labels:
- Flexor muscle tendons
- Abductor pollicis brevis tendon
- Ulnar artery
- Opponens pollicis muscle
- Flexor retinaculum
- Abductor pollicis longus muscle tendon
- Ulnar nerve
- Median nerve
- Abductor digiti minimi muscle
- Trapezium
- Trapezoid
- Radial artery
- Hamate
- Capitate
- Extensor muscle tendons

A / L — M / P

Sectional Anatomy of the Forearm

Transverse Section Through the Proximal Forearm.   Transverse sections through the upper part of the forearm show the radius and the ulna, with the interosseous membrane between them (Fig. 7-16). These structures separate the muscles into anterior flexor and posterior extensor compartments. In the anterior compartment, the ulnar artery and ulnar nerve are on the medial side, the median nerve is centrally located, and the radial artery is lateral and near the surface. The superficial branch of the radial nerve is adjacent to the brachioradialis muscle. The deep branch of the radial nerve is more posteriorly located. The medial basilic and lateral cephalic veins are situated in the superficial fascia.

Transverse Section Through the Distal Forearm.   Transverse sections through the most distal part of the forearm show little musculature, because this region consists primarily of tendons going to the hand and fingers. A transverse section through the distal radius and ulna is shown in

Fig. 7-17. The large distal radius dominates this section. It articulates with the small ulnar head at the inferior radioulnar joint. The styloid process of the ulna is medial to the ulnar head. The space posterior to the osseous components is filled with tendons of the extensor muscles and with fascia. Tendons of the flexor muscles, together with arteries and nerves, fill the anterior space. The ulnar artery and ulnar nerve are anterior to the ulnar head. The radial artery is just anterior to the lateral side of the radius. The median nerve is close to the surface, anterior to the midpoint of the radius. The superficial cephalic and basilic veins are on the lateral and medial sides, respectively.

Articulations Associated with the Upper Extremity

An articulation, or joint, is where two bones come together. Numerous joints in the body allow little, if any, movement. For example, the sutures in the skull are joints, but they permit no movement. The symphysis pubis and intervertebral disks permit limited movement because the fibrocartilage in these joints is somewhat flexible. Other joints, such as the shoulder, allow a wide range of motion; these are synovial joints, which are more complex in structure than other types of joints. Synovial joints are found principally in the appendicular skeleton, because it is the part of the skeleton involved in movement. The other, less movable, joints are more common in the axial skeleton, where they contribute rigidity to form and structure.

Synovial joints are characterized by a fibrous joint capsule lined with a synovial membrane. The synovial membrane secretes synovial fluid, which helps lubricate the joint. The ends of the bones comprising the joint are covered with a layer of hyaline cartilage called the *articular cartilage*. The synovial membrane lines all aspects of the joint except over the articular cartilage. Fig. 7-18 shows the structure of a "typical" synovial joint. In addition to the components common to all synovial joints, some have other features, such as articular disks and intracapsular ligaments. Frequently, the fibrous capsule itself is thickened in places, forming a type of ligament. It is impossible (and unnecessary in this chapter) to describe all the synovial joints found in the body. The few presented here have been selected because of their interest and/or importance in imaging.

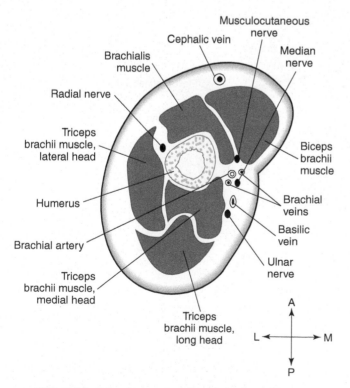

FIG. 7-15. Transverse section through the distal humerus.

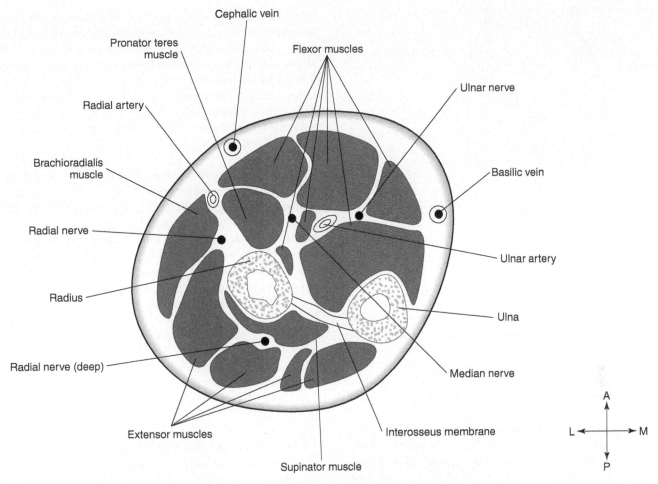

FIG. 7-16. Transverse section of the proximal forearm.

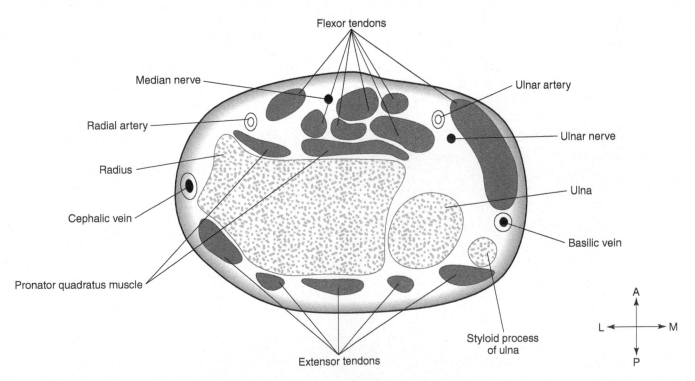

FIG. 7-17. Transverse section of the distal forearm.

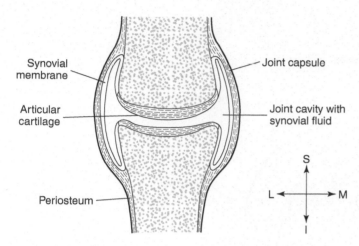

FIG. 7-18. Diagram of a "typical" synovial joint.

Description of the Shoulder Joint

The shoulder joint is a ball-and-socket joint in which the rounded head of the humerus articulates with the shallow concavity of the glenoid cavity (fossa) of the scapula. This joint has several names, each reflecting the osseous components of the joint. It may be called the *humeral*, the *glenohumeral*, or the *humeroscapular joint*. The clavicle and scapula form the pectoral girdle that attaches the upper extremity to the trunk. The shoulder joint offers a wide range of motion, but this is at the expense of stability. In other words, stability has been sacrificed for mobility. Although three ligaments help support the joint, most of the support for the joint comes from the strong muscle tendons that pass over it. For this reason, the shoulder is easily dislocated in young children before muscular strength is developed.

Articular Surfaces and the Joint Capsule. The shallow **glenoid fossa** is deepened by a fibrocartilage rim called the **glenoid labrum.** The joint capsule extends from the glenoid labrum to the anatomical neck of the humerus. The capsule is somewhat thin and loose, which contributes to the flexibility of the joint. An arch over the joint protects it from above and helps prevent superior displacement. The arch is formed by the acromion and the coracoid processes of the scapula and by the coracoacromial ligament between them. The deltoid muscle covers the joint. The radiograph in Fig. 7-19 shows the osseous components of the pectoral girdle and shoulder joint.

Capsular Ligaments of the Shoulder. Three ligaments help reinforce the joint capsule (Fig. 7-20). The transverse humeral ligament thickens the joint capsule between the greater and lesser tubercles of the humerus. This ligament holds the tendon from the long head of the biceps brachii muscle in place. The coracohumeral ligament strengthens the superior part of the capsule. This ligament extends from the coracoid process of the scapula to the anatomical neck of the humerus, near the greater tubercle. The glenohumeral ligament consists of three slight thickenings on the anterior side of the capsule. These thickenings extend from the margin of the glenoid fossa to the anatomical neck and lesser tubercle of the humerus. The glenohumeral ligaments may be indistinct or absent entirely. The coracoacromial ligament (Fig. 7-20) completes the arch over the shoulder.

Muscular Support for the Shoulder. The primary support for the shoulder joint comes from the muscles surrounding it. Four of these, the supraspinatus muscle, infraspinatus muscle, subscapularis muscle, and **teres minor muscle,** are collectively known as the **rotator cuff muscles.** These muscles, associated with the scapula, pull the head of the humerus upward and medially into the glenoid fossa. The tendon of the long head of the biceps brachii muscle also helps hold the humeral head in place. This tendon attaches to the supraglenoid tubercle of the scapula, passes over the head of the humerus within the joint capsule, and descends along the intertubercular groove. The shoulder

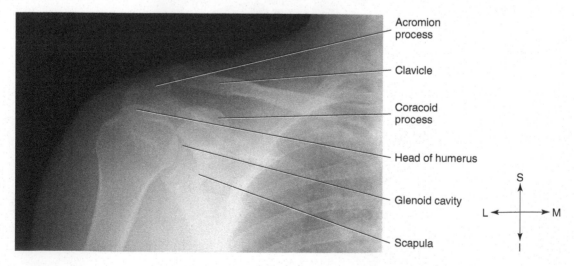

FIG. 7-19. Radiograph of the shoulder.

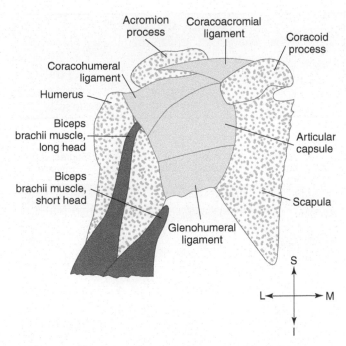

FIG. 7-20. Anterior surface view of the humeroscapular joint showing the joint capsule and reinforcing ligaments.

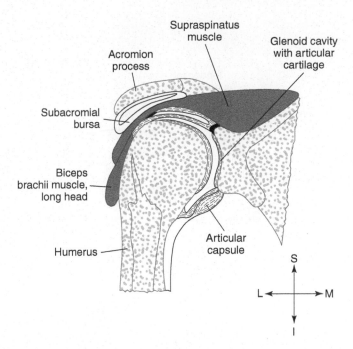

FIG. 7-21. Subacromial bursa in a coronal view of the shoulder joint.

joint has little support inferiorly, consequently, most dislocations are in that direction.

Bursae. Several **bursae** are associated with the shoulder. Bursae are synovial membrane sacs filled with synovial fluid. They are found where tendons cross bones, ligaments, or other tendons. Bursae act as cushions to reduce the friction between the moving parts. Four of the shoulder bursae are the subdeltoid, subacromial, subscapularis, and subcoracoid bursae. The subacromial bursa is shown in Fig. 7-21, which represents a coronal view of the shoulder.

QUICK CHECK

7.24 What structures form an arch over the shoulder joint to help prevent superior displacement?

7.25 What are the three capsular ligaments that reinforce the joint capsule of the shoulder?

7.26 Most shoulder dislocations occur in what direction—superiorly, inferiorly, medially, or laterally? Why?

Sectional Anatomy of the Shoulder Joint

There are relatively few components to look for when examining the sectional anatomy of the shoulder. The osseous elements are the humerus, scapula, and clavicle. The acromion process, spine, coracoid process, and glenoid cavity of the scapula contribute to the joint. Superiorly, the clavicle contributes to the coracoclavicular articulation. The muscular elements are the rotator cuff muscles and tendons of the biceps brachii muscle. The deltoid muscle

covers the joint anteriorly, laterally, and posteriorly. Representative sections showing the osseous and muscular components are presented in Figs. 7-22 and 7-23.

Transverse Section Through the Humeral Head. Fig. 7-22 illustrates a transverse section through the superior portion of the head of the humerus. The coracoid process of the scapula and the clavicle are close together, separated only by the coracoclavicular ligament. The other osseous component, the **spine of the scapula,** is situated more posteriorly. The muscular components at this level are the infraspinatus,

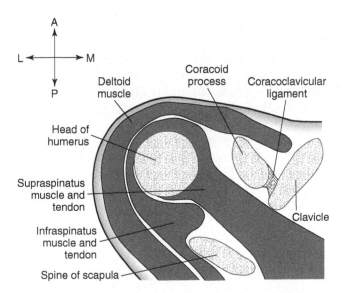

FIG. 7-22. Transverse section of the shoulder joint through the humeral head.

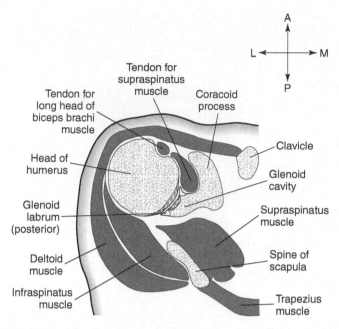

FIG. 7-23. Transverse section of the shoulder joint through the glenoid cavity.

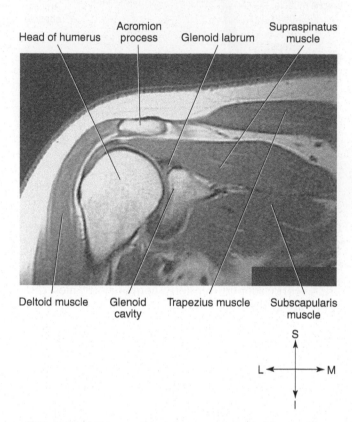

FIG. 7-24. MR image showing a coronal view of the shoulder.

supraspinatus, and deltoid muscles. The **supraspinatus muscle** occupies the space between the coracoid and the spine, and its tendon extends to the greater tubercle of the humeral head. The **infraspinatus muscle** is evident posterior to the spine, actually in the infraspinous fossa. The tendon of this muscle also extends to the greater tubercle of the humeral head, but it is more posterior. The deltoid muscle encloses the joint on the anterior, lateral, and posterior sides.

Transverse Section Through the Glenoid Cavity. In transverse sections through the glenoid cavity, the glenoid labrum appears at the edges of the glenoid cavity. The tendon for the supraspinatus muscle occupies the space between the coracoid process of the scapula and the head of the humerus. The tendon for the long head of the biceps brachii muscle is in the bicipital groove of the humerus. The supraspinatus and the infraspinatus muscles are associated with the spine of the scapula. The deltoid muscle continues to enclose the joint anteriorly, laterally, and posteriorly. These features are illustrated in Fig. 7-23.

Coronal Section Through the Shoulder. The magnetic resonance (MR) image in Fig. 7-24 is similar to the line drawing in Fig. 7-21 and shows a coronal view of the shoulder. This view shows the head of the humerus articulating with the glenoid cavity of the scapula. The glenoid labrum is around the periphery of the glenoid cavity and deepens the fossa. The **acromion process of the scapula** is superior to the articulation. The muscular components include the deltoid, supraspinatus, and subscapularis muscles. The trapezius muscle is present, but it does not contribute to the shoulder joint.

Description of the Elbow Joint

The joint capsule at the elbow encloses three separate articulations. Two of the articulations are uniaxial hinge joints that allow flexion and extension of the forearm. The third is a pivot joint that permits pronation and supination of the forearm. The radiographs in Figs. 7-25 and 7-26 show these articulations.

Humeroulnar Articulation. On the medial side, the trochlear notch of the ulna articulates with the **trochlea of the humerus,** forming the humeroulnar joint. This is a uniaxial hinge joint that permits flexion and extension. On the distal posterior surface of the humerus is a deep concavity called the **olecranon fossa of the humerus,** which accommodates the **olecranon process of the ulna.** On the distal anterior surface of the humerus is a shallow depression, called the **coronoid fossa of the humerus,** which accommodates the **coronoid process of the ulna.**

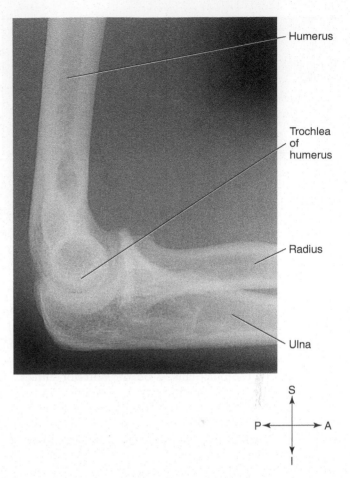

FIG. 7-25. Radiograph of the elbow in an extended position showing the relationship among the humerus, the radius, and the ulna.

FIG. 7-26. Radiograph of the elbow in a flexed position showing the relationship among the osseous components.

Humeroradial Articulation. The humeroradial articulation is on the lateral side of the elbow. The articulating surfaces are the head of the radius and the **capitulum of the humerus.** This is also a uniaxial hinge joint that permits flexion and extension. The humeroulnar and the humeroradial articulations make up what is commonly called the "elbow joint."

Radioulnar Articulation. The third articulation, enclosed within the elbow joint capsule, is between the head of the radius and the radial notch of the ulna. This is the proximal radioulnar joint. It is a pivot joint, which allows rotation of the radius. The **annular ligament** wraps around the head of the radius and attaches to the anterior and posterior margins of the radial notch to help hold the radial head in place.

Joint Capsule of the Elbow. The fibrous joint capsule of the elbow is relatively weak anteriorly and posteriorly, but it is strengthened laterally and medially by two collateral ligaments. Proximally, the fibrous capsule is attached to the superior margins of the radial and coronoid fossae on the anterior surface and to the olecranon fossa posteriorly. The distal attachments are to the margins of the trochlear notch, the coronoid process, and the annular ligament. The lateral (radial) collateral and medial (ulnar) collateral ligaments strengthen the joint capsule on the sides. The stability of the joint depends on these two ligaments.

Muscular Action of the Elbow. The primary flexor of the forearm at the elbow is the brachialis muscle. The biceps brachii is also an important flexor when resistance to movement occurs. Flexion is limited by the presence of the collateral ligaments, the tension in the antagonistic muscles, and the opposing surfaces of the arm and forearm. The principal extensor muscle acting on the elbow is the triceps brachii. Extension is limited by the collateral ligaments, the tension in the antagonistic muscles, and the olecranon process of the ulna in the olecranon fossa of the humerus.

Sectional Anatomy of the Elbow Joint

The musculoskeletal features of the elbow are probably best illustrated by sagittal sections through the humeroulnar and humeroradial articulations and by a transverse section through the radioulnar articulation.

Sagittal Section Through the Humerus and the Ulna.   Fig. 7-27 illustrates the medial portion of the elbow joint. In this region, the trochlear notch of the ulna articulates with the trochlea of the humerus. The powerful flexor muscle, the brachialis, is on the anterior surface of the joint. The biceps brachii, which also acts as a flexor, is superficial to the brachialis. These muscles are opposed by the triceps brachii, a powerful extensor located on the posterior surface of the humerus. These muscles insert on the ulna.

Sagittal Section Through the Humerus and the Radius.   In sagittal sections through the lateral portion of the elbow, the capitulum of the humerus and the radius are evident (Fig. 7-28). The triceps brachii and brachialis muscles are less apparent. However, because they insert on

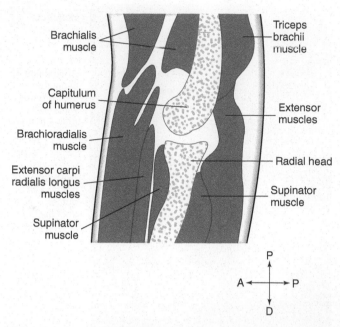

FIG. 7-28. Sagittal section through the lateral portion of the elbow showing the articulation of the humerus and the radius.

the ulna, only their association with the humerus is evident in lateral sections through the radius. More muscles associated with the forearm are visible in this section.

Transverse Section Through the Radius and the Ulna.   Fig. 7-29 illustrates a transverse section through the head of the radius as it articulates in the radial notch of the ulna. This is a pivot joint that allows rotation of the forearm. The annular ligament holds the radial head in place. The ulnar nerve and a branch of the ulnar artery are near the surface on the medial side. The extensor and flexor muscles are evident at this level.

Working with Images of the Upper Extremity

The computed tomography (CT) image in Fig. 7-30 is a reconstruction of the wrist and shows the bones of the distal forearm, the carpals, and the metacarpals. The distal radius is larger than the distal ulna. The styloid processes of both the radius and ulna are evident. Note the two rows of carpals and the five metacarpals. The metacarpals are numbered consecutively from lateral to medial.

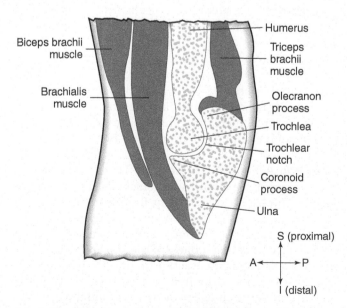

FIG. 7-27. Sagittal section through the medial portion of the elbow showing the articulation of the humerus and the ulna.

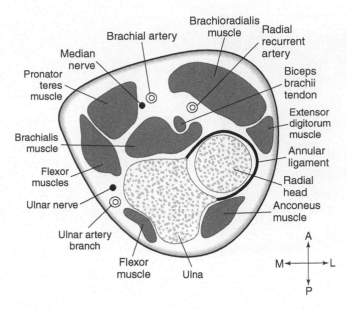

FIG. 7-29. Transverse section through the proximal portion of the forearm showing the relationship of the head of the radius to the ulna.

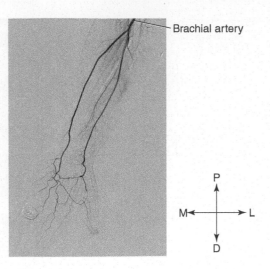

FIG. 7-31. Arteriogram of the vessels in the forearm.

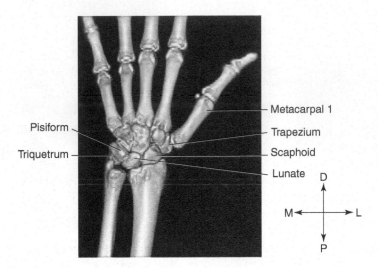

FIG. 7-30. CT image of the wrist.

The arteriogram in Fig. 7-31 shows the brachial artery as it divides into the radial and ulnar arteries in the region of the elbow. Branches of the radial and ulnar arteries anastomose to form the palmar aches in the hand.

The MR image in Fig. 7-32 is a transverse section through the shoulder. This image shows the scapula with the head of the humerus and the glenoid fossa. The tendon for the long head of the biceps brachii muscle is in the bicipital groove of the humeral head. The deltoid muscle covers the shoulder. The subscapularis and infraspinatus muscles are associated with the scapula. The teres minor muscle is between the deltoid and the infraspinatus muscles. Anteriorly the coracobrachialis and the short head of the biceps brachii muscle appear as one entity. Blood vessels in the region are the axillary artery and vein.

The coronal oblique MR image in Fig. 7-33 is in the region of the shoulder joint and shows the head of the humerus articulating with the glenoid cavity of the scapula. The acromion process of the scapula is superior to the joint. The glenoid cavity is deepened by the glenoid labrum. The deltoid muscle is superficial over the shoulder. The supraspinatus and subscapularis muscles are associated with the scapula.

The sagittal MR image in Fig. 7-34 is through the humeroulnar articulation. The trochlea of the humerus articulates with the trochlear notch of the ulna. The triceps brachii muscle inserts on the olecranon process of the ulna. Anteriorly, the biceps brachii muscle is superficial, and the deeper brachialis muscle inserts on the ulna.

Long head of
biceps brachii
tendon

Short head of
biceps brachii and
coracobrachialis muscles

Axillary vessels

Teres minor muscle

A
L ← → M
P

FIG. 7-32. Transverse MR image through the shoulder. (Modified from Bo WJ et al: *Basic atlas of sectional anatomy: with correlated imaging,* ed 4, St Louis, 2007, Elsevier/Saunders.)

Acromion
of scapula

Glenoid
labrum

S
L ← → M
I

FIG. 7-33. Coronal oblique MR image through the shoulder. (Modified from Weir J, Abrahams PH: *Imaging atlas of human anatomy,* ed 3, St Louis, 2003, Elsevier/Mosby.)

Shaft of humerus

Coronoid process of ulna

Brachialis muscle

S
A ← → P
I

FIG. 7-34. Sagittal MR image through the elbow. (Modified from Weir J, Abrahams PH: *Imaging atlas of human anatomy,* ed 3, St Louis, 2003, Elsevier/Mosby.)

Important Anatomical Relationships in the Upper Extremity

- The biceps brachii muscle is in the anterior compartment of the arm, and the triceps brachii is in the posterior compartment (see Figs. 7-14 and 7-15).
- The basilic vein is a superficial vein on the medial side of the arm (see Figs. 7-14 and 7-15).
- The cephalic vein is a superficial vein on the anterolateral side of the arm (see Figs. 7-14 and 7-15).
- The radius on the lateral side of the forearm and the ulna on the medial side of the forearm are connected by an interosseous membrane (see Fig. 7-16).
- The flexor retinaculum extends between the hamate and the trapezium to form a roof over the carpal tunnel (see Fig. 7-13).

- The median nerve is located within the carpal tunnel (see Fig. 7-13).
- The ulnar artery and nerve are superficial to the flexor retinaculum and are on the anteromedial side of the forearm (see Fig. 7-13).
- The infraspinatus muscle is below the spine of the scapula; the supraspinatus muscle is anterior and above the spine (see Figs. 7-21 to 7-24).
- The subscapularis muscle is deep to the plate, or body, of the scapula (see Fig. 7-24).
- The trochlea of the humerus articulates with the trochlear (semilunar) notch of the ulna (see Figs. 7-25 to 7-27).

Summary

- The clavicle and scapula make up the pectoral girdle.
- Three groups of muscles attach the pectoral girdle to the trunk of the body: one group extends from the trunk to the scapula and moves the scapula; another group extends from the scapula to the humerus and moves the arm; the third group extends from the trunk to the humerus and moves the humerus.
- The anterior wall of the axilla is the pectoralis major muscle. The posterior wall is the scapula and subscapularis muscle. The lateral wall is the head of the humerus. The axilla contains vessels and nerves that pass from the neck to the arm, as well as numerous lymph nodes.
- The only bone in the arm is the humerus.
- The muscles in the arm are the triceps brachii on the posterior side and the biceps brachii, coracobrachialis, and brachialis in the anterior compartment.
- The primary vascular supply to the arm is from the brachial artery. One or two brachial veins accompany the artery.
- The major nerves in the arm are the musculocutaneous, median, ulnar, radial, and axillary nerves, which are branches of the brachial plexus.
- The cubital fossa is a triangular arch on the anterior side of the elbow joint. The base of the triangle is a line between the medial and lateral epicondyles of the humerus. The sides are the brachioradialis and pronator teres muscles. The apex is where the two muscles intersect.
- The contents of the fossa are the median nerve, brachial artery, and veins, biceps brachii tendon, and radial nerve. The medial cubital vein is in the superficial fascia that overlies the cubital fossa.
- The bones in the forearm are the radius and the ulna.
- In general, the muscles in the forearm act on the wrist. The anterior compartment contains the flexor/pronator group and the posterior compartment contains the extensor/supinator group.
- Vascular supply in the forearm is from the radial and ulnar arteries, which are branches of the brachial artery in the arm. Veins accompany the arteries.
- The largest nerve in the forearm is the median nerve. The ulnar nerve is on the medial side, and the radial nerve is on the lateral side.
- The wrist has two irregular rows of carpals. The proximal row, from lateral to medial, contains the scaphoid, lunate, triquetral, and pisiform. The distal row, from later to medial, has the trapezium, trapezoid, capitate, and hamate.
- The carpal tunnel is filled with flexor tendons from the forearm, and these tendons may compress the median nerve, which is in the tunnel.
- The shoulder joint is a ball-and-socket joint in which the head of the humerus articulates with the glenoid fossa of the scapula.
- Three capsular ligaments and the rotator cuff muscle tendons provide support for the shoulder joint.
- Bursae reduce friction between the moving parts in the shoulder. Four of these are the deltoid, subacromial, subscapularis, and subcoracoid bursae.
- The capsule of the elbow joint encloses the humeroulnar, humeroradial, and radioulnar articulations.
- The lateral (radial) collateral and medial (ulnar) collateral ligaments strengthen the joint capsule on the sides.

• REVIEW QUESTIONS •

1. What bones make up the pectoral girdle?
2. What muscles form the anterior boundary of the axilla?
3. What are the three muscles in the anterior compartment of the arm?
4. What are the four terminal branches of the brachial plexus that traverse the arm?
5. What are the two superficial veins found in the arm and where are they located?
6. What muscle forms the lateral boundary of the cubital fossa? What muscle forms the medial boundary?
7. List the contents of the cubital fossa in sequence from medial to lateral.
8. What significant vein is located in the superficial fascia overlying the cubital fossa?
9. What two bones are in the forearm and what are their relative positions?
10. What is the function of the muscles in the anterior compartment of the forearm? What is the function of the muscles in the posterior compartment?
11. What nerve supplies the muscles of the posterior compartment of the forearm?
12. Name the four bones in the proximal row of carpals. Name the four bones in the distal row.
13. What nerve is just beneath the flexor retinaculum and is implicated in carpal tunnel syndrome?
14. Name four features of all synovial joints.
15. Name the three structures that form an arch over the glenohumeral joint.
16. Name the four rotator cuff muscles.
17. What ligament strengthens the superior part of the fibrous capsule around the glenohumeral joint? What ligament strengthens the anterior portion?
18. Name three different articulations enclosed by the fibrous capsule of the elbow. Which one is a pivot joint?
19. What muscle is the primary flexor of the forearm at the elbow? What muscle is the primary extensor?
20. What is the significance of the biceps brachii muscle in action at the elbow?

• CHAPTER QUIZ •

Name the Following:

1. The space at the junction of the arm and the thorax
2. The tendon in the bicipital (intertubercular) groove
3. The superficial vein on the medial side of the arm
4. The nerve plexus from which the nerves in the arm originate
5. The vein in the superficial fascia over the cubital fossa
6. The bone on the lateral side of the forearm
7. The bone with an olecranon process and a coronoid process
8. The nerve that supplies the muscles in the posterior compartment of the forearm
9. The fibrous connective tissue sheet that bridges the carpal groove
10. The fibrocartilaginous rim around the glenoid cavity

True/False:

1. The transverse humeral ligament connects the two ends of the glenoid labrum.
2. The rotator cuff muscles pull the head of the humerus upward and medially into the glenoid cavity.
3. In transverse sections through the head of the humerus, the infraspinatus muscle appears posterior (superficial) to the spine of the scapula.
4. The radioulnar articulation is a pivot joint.
5. The ulnar collateral ligament strengthens the fibrous capsule of the elbow on the lateral side.
6. The annular ligament holds the head of the radius in the radial notch of the ulna.
7. The pectoralis major and latissimus dorsi muscles extend from the trunk of the body to the scapula.
8. Muscles that extend between the scapula and the humerus tend to move the scapula.
9. The anterior muscles in the forearm are extensors and the posterior muscles are flexors.
10. The coracobrachialis muscle, located in the arm, acts primarily on the shoulder joint.

Answers to the Review Questions and Chapter Quiz questions can be found at http://evolve.elsevier.com/Applegate/SAlearning/

CHAPTER EIGHT

The Lower Extremity | 8

Anatomical Review of the Lower Extremity
Attachment of the Lower Extremity to the Trunk
Gluteal Region
General Anatomy of the Thigh
General Anatomy of the Leg
General Anatomy of the Foot
Sectional Anatomy of the Lower Extremity
Sectional Anatomy of the Thigh
Sectional Anatomy of the Leg

Articulations Associated with the Lower Extremity
Description of the Hip (Coxal) Joint
Sectional Anatomy of the Hip Joint
Description of the Knee Joint
Sectional Anatomy of the Knee Joint
Description of the Ankle Joint
Important Anatomical Relationships in the Lower Extremity
Working with Images of the Lower Extremity

OBJECTIVES

Upon completion of this chapter, the student should be able to do the following:
- Name the bones that make up the pelvic girdle.
- Name the muscles in the gluteal region and describe their anatomical relationships with other body structures.
- Identify the skeletal, muscular, vascular, and nerve components of the thigh and describe the location, boundaries, and contents of the femoral triangle.
- Identify the structural components of the thigh in transverse sections.
- Identify the skeletal, muscular, vascular, and nerve components of the leg and describe the location, boundaries, and contents of popliteal fossa.
- Identify the structural components of the leg in transverse sections.
- Identify the bones of the foot.
- Describe the structure of the hip (coxal) joint and discuss the anatomical relationships of its components.
- Identify the structural components of the hip (coxal) joint in transverse, sagittal, and coronal sections.
- Describe the structure of the knee joint and discuss the anatomical relationships of its components.
- Identify the structural components of the knee in sagittal and coronal sections.
- Describe the structure of the ankle joint, including the talocrural and talocalcaneal articulations and musculotendinous structures.

Key Terms, Structures, and Features to Be Identified and/or Described

Acetabulum
Adductor brevis muscle
Adductor longus muscle
Adductor magnus muscle
Calcaneal tendon
Calcaneus
Common peroneal nerve
Coxal joint
Femoral artery and vein
Femoral nerve
Femoral triangle
Femur
Fibula

Gastrocnemius muscle
Gluteus maximus muscle
Gluteus medius muscle
Gluteus minimus muscle
Gracilis muscle
Great saphenous vein
Hallux
Hamstring muscles
Iliopsoas muscle
Interosseous membrane
Lateral and medial menisci
Obturator externus muscle
Obturator internus muscle

Os coxae
Patella
Pectineus muscle
Peroneus muscle
Piriformis muscle
Popliteal fossa
Quadriceps femoris muscle group
Sartorius muscle
Sciatic nerve
Small saphenous vein
Soleus muscle
Subtalar articulations
Talocalcaneal joint

Anatomical Review of the Lower Extremity

The lower extremity consists of the thigh, the leg, and the foot. The thigh is the superior portion of the lower extremity and articulates with the axial skeleton. The single bone in the thigh is the **femur.** Two bones form the framework of the leg: the **fibula** on the lateral side and the **tibia** on the medial side. The leg articulates with the thigh and the foot by hinge joints at the knee and ankle. The foot constitutes the most distal part and includes the tarsals, metatarsals, and phalanges. The lower extremity supports the weight of the body; thus some freedom of movement in the joints has been sacrificed to acquire strength and stability. Note that in common use, the terms "lower extremity" and "leg" are often used synonymously. Anatomically, this is not correct. "Leg" refers only to the portion of the lower extremity between the knee and the ankle.

Attachment of the Lower Extremity to the Trunk

The pelvic girdle provides the connection between the lower extremity and the axial skeleton. In the child, the ilium, ischium, and pubis are separate bones, each with its own ossification center. These three bones on each side are connected by hyaline cartilage to form the two halves of the pelvic girdle. In the adult, when ossification is complete, the three bones (ilium, ischium, and pubis) are fused together into a single unit called the *os coxa*, or innominate bone. Posteriorly, each os coxa meets the sacrum, which is a part of the axial skeleton, at the sacroiliac joint. Each os coxa has a deep fossa, called the **acetabulum,** which articulates with the head of the femur at the hip. Numerous muscles extend over the articulation between the head of the femur and the acetabulum to strengthen the joint and provide stability. The radiograph in Fig. 8-1 shows the two **os coxae** and their articulation with the femur on each side.

Gluteal Region

The gluteal, or buttock, region is bounded superiorly by the iliac crest and inferiorly by the lower margin of the gluteus maximus muscle, which is marked by a crease or groove just below the gluteal fold. It is an intermediate region that is continuous with the lower trunk superiorly above and with the posterior surface of the thigh inferiorly. It is included here because the muscles appear in sections through the

Os coxa

Sacroiliac joint

Head of femur in the acetabulum

Obturator foramen

Pubic symphysis

FIG. 8-1 Radiograph of the pelvic girdle.

upper thigh and hip. The muscles of the gluteal region are summarized in Table 8-1.

The **tensor fasciae latae muscle is** the most lateral muscle in the gluteal region. This muscle flexes the thigh, but it also helps extend the leg at the knee by putting tension on the fascia lata. The three gluteus muscles account for the bulk and contour of the region. These muscles act on the hip joint to move the thigh. The largest and most superficial of the gluteus muscles is the **gluteus maximus muscle.** It is a powerful extensor of the thigh. The **gluteus medius muscle** lies deep to the gluteus maximus muscle; however, a portion of the gluteus medius muscle usually extends more superiorly than the gluteus maximus muscle. The **gluteus minimus muscle** is the smallest and the deepest of the three muscles. Both the gluteus medius and the gluteus minimus muscles abduct and medially rotate the thigh.

The deep gluteal muscles (Fig. 8-2) include the piriformis, obturator internus, superior and inferior gemellus, and quadratus femoris muscles. In general, the deep gluteal muscles laterally rotate the thigh at the hip. The **piriformis muscle** is the most superior of these and serves as a landmark for structures that enter the gluteal region deep to the gluteus maximus. Nerves, vessels, and other muscles are described as entering the region either above or below the piriformis muscle. The piriformis muscle originates on the anterior surface of the sacrum, passes through the greater sciatic notch, and inserts on the greater trochanter of the femur. The sciatic nerve, the largest nerve in the region, enters the gluteal region through the greater sciatic notch, just inferior to the piriformis muscle. Muscles inferior to the piriformis are the obturator internus, the gemellus, and the quadratus femoris.

The **obturator internus muscle** is an intrapelvic muscle that covers the space of the obturator foramen on the internal side, but its tendon passes through the lesser sciatic notch and becomes extrapelvic in the gluteal region.

The superior and inferior gemellus muscles are closely associated with the obturator internus muscle and often obscure the extrapelvic portion of the obturator internus. Some anatomists consider the three muscles to be three parts of one muscle. The gaster, or belly, of the superior

FIG. 8-2 Muscles in the deep gluteal region. (Modified from Drake R, Vogl W, Mitchell AW: *Gray's anatomy for students,* London, 2005, Elsevier/Churchill Livingstone.)

TABLE 8-1   Muscles Located in the Gluteal Region

Muscle	Origin	Insertion	Action	Innervation
Tensor fascia latae	Iliac crest	Iliotibial tract	Flex thigh; tense fascia lata	Superior gluteal
Gluteus maximus	Ilium, sacrum, coccyx	Gluteal tuberosity; iliotibial tract	Extend thigh	Inferior gluteal
Gluteus medius	Ilium	Greater trochanter	Abduct thigh	Superior gluteal
Gluteus minimus	Ilium	Greater trochanter	Abduct thigh	Superior gluteal
Piriformis	Sacrum	Greater trochanter	Laterally rotate thigh	Branches from S1 and S2
Obturator externus	Margin of obturator foramen	Trochanteric fossa	Laterally rotate thigh	Obturator
Obturator internus	Margin of obturator foramen	Greater trochanter	Laterally rotate thigh	L5 and S1
Gemellus, superior and inferior	Ischium; margin of lesser sciatic notch	Obturator internus tendon; greater trochanter	Laterally rotate thigh	Sacral plexus
Quadratus femoris	Ischial tuberosity	Greater trochanter and shaft of femur	Laterally rotate thigh	L4, L5, S1

gemellus muscle is superior to the obturator internus tendon, whereas the inferior gemellus muscle is inferior to the tendon. The quadratus femoris is the most inferior muscle in the deep gluteal region.

The **obturator externus muscle** is often described with the adductor group of thigh muscles because of its location. It is included with the deep gluteal muscles because it is closely related to them functionally as a lateral rotator of the thigh. The obturator externus originates around the margin of the obturator foramen and inserts on the trochanteric fossa of the femur. It covers the space of the obturator foramen on the external side.

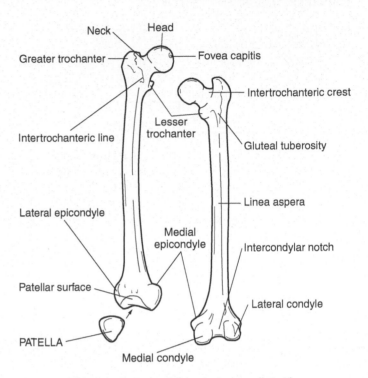

FIG. 8-3 Features of the right femur and patella.

> ### QUICK CHECK
>
> 8.1 In the adult, what bones provide the connection between the lower extremity and the axial skeleton?
> 8.2 What are the boundaries of the gluteal region?
> 8.3 What is the most lateral muscle in the gluteal region?
> 8.4 What muscle in the gluteal region originates in the pelvis and then passes through the greater sciatic notch to insert on the femur?

General Anatomy of the Thigh

The thigh is the most proximal portion of the lower extremity. Anterior, posterior, and medial muscle compartments surround the femur, which is the only bone in the thigh. A neurovascular bundle accompanies each muscle compartment. The muscles are invested by deep fascia, which also projects inward to create intermuscular septa. On the lateral side of the thigh, the deep fascia thickens to form the iliotibial tract, which extends from the ilium to the tibia. The tensor fasciae latae and gluteus maximus muscles are attached to the upper part of the iliotibial tract. Superficial fascia and skin complete the coverings of the thigh. The superficial fascia contains the great (long) saphenous vein and its tributaries. Numerous lymph nodes are located in the superficial fascia of the inguinal region near the great (long) saphenous vein. The great (long) saphenous vein penetrates the fascia to drain into the femoral vein.

Osseous Components. The only bone in the thigh is the femur, which is the longest and heaviest bone in the body. The proximal end of the femur consists of a rounded head that fits into the acetabulum of the os coxa, a slender neck that projects laterally away from the head, and the greater and lesser trochanters, which provide points of attachment for muscles. The distal end of the femur, at the knee joint, is broadened with two large condyles for articulation with the tibia in the leg. Between the two ends of the bone is a long, fairly smooth shaft. A rough ridge on the posterior surface, the linea aspera, provides attachment for muscles. Superiorly, the linea aspera expands and becomes the gluteal tuberosity. Some of the features of the femur are shown in Fig. 8-3.

Muscular Components. Some muscles in the thigh region have origins on the pelvic girdle and insertions on the femur. These muscles move the thigh by acting on the hip joint. Other muscles seen in sections of the thigh originate on the femur and insert on the tibia or fibula of the leg. These muscles move the leg by acting on the knee joint. Another muscle group extends from the pelvic girdle to the leg and acts on both the hip and the knee joints. The muscles of the thigh are divided into three compartments by intermuscular septa of deep fascia (Fig. 8-4). The muscles in each compartment have similar functions, and each compartment has its own neurovascular bundle. The muscles of the thigh are summarized in Table 8-2.

Anterior Muscle Compartment. The largest muscle mass in the anterior compartment of the thigh is the **quadriceps femoris muscle group.** This compartment also contains the terminal portion of the iliopsoas muscle, from the posterior abdominopelvic wall, and the sartorius muscle. In general, the femoral nerve innervates the muscles in the anterior compartment.

The iliopsoas muscle inserts on the lesser trochanter of the femur and flexes the thigh. This muscle is discussed in more detail with the musculature of the posterior abdominal wall. The **sartorius muscle** is a long, straplike muscle that courses obliquely across the anterior part of the thigh. It is superficial to the other anterior thigh muscles and is the longest muscle in the body. It extends over the hip and the knee and therefore has an effect on both joints.

The quadriceps femoris muscle group occupies the major portion of the anterior compartment. As the name implies, the group comprises four muscles: namely, the rectus femoris, the vastus lateralis, the vastus medialis, and the vastus intermedius. These muscles cover the front and sides of the femur. The vastus lateralis is on the lateral side, the vastus medialis on the medial side, and the vastus intermedius between the other two on the anterior portion of the shaft. These three muscles make a groove, or trough, that holds the rectus femoris. The four muscles of the quadriceps femoris group have a common tendinous insertion, the quadriceps tendon, on the superior part of the **patella.** The tendon continues over the patella as the patellar ligament and finally attaches to the tibial tuberosity. All four parts of the quadriceps femoris act as extensors of the leg at the knee joint and are used in climbing, walking, running, and rising from a chair. The rectus femoris extends over the hip joint, and it also affects that joint by flexing the thigh.

Medial Muscle Compartment. The main action of the muscles in the medial compartment is to adduct the thigh. Almost all the muscles in this compartment originate on either the pubis or the ischium and insert on the femur. The exception to this is the **gracilis muscle,** which inserts on the tibia. The muscles in the medial compartment are innervated by the obturator nerve, except for portions of the pectineus and adductor magnus, which are supplied by the femoral and sciatic nerves, respectively. The muscles are arranged in three levels or layers. The superficial, or anterior, layer consists of the pectineus, the adductor longus, and the gracilis. The pectineus is a rectangular muscle just medial to the iliopsoas in the floor of the femoral triangle. The **adductor longus muscle** is medial to the pectineus. The most medial muscle of the anterior layer is the

FIG. 8-4 Muscle compartments of the thigh. (Modified from Drake R, Vogl W, Mitchell AW: *Gray's anatomy for students,* London, 2005, Elsevier/Churchill Livingstone.)

TABLE 8-2   Muscles Located in the Thigh

Muscle	Origin	Insertion	Action	Innervation
Anterior Compartment				
Iliopsoas	Lumbar vertebrae and iliac fossa	Lesser trochanter	Flex thigh	Femoral
Sartorius	Anterior superior iliac spine	Superior medial tibia	Flex thigh and leg	Femoral
Quadriceps femoris				
Rectus femoris	Anterior superior iliac spine	Tibial tuberosity	Extend leg and flex thigh	Femoral
Vastus lateralis	Lateral shaft of femur	Tibial tuberosity	Extend leg	Femoral
Vastus medialis	Medial shaft of femur	Tibial tuberosity	Extend leg	Femoral
Vastus intermedius	Anterior shaft of femur	Tibial tuberosity	Extend leg	Femoral
Medial (Adductor) Compartment				
Pectineus	Pubis	Femur	Adduct thigh	Obturator and femoral
Adductor longus	Pubis	Linea aspera of femur	Adduct thigh	Obturator
Adductor brevis	Pubis	Linea aspera of femur	Adduct thigh	Obturator
Adductor magnus	Pubis	Extensive on linea aspera	Adduct thigh	Obturator and sciatic
Gracilis	Pubis	Superior medial tibia	Adduct thigh	Obturator
Posterior (Hamstring) Compartment				
Biceps femoris	Ischial tuberosity	Fibula	Flex leg at knee	Sciatic
Semitendinosus	Ischial tuberosity	Medial surface of tibia	Flex leg at knee	Sciatic
Semimembranosus	Ischial tuberosity	Medial condyle of tibia	Flex leg at knee	Sciatic

gracilis. It is also the longest muscle of the group; it extends down the medial side of the thigh from the pubis bone to the upper part of the medial surface of the tibia.

The middle, or intermediate, layer of the middle compartment is occupied by the **adductor brevis muscle.** The deep, or posterior, layer consists of the **adductor magnus muscle.**

Posterior Muscle Compartment. The posterior muscle compartment consists of the hamstring muscle group. The **hamstring muscles** are the biceps femoris, the semitendinosus, and the semimembranosus, and all arise from the ischial tuberosity. The biceps femoris is the most lateral of the three muscles as it descends to insert on the upper part of the fibula. The middle muscle is the semitendinosus, which inserts on the upper part of the medial surface of the tibial shaft. The most medial of the three muscles is the semimembranosus, which inserts on the posteromedial surface of the medial condyle of the tibia. Near their origin on the ischial tuberosity, the tendons of the biceps femoris and the semitendinosus overlie the tendon of the semimembranosus. The hamstring muscles extend over the hip and the knee joints and consequently have an effect on both. These muscles extend the thigh at the hip and flex the leg at the knee. All three of the hamstring muscles are innervated by the sciatic nerve.

QUICK CHECK

8.5 What is the osseous component of the thigh?

8.6 What are the four muscles of the quadriceps femoris?

8.7 What is the general function of the muscles in the medial compartment of the thigh?

8.8 What is the most lateral muscle in the hamstring group?

Vascular Components. The primary blood supply to the lower limb is the **femoral artery,** which is a continuation of the external iliac artery. It begins at the midpoint of the inguinal ligament and descends in the anteromedial part of the thigh to the knee, where it continues as the popliteal artery. A **femoral vein** accompanies the femoral artery throughout the region. The **great saphenous vein** is a superficial vein that begins on the dorsal and medial side of the foot and ascends through the leg and thigh. In the upper region of the thigh, it empties into the femoral vein. The great saphenous vein is the longest vein in the body.

Nerves in the Thigh. The **femoral nerve,** which supplies the quadriceps femoris muscle group and the sartorius, begins in the abdomen as the largest branch of the lumbar plexus. It passes under the inguinal ligament, lateral to the femoral artery and femoral vein, to enter the thigh where it divides into numerous terminal branches that supply the anterior thigh muscles.

The **sciatic nerve** is the largest nerve in the body. It begins in the pelvis as a branch of the sacral plexus, leaves the pelvis through the greater sciatic notch (foramen),

enters the gluteal region inferior to the piriformis muscle, and continues into the posterior region of the thigh. The sciatic nerve is really two nerves, the tibial nerve and the common peroneal nerve, which are wrapped in the same connective tissue sheath. In the distal thigh, the two nerves separate and continue into the leg. The sciatic nerve and its branches supply the hamstring muscles in the posterior region of the thigh.

Femoral Triangle. The **femoral triangle** is in the upper, medial part of the anterior muscle compartment of the thigh. The base of the triangle (superior margin) is formed by the inguinal ligament. The lateral margin is the medial border of the sartorius muscle, and the medial margin is the lateral border of the adductor longus muscle. The **iliopsoas muscle** and the **pectineus muscle** make up the floor of the triangle. The femoral artery and femoral vein, which are enclosed within a femoral sheath made of tough connective tissue, pass through the femoral triangle. The artery is lateral to the vein in the sheath. Fat and lymphoid tissue, also in the sheath, are medial to the artery and vein. The femoral nerve is not enclosed in the sheath, but it passes through the femoral triangle lateral to the sheath. Fig. 8-5 illustrates the components of the femoral triangle.

A subsartorial canal (Hunter's canal) links the apex of the femoral triangle to the popliteal fossa. The canal is really an intermuscular groove beneath the sartorius muscle. The subsartorial canal contains connective tissue in addition to the femoral artery and vein, which continue their descent to the popliteal fossa.

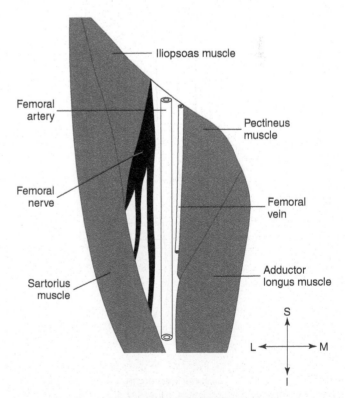

FIG. 8-5 Surface view of the femoral triangle.

QUICK CHECK

8.9   What provides most of the arterial blood supply to the thigh?

8.10 What are the two major nerves in the thigh?

8.11 What structures form the boundaries of the femoral triangle?

General Anatomy of the Leg

Osseous Components.   Anatomically, the leg is the portion of the lower extremity between the knee and the foot. Its framework consists of two bones, the tibia and the fibula (Fig. 8-6). The tibia, on the medial side, is the larger of the two bones and is the weight-bearing bone. The tibia articulates proximally with the condyles of the femur at the knee and distally with the talus, which is one of the tarsal bones. The distal end of the tibia is the medial malleolus. This is near the surface and can be palpated as a subcutaneous bump on the medial side of the ankle. The fibula, on the lateral side, is a long, slender bone that functions primarily as an attachment for muscles and to lend stability. The distal end of the fibula is the lateral malleolus, which can be palpated as a subcutaneous bump on the lateral side of the ankle. The shafts of the tibia and fibula are connected by strong, oblique, connective tissue fibers that form an **interosseous membrane.** The interosseous membrane is

continuous inferiorly with the interosseous ligament, which forms the principal connection between the distal tibia and distal fibula. The inferior tibiofibular joint is strengthened also by the anterior and posterior tibiofibular ligaments. They extend from the borders of the fibular notch on the tibia to the anterior and posterior surfaces of the lateral malleolus of the fibula.

Muscular Components.   The muscles of the leg are divided into anterior, lateral, and posterior compartments (Fig. 8-7) by intermuscular septa, by the interosseous membrane, and by the tibia and fibula. A partition formed by the tibia, the fibula, and the interosseous membrane separates the anterior and posterior compartments. Intermuscular septa separate the lateral compartment from the anterior and posterior compartments. The muscles of the leg act on the foot and toes. In general, the muscles in the anterior compartment dorsiflex the foot and extend the toes. The posterior muscles plantarflex the foot and flex the toes. The lateral muscle compartment everts the foot. Inversion of the foot is accomplished by the **tibialis posterior muscle** in the posterior compartment. The muscles of the leg are summarized in Table 8-3.

Anterior Muscle Compartment.   Anterior to the interosseous membrane, the muscles of the anterior compartment function primarily in dorsiflexion of the foot at the ankle joint and in extension of the toes. The four muscles in the anterior compartment are the **tibialis anterior muscle,** the extensor digitorum longus, the extensor hallucis longus, and the peroneus tertius. Both the tibialis anterior and the extensor digitorum longus originate on the lateral condyle of

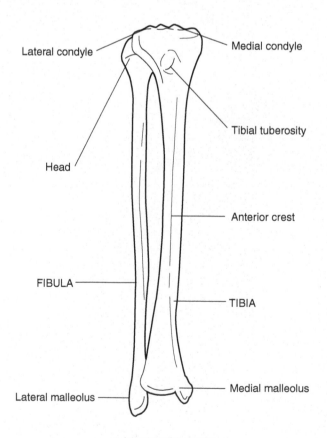

Anterior view (right)

FIG. 8-6 Features of the tibia and fibula.

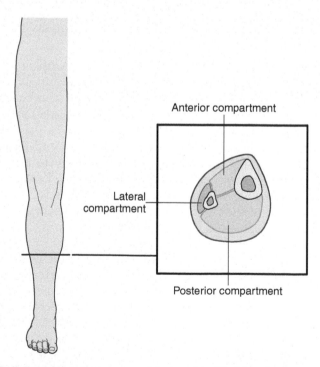

FIG. 8-7 Muscle compartments of the leg. (Modified from Drake R, Vogl W, Mitchell AW: *Gray's anatomy for students,* London, 2005, Elsevier/Churchill Livingstone.)

TABLE 8-3 Muscles Located in the Leg

Muscle	Origin	Insertion	Action	Innervation
Anterior Compartment				
Tibialis anterior	Lateral condyle of tibia	First cuneiform and metatarsal	Dorsiflex foot	Deep peroneal
Extensor digitorum longus	Lateral condyle of tibia	Phalanges of second to fifth toes	Extend toes	Deep peroneal
Extensor hallucis longus	Middle fibula	Distal phalanx of great toe	Extend great toe	Deep peroneal
Peroneus tertius	Distal fibula	Fifth metatarsal	Dorsiflex foot	Deep peroneal
Posterior Compartment				
Superficial layer				
Gastrocnemius	Lateral and medial condyles of femur	Posterior calcaneus	Plantarflex foot; flex knee	Tibial
Soleus	Tibia and fibula	Posterior calcaneus	Plantarflex foot	Tibial
Plantaris	Popliteal surface of femur	Posterior calcaneus	Plantarflex foot	Tibial
Deep layer				
Tibialis posterior	Tibia and fibula	Tarsals and metatarsals	Plantarflex and invert foot	Tibial
Flexor digitorum longus	Middle tibia	Distal phalanges of lateral four toes	Flex lateral four toes	Tibial
Flexor hallucis longus	Distal fibula	Distal phalanx of great toe	Flex great toe	Tibial
Popliteus	Lateral condyle of femur	Tibia	Medially rotate leg	Tibial
Lateral Compartment				
Peroneus longus	Lateral condyle of tibia; proximal fibula	First metatarsal	Evert and plantarflex foot	Superficial peroneal
Peroneus brevis	Distal fibula	Fifth metatarsal	Evert and plantarflex foot	Superficial peroneal

the tibia and extend throughout the entire length of the leg. They are seen in transverse sections through the proximal leg with the tibialis anterior muscle medial to the extensor digitorum longus muscle. The extensor hallucis longus and the peroneus tertius originate on the middle and distal portions of the fibula and interosseous membrane. In distal sections of the leg, the sequence of these muscles, from medial to lateral, is as follows: tibialis anterior, extensor hallucis longus, extensor digitorum longus, and peroneus tertius.

Lateral Muscle Compartment.   The lateral muscle compartment is separated from the other compartments by the anterior and posterior intermuscular septa and the lateral surface of the fibula. The peroneus longus and peroneus brevis are the major muscles in the compartment. The peroneus longus is the more superficial of the two muscles. It originates on the proximal part of the fibula and on the lateral condyle of the tibia. Its tendon continues down the leg, passes behind and below the lateral malleolus, and then curves medially under the foot to attach to the first metatarsal. The peroneus brevis muscle originates on the distal half of the fibula. Its tendon also curves around the lateral malleolus, but the peroneus brevis muscle inserts on the fifth metatarsal. Both muscles evert the foot and are weak plantarflexors at the ankle.

Posterior Muscle Compartment.   Of the three muscle compartments in the leg, the posterior compartment has the greatest bulk because of the mass of the gastrocnemius and soleus muscles. From medial to lateral, the anterior

delineation of the compartment is as follows: the tibia, the interosseous membrane, the fibula, and the posterior intermuscular septum. The posterior compartment is subdivided into superficial and deep muscles by a transverse intermuscular septum. The subdivisions of the posterior muscle compartment are illustrated in Fig. 8-8.

The principal superficial muscles of the posterior compartment are the gastrocnemius and the soleus, which form most of the contour of the calf of the leg. The **gastrocnemius muscle** originates by two heads from the lateral and medial condyles of the femur. The two heads come together at the inferior margin of the popliteal fossa to form a single gaster of the muscle. From the gaster, a long, tough tendon descends to insert on the posterior surface of the calcaneus. The gastrocnemius muscle is a strong plantarflexor of the foot at the ankle. Because of its origin on the femur, it is also a weak flexor of the knee. The broad, flat, fleshy **soleus muscle** lies deep to the gastrocnemius and is attached to the posterior surface of the tibia and fibula. The tendons of the gastrocnemius and soleus muscles join, forming a single common tendon that inserts on the posterior surface of the calcaneus. This common tendon is the calcaneal, or Achilles, tendon. The soleus muscle works with the gastrocnemius muscle in plantarflexing the joint, but it has no action on the knee. Because the gastrocnemius and soleus muscles together have three heads of origin but a single common insertion and because they function together, they sometimes are collectively called the *triceps surae muscle.*

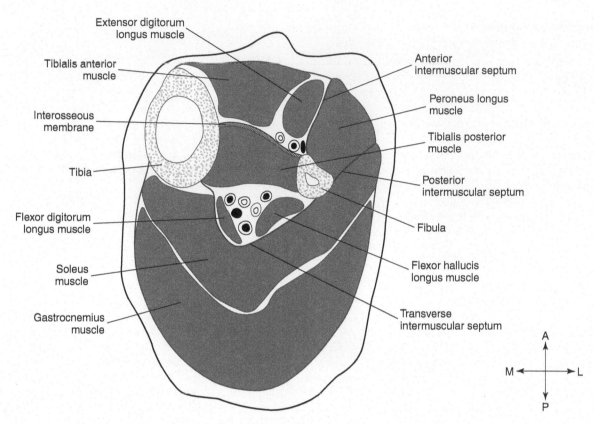

FIG. 8-8. Subdivisions of the posterior muscle compartment of the leg.

From medial to lateral, the deep muscles in the posterior compartment are the flexor digitorum longus, the tibialis posterior, and the flexor hallucis longus. The tendons of these muscles curve to the sole of the foot and insert on the tarsals, metatarsals, or phalanges. The flexor hallucis longus muscle flexes the great toe **(hallux),** whereas the flexor digitorum longus muscle flexes the lateral four toes. Both of these muscles also assist in plantarflexing the foot. A fourth deep muscle, the popliteus, is a thin muscle in the popliteal region. It forms the floor of the popliteal fossa and acts on the knee joint to medially rotate the leg.

The small plantaris is a weak muscle at the superior border of the lateral head of the gastrocnemius. It has a long, thin tendon, which may become part of the Achilles tendon or may insert directly on the calcaneus. The plantaris muscle varies in size and may be absent with no apparent effect. The weak tendon may rupture during violent ankle movements and cause severe pain in the calf of the leg. Because the muscle is of little practical use in movement of the knee and ankle, its long tendon sometimes is used as a graft in reconstructive hand surgery.

Vascular Components.   In the superior region of the leg, the popliteal artery, which is the continuation of the femoral artery, branches into anterior and posterior tibial arteries. The anterior tibial artery, the smaller of the two branches, passes through the interosseous membrane and descends the leg on the anterior surface of this membrane. It supplies the muscles of the anterior compartment. The posterior tibial artery is the larger of the two branches. It descends through the leg on the posterior surface of the tibialis posterior muscle and supplies the muscles of the posterior compartment. The peroneal artery is the largest and most important branch of the posterior tibial artery. It supplies the lateral muscle compartment in addition to giving off branches to some of the muscles in the posterior compartment. One or more deep veins accompany each of the arteries. The superficial great saphenous vein, on the medial side, and the **small saphenous vein,** on the lateral side, also ascend through the leg.

Nerves in the Leg.   The **tibial nerve,** which is the larger terminal branch of the sciatic nerve, provides the nerve supply for all the muscles in the posterior compartment of the leg. It descends, with the posterior tibial artery, between the soleus muscle and the posterior tibialis muscle. The deep peroneal nerve, one of the two terminal branches of the **common peroneal nerve,** accompanies the anterior tibial artery and vein as they descend the leg, anterior to the interosseous membrane. This nerve supplies the muscles of the anterior compartment. The second terminal branch of the common peroneal nerve is the superficial peroneal

---

QUICK CHECK

8.12   What two bones provide the osseous structure of the leg?

8.13   What is the function of the muscles in the anterior compartment of the leg?

8.14   Name the two muscles in the superficial layer of the posterior compartment of the leg.

nerve, which lies anterior and lateral to the fibula and provides the nerve supply for the lateral compartment.

Popliteal Fossa. The **popliteal fossa** is the diamond-shaped, fat-filled region behind the knee joint. The vessels and nerves that continue from the thigh into the leg pass through this area. The upper two margins are formed by the diverging tendons of the hamstring muscles. The lateral and medial heads of the gastrocnemius muscle form the inferior two margins. The small plantaris muscle also contributes to the inferior lateral margin. The roof of the fossa consists of the deep fascia that envelops the muscles of the thigh and the leg. From superior to inferior, the floor of the fossa is formed by the popliteal surface of the femur, the capsule of the knee joint, and the popliteus muscle.

When the femoral artery and vein enter the fossa, they become the popliteal artery and vein. Lymph nodes usually are in the region of the popliteal artery. The popliteal vein is superficial to the artery. The tibial and common peroneal nerves, which are terminal branches of the sciatic nerve, also pass through the fossa. These two nerves are superficial to the popliteal vessels. The contents of the fossa are embedded in the fat. The popliteal fossa is illustrated in Fig. 8-9.

QUICK CHECK

8.15 What artery and nerve descend through the leg between the tibialis posterior and soleus muscles?

8.16 Where is the popliteal fossa located?

8.17 What structures form the margins of the popliteal fossa?

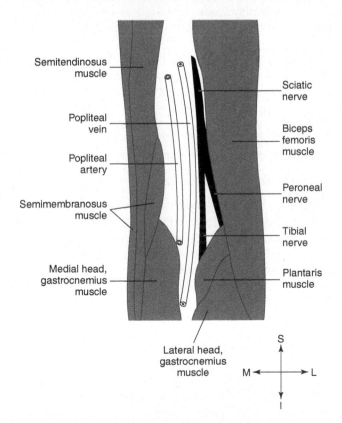

FIG. 8-9. Surface view of the popliteal fossa.

General Anatomy of the Foot

The foot (Fig. 8-10) is composed of the ankle, instep, and five toes. The ankle, or **tarsus,** has seven tarsal bones. The largest tarsal bone is the **calcaneus,** or heel bone. The **talus,** another tarsal bone, rests on top of the calcaneus and articulates with the tibia and fibula to form the talocrural joint. The articulation between the talus and calcaneus forms the talocalcaneal joint. The other tarsal bones are the navicular, the cuboid, and the medial, intermediate, and lateral cuneiform.

The instep of the foot, or metatarsus, contains five metatarsal bones, one in line with each toe. The distal ends of these bones form the ball of the foot. These bones are not named but are numbered 1 through 5, starting on the medial side. The tarsals and metatarsals, together with strong tendons and ligaments, form the arches of the foot.

The 14 bones of the toes are called *phalanges*. Each toe has three phalanges except for the great (or big) toe (the hallux), which has only two. The proximal phalanx of each toe articulates with a metatarsal. The distal phalanx is at the tip of the toe, under the toenail, and the middle phalanx is between the other two. The hallux does not have a middle phalanx. The radiograph in Fig. 8-11 shows some of the bones of the foot.

QUICK CHECK

8.18 What is the largest bone in the tarsus?

8.19 How many bones form the instep of the foot?

8.20 What is the hallux?

Sectional Anatomy of the Lower Extremity

Sectional Anatomy of the Thigh

Transverse Section Through the Proximal Femur. A transverse section through the proximal femur (illustrated in Fig. 8-12) shows the three muscle compartments of the thigh. The anterior compartment contains the quadriceps femoris muscle group and the sartorius muscle. Just deep to the sartorius muscle, the femoral artery and vein descend in the subcutaneous tissue near the medial boundary of this compartment. The medial compartment contains the adductor longus, adductor brevis, and adductor magnus muscles and the gracilis muscle, which is more superficial than the adductors. The posterior compartment contains the hamstring muscles. At superior levels of the thigh, the gluteus maximus muscle may be evident before it inserts on the iliotibial tract and gluteal tuberosity of the femur. The sciatic nerve supplies the posterior compartment.

Transverse Section Through the Distal Femur. The adductor muscles in the medial compartment are absent in sections through the distal femur because these muscles insert at more superior levels. Only muscles that extend

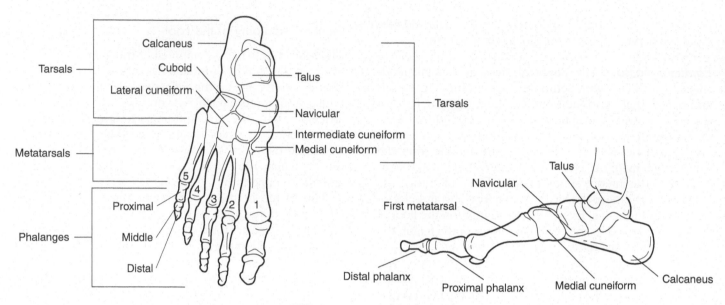

FIG. 8-10. Bones of the foot.

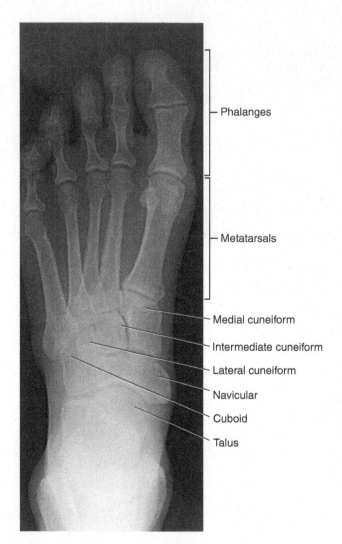

FIG. 8-11. Radiograph of the foot.

over the knee joint are evident. The three vastus muscles with the quadriceps femora tendon occupy the anterior compartment. In proximal regions of the femur, the sartorius muscle is superficial in the anterior compartment. As the sartorius muscle descends, it crosses obliquely over the thigh to insert on the medial tibia. In sections through the distal thigh, the sartorius muscle is next to the gracilis muscle on the medial side. The three muscles of the hamstrings occupy the posterior compartment. The tibial nerve, a branch of the sciatic nerve, is between the biceps femoris and semimembranosus muscles. A transverse section through the distal femur is illustrated in Fig. 8-13.

QUICK CHECK

8.21   In transverse sections through the proximal femur, what is the most superficial muscle in the medial compartment?

8.22   Describe how the position of the sartorius muscle changes in proximal and distal regions.

Sectional Anatomy of the Leg

Transverse Section Through the Proximal Leg.   The appearance of sections through the leg, the region between the knee and the ankle, varies because the muscles originate and insert in different regions. A transverse section through the proximal leg, near the lower region of the popliteal fossa, shows the lateral and medial condyles of the tibia and the head of the fibula. Muscle mass is minimal at this level, especially in the anterior and lateral compartments. The two heads of the gastrocnemius muscle are evident in the posterior compartment (Fig. 8-14).

Transverse Section Through the Midcalf Region.   At more inferior levels of the leg, through the shafts of the tibia and fibula in the midcalf region, more muscle mass is

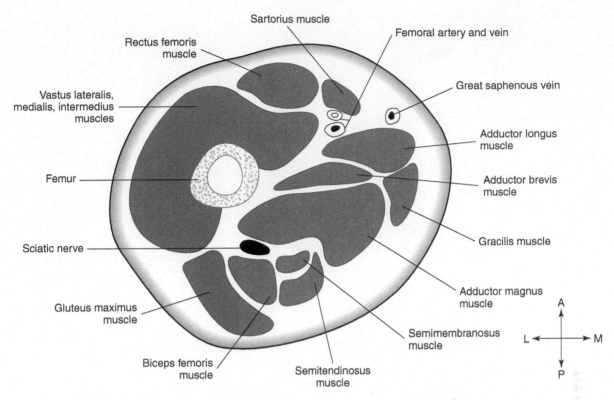

FIG. 8-12. Transverse section through the proximal portion of the femur.

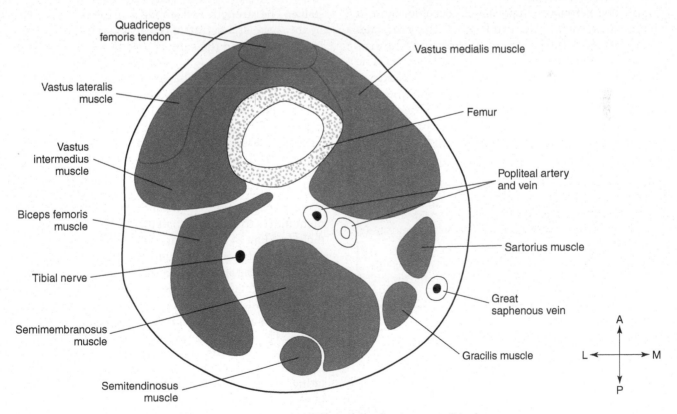

FIG. 8-13. Transverse section through the distal portion of the femur.

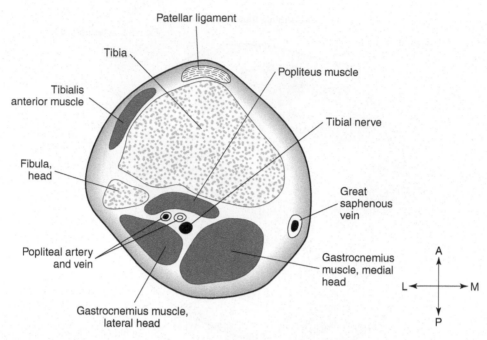

Patellar ligament

Tibia

Popliteus muscle

Tibialis anterior muscle

Tibial nerve

Fibula, head

Great saphenous vein

Popliteal artery and vein

Gastrocnemius muscle, medial head

Gastrocnemius muscle, lateral head

A
L ←→ M
P

FIG. 8-14. Transverse section through the proximal portion of the leg.

present and the intermuscular septa are more evident than in the proximal leg. The tibialis anterior and the extensor digitorum longus muscles are anterior to the interosseous membrane. The peroneus longus muscle occupies most of the lateral compartment. The two heads of the gastrocnemius muscle merge in the posterior compartment. The mass of the soleus muscle is just beneath the gastrocnemius. The tibialis posterior muscle is the most obvious deep muscle in this region. At more distal levels, near the ankle, the muscles become smaller and more tendinous. Here, the anterior tibial artery is near the surface along the anterior margin of the tibia. A transverse section through the midcalf region is illustrated in Fig. 8-15.

QUICK CHECK

8.23   In transverse sections through the proximal leg, near the popliteal fossa, what osseous elements are present?

8.24   In transverse sections through the midcalf region, what two muscles are anterior to the interosseous membrane?

Articulations Associated with the Lower Extremity

Description of the Hip (Coxal) Joint

The hip (coxal) joint is formed by the articulation of the head of the femur in the acetabulum of the os coxa (hip bone). The hip joint is a multiaxial ball-and-socket joint,

which allows flexion, extension, abduction, adduction, medial and lateral rotation, and circumduction. This joint bears the weight of the body; therefore it is strong and stable. The strength and stability of the hip are enhanced by the shape and nature of the articular surfaces, the dense joint capsule, and the capsular ligaments.

Articular Surfaces.   The articular surface of the femur is the head, which represents about two thirds of a sphere. The femoral head is covered by articular cartilage, except at a small depression, or pit, called the *fovea capitis femoris.* The ligamentum teres femoris (ligament of the head of the femur) attaches to the femoral head at the fovea. The femoral head fits into the acetabulum, a deep, cup-shaped socket in the os coxa. The shaft of the femur is displaced about 2 inches from the head by the neck. This displacement moves the femoral shaft away from the pelvis to allow more freedom of movement.

The rim of the acetabulum is incomplete at the inferior margin, leaving an acetabular notch, which is closed by the transverse acetabular ligament. The concavity of the acetabulum is further deepened by the acetabular labrum, a fibrocartilaginous rim attached to the bony margin of the socket. The articulating surface of the acetabulum, the lunate surface, consists of a C-shaped area covered by articular cartilage that surrounds a centrally located, nonarticulating, acetabular fossa. The acetabular fossa contains a pad of fat that is covered by a synovial membrane and represents the coxal attachment of the ligamentum teres femoris. This ligament helps hold the femoral head in the acetabulum. Fig. 8-16 illustrates features of the acetabulum.

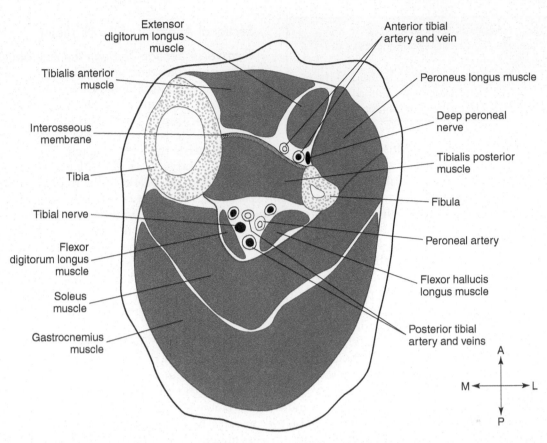

FIG. 8-15. Transverse section through the midcalf region.

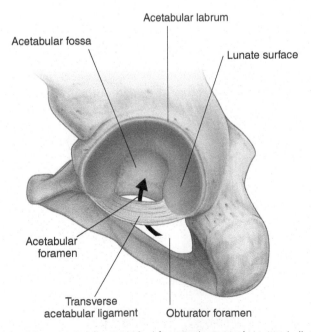

FIG. 8-16. Features of the acetabulum. (Modified from Drake R, Vogl W, Mitchell AW: *Gray's anatomy for students,* London, 2005, Elsevier/Churchill Livingstone.)

Joint Capsule and Associated Muscles.   A dense, fibrous joint capsule forms a cylinder that extends from the margin of the acetabulum to the neck of the femur near the trochanters. Synovial membrane lines the fibrous joint capsule. The capsule is thickened and reinforced by the iliofemoral, pubofemoral, and ischiofemoral ligaments.

Most of the muscles associated with the hip joint function to move the thigh as well as stabilize the joint. All these muscles originate on some part of the pelvic girdle, and most of them insert on some part of the femur. Exceptions to this are the gracilis and sartorius muscles, which extend down to the tibia and move the knee in addition to the hip. The muscles may be divided into anterior, posterior, and medial groups. The iliopsoas and the sartorius belong to the anterior group and flex the thigh. The posterolateral group is more extensive and contains the buttock muscles and the deep lateral rotators. The buttock muscles include the gluteus maximus, the gluteus medius, and the gluteus minimus. The deep rotators are located directly over the posterior portion of the joint. These muscles are the piriformis, the gemelli, the obturators, and the quadratus femoris. The medial muscle group is responsible for adduction of the thigh and includes the pectineus and the gracilis in addition to the adductor longus, the adductor brevis, and the adductor magnus. All the muscles associated with the hip have been described in the sections dealing with the gluteal region and the thigh.

Neurovascular Structures.   The principal neurovascular structures visible in sections of the hip are the femoral artery, the femoral vein, the femoral nerve, and the sciatic nerve. The femoral vessels and the femoral nerve are closely associated with and superficial to the iliopsoas muscle. The sciatic nerve, a branch of the sacral plexus, is the largest peripheral nerve in the body. It begins in the pelvis, deep to the piriformis muscle. The sciatic nerve exits the pelvis through the greater sciatic notch, just inferior to the piriformis. It then descends superficial to the gemelli muscles but deep to the gluteus maximus.

Sectional Anatomy of the Hip Joint

Transverse Section Through the Acetabulum.   Fig. 8-17 illustrates a transverse section through the upper portion of the hip. The gluteal muscles are clearly evident in the posterior compartment. The piriformis muscle, one of the deep rotators, is deep to the gluteus maximus muscle. The piriformis muscle is closely related to the sciatic nerve; they both traverse the sciatic notch. The obturator internus muscle, another of the deep lateral rotators, is medial to the bones of the pelvic girdle. In the anterior muscle compartment, the sartorius and tensor fasciae latae muscles are located superficially, with the iliopsoas and rectus femoris muscle just deep to the sartorius muscle. The pectineus muscle is medial to the iliopsoas muscle.

In the acetabulum, the humeral head articulates at the periphery of the socket, leaving a space, the acetabular fossa, in the center. The ligamentum teres femoris attaches the femoral head to the acetabular fossa.

Sagittal Section Through the Acetabulum.   A sagittal section through the acetabulum (illustrated in Fig. 8-18) shows the arrangement of the deep lateral rotators associated with the hip. The piriformis muscle, at the margin of the gluteus medius muscle, is the most superior of these muscles, followed by the gemellus and the quadratus femoris muscles. The tendon for the obturator internus muscle merges with the superior and inferior gemelli muscles. The obturator externus muscle is deep to the gluteus maximus muscle and inferior to the piriformis muscle. Recall that the piriformis muscle is a landmark for structures found deep to the gluteus maximus muscle. The three layers of the adductor muscles in the medial compartment, as well as the pectineus muscle, are evident.

Coronal Section Through the Acetabulum.   Fig. 8-19 illustrates a coronal section through the acetabulum. This shows the obturator foramen, which is an opening between the ilium and the pubis, closed off by the obturator internus and obturator externus muscles. The lateral to medial sequence of the iliopsoas, pectineus, adductor brevis, and gracilis muscles is well represented. The magnetic resonance (MR) image in Fig. 8-20 illustrates similar features.

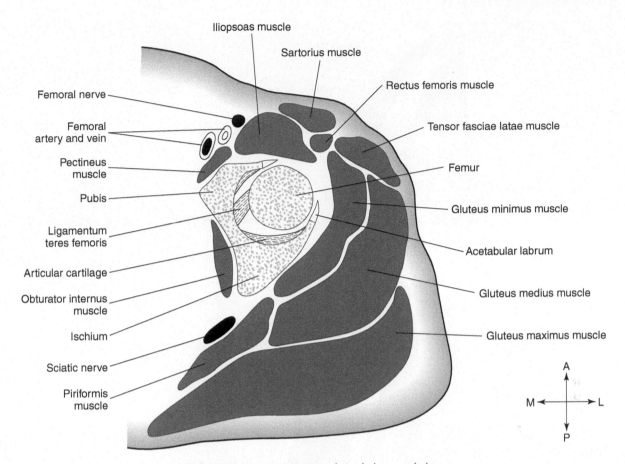

FIG. 8-17. Transverse section through the acetabulum.

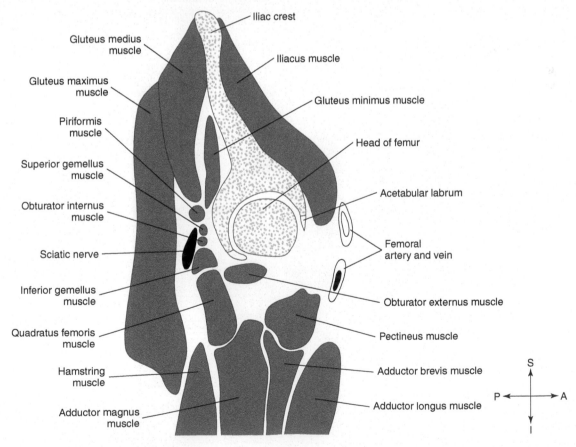

FIG. 8-18. Sagittal section through the acetabulum.

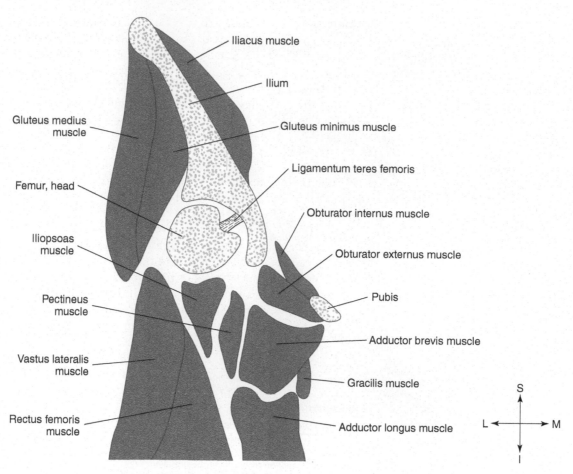

FIG. 8-19. Coronal section through the acetabulum.

FIG. 8-20. MR image of a coronal section through the acetabulum.

Description of the Knee Joint

Articular Surfaces of the Knee Joint. The knee **(tibiofemoral joint)** is probably the most complex yet most vulnerable joint in the body. It is principally a hinge joint, but it also allows some gliding motion. The bony components are the femur, the tibia, and the patella. The large, rounded condyles on the femur articulate with the rather flattened tibial plateaus. Anteriorly, the patella fits between the lateral and the medial condyles of the femur to form the patellofemoral articulation. The articulating surfaces are covered with hyaline articular cartilage. The radiographs in Figs. 8-21 and 8-22 show the articular surfaces of the knee joint.

Ligaments Associated with the Joint Capsule. A fibrous capsule forms a sleeve that encloses the knee joint. The capsule extends from a region on the femur just proximal to the lateral and medial condyles down to the tibia, just distal to the articulating surfaces. The fibrous capsule is lined with a synovial membrane, which secretes a lubricating synovial fluid into the joint cavity. Numerous ligaments and tendons add stability to the joint.

Concave, fibrocartilaginous pads called *menisci* (singular, meniscus) are interposed between the femoral condyles and the tibial plateaus. These lateral and medial menisci make shallow sockets for the rounded condyles. Anteriorly, the two menisci are joined together by a transverse ligament.

The fibrous capsule is strengthened by five ligaments; these are called *external* or *extracapsular ligaments* to distinguish them from those inside the capsule. Thickenings of the capsule on the lateral and medial side form lateral (fibular) and medial (tibial) collateral ligaments. Anteriorly, the continuation of the quadriceps femoris tendon forms the patellar ligament. Posterior to the joint, in the popliteal region, the capsule is strengthened by the oblique popliteal and arcuate popliteal ligaments. The oblique popliteal ligament is a broad expansion of the semimembranosus tendon. It arises from the posterior aspect of the medial tibial condyle and attaches near the center of the capsule. The Y-shaped arcuate popliteal ligament arises from the head of the fibula, then spreads out to attach to the lateral condyle of the femur and the intercondylar area of the tibia.

Intracapsular ligaments are inside the fibrous capsule rather than external to it. The anterior and posterior cruciate ligaments are intracapsular. They are located between the lateral and medial condyles of the femur, and they attach the femur to the tibia. The anterior cruciate ligament extends anteriorly from the lateral condyle of the femur to a point on the anterior surface of the tibia on the medial side of the intercondylar eminence. The posterior cruciate ligament extends between the medial condyle of the femur and the posterior surface of the tibia. Note that the anterior cruciate ligament attaches to the anterior tibial surface and that the posterior cruciate ligament attaches to the posterior surface of the tibia.

Muscular Support for the Knee Joint. Muscles and their tendons form the major support for the knee joint. Therefore proper muscle conditioning can reduce the likelihood and severity of knee injuries. Conversely, weakened muscles contribute to instability of the knee joint. The primary muscles that contribute strength to the joint are the quadriceps femoris, the hamstrings, the sartorius, the gracilis, and the gastrocnemius. In addition to stabilizing the knee, these muscles move the leg by their action on the knee joint. (See Tables 8-2 and 8-3 for a review of these muscles and their actions.)

Neurovascular Structures Associated with the Knee Joint. The principal neurovascular supply to the knee comes from the vessels and nerves in the popliteal fossa, which from medial to lateral include the popliteal artery, the popliteal vein, the tibial nerve, and the common peroneal nerve. The popliteal artery is a continuation of the femoral artery. In the popliteal fossa, it gives off several genicular arteries, which course around the bones to supply the components of the joint. The tibial and common peroneal nerves are terminal branches of the sciatic nerve.

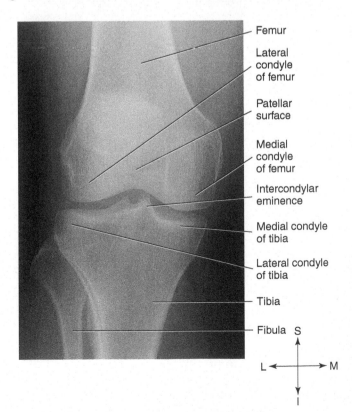

Femur

Lateral
condyle
of femur

Patellar
surface

Medial
condyle
of femur

Intercondylar
eminence

Medial condyle
of tibia

Lateral condyle
of tibia

Tibia

Fibula   S

L ← → M

I

FIG. 8-21. Radiograph of the knee.

QUICK CHECK

8.35   What type of cartilage covers the articulating surfaces of the knee joint?

8.36   Where are the menisci located in the knee?

8.37   What ligaments of the knee are intracapsular?

8.38   In addition to stabilizing the joint, muscular support associated with the knee has what junction?

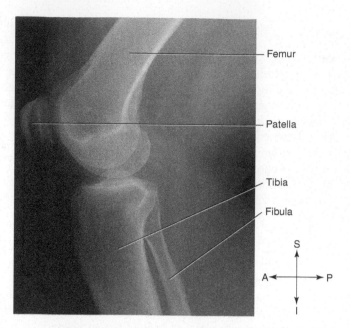

FIG. 8-22. Radiograph of the knee, lateral view.

Sectional Anatomy of the Knee Joint

Sagittal Section Through the Lateral Femur and the Tibia.

Fig. 8-23 illustrates a sagittal section of the knee joint, showing the articulation of the lateral condyle of the femur with the tibia and the lateral meniscus between the two bones. The patella is anterior to the femur. The patellar ligament extends from the patella down to the tibial tuberosity as an extension of the quadriceps femoris tendon. Three bursae associated with the patella, two subcutaneous and one deep, are also shown. A magnetic resonance (MR) image of a similar region is shown in Fig. 8-24.

Coronal Section Through the Knee Joint.

A coronal (frontal) section through the knee joint (Fig. 8-25) shows both the **lateral and the medial menisci.** The joint capsule is reinforced at the sides by the lateral and the medial collateral ligaments. The intracapsular anterior and posterior cruciate ligaments are in the space between the two femoral condyles.

QUICK CHECK
8.39　In sagittal sections through the lateral region of the knee joint, what ligament extends from the patella to the tibial tuberosity?
8.40　In coronal sections through the knee joint, what ligaments are located in the space between the lateral and medial condyles of the femur?

Description of the Ankle Joint

The ankle, or **talocrural joint,** consists of the articulation between the distal tibia and fibula of the leg and the talus of the tarsal bones. In addition, some attention is given to

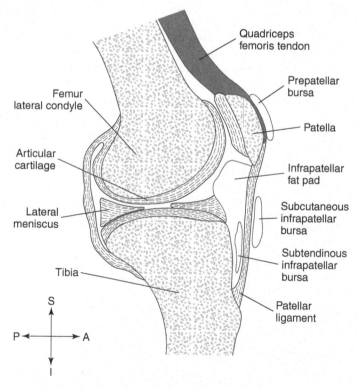

FIG. 8-23. Sagittal section through the lateral femur and tibia.

the relationships of the talus to the calcaneus. The articular surfaces of the talus are shown in Fig. 8-26, which illustrates a coronal section through the ankle.

Talocrural Articulation.

The talocrural joint is a hinge-type synovial joint, which permits dorsiflexion and plantarflexion of the foot. Medial and lateral movement is

FIG. 8-24. MR image of a sagittal section through the lateral femur.

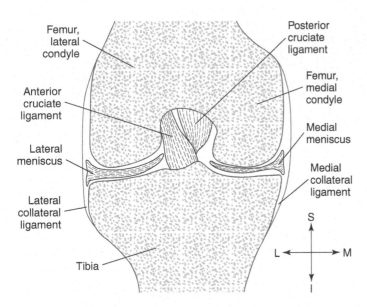

FIG. 8-25. Coronal section through the knee joint.

restricted by the medial malleolus of the tibia and the lateral malleolus of the fibula. The talus has three articular surfaces that contribute to the joint. The largest is the superior rounded surface, the trochlea, which rests in the inferior concave surface of the distal tibia. Laterally and medially on the talus are facets for articulation with the malleoli of the fibula and tibia. The radiograph in Fig. 8-27 shows the three articular surfaces of the talocrural joint.

The talocrural joint is enclosed in a thin, fibrous capsule that is strengthened on the sides by ligaments. The lateral (fibular) ligament extends from the lateral malleolus to the talus and the calcaneus and provides lateral support. Distally, the ligament is divided into three parts, according to the area of attachment. The anterior and posterior talofibular ligaments attach to the anterior and posterior regions of the talus. The calcaneofibular ligament forms a cord that extends from the lateral malleolus to the lateral surface of the calcaneus. The ligament on the medial side is much stronger than the lateral ligament. The medial (deltoid or tibial) ligament arises from the medial malleolus and provides medial support. The fibers of the ligament fan out to form a broad base of attachment on the anterior and posterior regions of the talus, the calcaneus, and the navicular. The four individual portions of the ligament are named according to their distal attachments as the anterior and posterior tibiotalar, the tibiocalcaneal, and the tibionavicular ligaments. The ligaments of the ankle are summarized in Table 8-4.

Talocalcaneal Articulations. Inferiorly, in the subtalar region, three facets of the talus articulate with the calcaneus. This subtalar, or talocalcaneal, joint has a fibrous capsule that is distinct from that of the ankle. The interosseous ligament, located in a space called the *tarsal sinus*, extends from the midtalar region to the calcaneus and provides support for the joint. The **talocalcaneal joint** is a gliding synovial joint that allows inversion and eversion of the foot. The radiograph in Fig. 8-28 shows the **subtalar articulations.** Fig. 8-29 is an MR image of a sagittal section through the talocrural and subtalar articulations.

FIG. 8-26. Coronal section through the ankle.

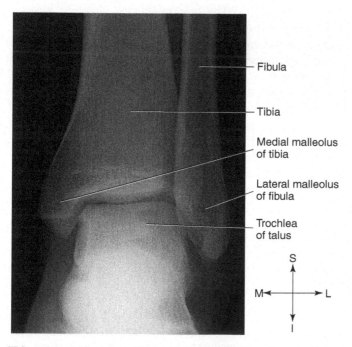

FIG. 8-27. Radiograph of the ankle showing the articulating surfaces of the talocrural joint.

TABLE 8-4   Ligaments of the Ankle

Ligament Name	Origin	Insertion
Lateral (Fibular) Ligament		
Anterior talofibular	Lateral malleolus of fibula	Anterior talus
Posterior talofibular	Lateral malleolus of fibula	Posterior talus
Calcaneofibular	Lateral malleolus of fibula	Lateral surface of calcaneus
Medial (Tibial) Ligament (Also called *deltoid ligament*)		
Anterior tibiotalar	Medial malleolus of tibia	Anterior surface of talus
Posterior tibiotalar	Medial malleolus of tibia	Posterior surface of talus
Tibiocalcaneal	Medial malleolus of tibia	Calcaneus
Tibionavicular	Medial malleolus of tibia	Navicular bone

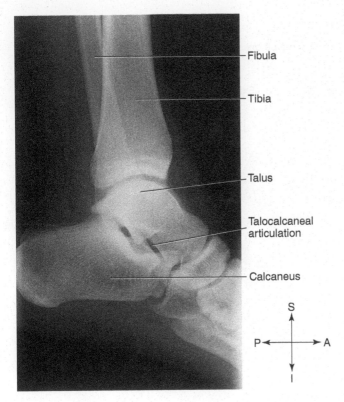

FIG. 8-28. Radiograph of the ankle showing the subtalar articulations.

Musculotendinous Structures Associated with the Ankle. In addition to the ligaments summarized in Table 8-4, support for the ankle comes from the musculotendinous structures in the region. These may be divided into medial, lateral, anterior, and posterior groups. The relationships of the musculotendinous structures of the ankle are shown in Fig. 8-30, which illustrates a transverse section just superior to the joint cavity.

The medial group includes the tibialis posterior, the flexor digitorum longus, and the flexor hallucis longus muscles. The tibialis posterior muscle is the most anterior of the three, and the flexor hallucis longus muscle is the most posterior. The posterior tibial artery and tibial nerve are located between the flexor digitorum longus and the flexor hallucis longus. Posterior to the medial malleolus, the tibial nerve divides into the medial and lateral plantar nerves.

The lateral group consists of the peroneus longus and peroneus brevis muscles. As the muscles descend the leg, the peroneus brevis is anterior to the peroneus longus. The two muscles follow a groove in the lateral malleolus, then curve forward under the malleolus and extend anteriorly to the metatarsals. In the foot, the peroneus brevis muscle is superior to the peroneus longus (see Fig. 8-26).

The anterior muscle group consists of the tibialis anterior, the extensor hallucis longus, the extensor digitorum longus, and the peroneus tertius muscles. The tibialis anterior is the most prominent and most medial of these muscles. The extensor digitorum longus and peroneus tertius muscles are difficult to separate and are the most lateral muscles of the group. The anterior tibial artery and deep peroneal nerve are deep to the extensor hallucis muscle.

The **calcaneal tendon** (Achilles tendon) constitutes the only musculotendinous structure in the posterior group. This tendon arises from the gastrocnemius and soleus muscles and attaches to the posterior surface of the calcaneus. The calcaneal tendon is the thickest and strongest tendon in the body.

QUICK CHECK

8.41   What are the articulating surfaces of the talocrural articulation?

8.42   What are the articulating surfaces of the subtalar joint of the ankle?

8.43   What musculotendinous structure provides support in the posterior region of the ankle?

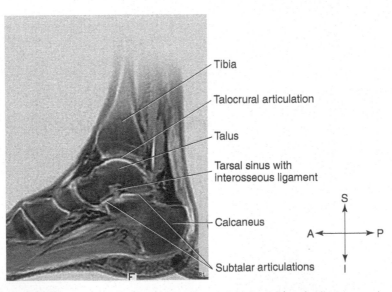

FIG. 8-29. MR image of a sagittal section through the talocrural and subtalar articulations.

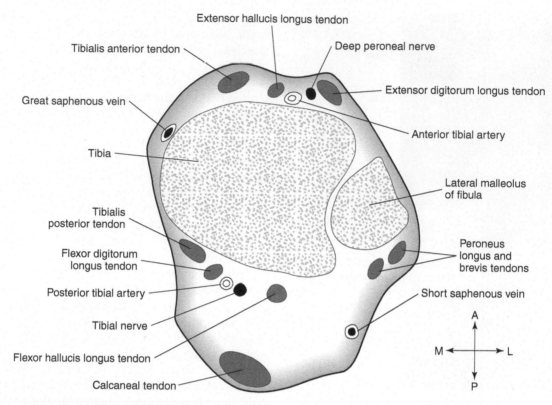

FIG. 8-30. Transverse section through the lateral malleolus of the fibula showing the relationship of the musculotendinous structures passing through the ankle joint.

Working with Images of the Lower Extremity

The transverse computed tomography (CT) image in Fig. 8-31 shows the proximal femur and the muscle compartments of the thigh. It is similar to the line drawing in Fig. 8-12. The anterior muscle compartment contains the quadriceps femoris group and the sartorius muscle. The medial muscles are the three adductors and the gracilis muscle. The posterior compartment contains the hamstring muscles. In this image a small portion of the gluteus maximus muscle is also present in the posterior compartment.

The transverse CT image in Fig. 8-32 shows the distal region of the shaft of the femur and the muscles associated with this region. It is similar to the line drawing in Fig. 8-13. The adductor muscles are absent because they insert at more superior levels. The three vastus muscles and the quadriceps femoris tendon are in the anterior compartment. The tendon is what remains of the rectus femoris muscle. In this distal region, the sartorius muscle is adjacent to the gracilis muscle. The three hamstring muscles occupy the posterior compartment. The deep vessels are the popliteal artery and vein. The great saphenous vein is superficial.

The transverse CT image in Fig. 8-33 shows the tibia and fibula in the proximal region of the leg. This image is similar to the line drawing in Fig. 8-14. The tibialis

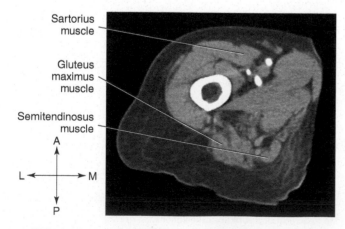

FIG. 8-31. Transverse CT image through the proximal femur.

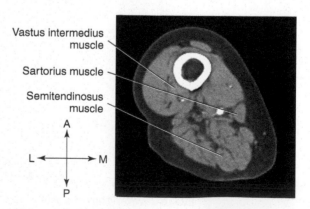

FIG. 8-32. Transverse CT image through the distal femur.

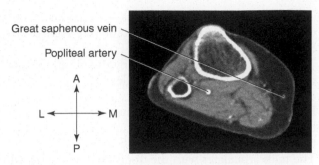

FIG. 8-33. Transverse CT image through the proximal portion of the leg.

anterior muscle is adjacent to the tibia. The two heads of the gastrocnemius muscle are in the superficial posterior compartment, and the popliteus is a deep posterior muscle. The popliteal vessels are between the superficial and deep layers, and the great saphenous vein is superficial on the medial side.

The transverse CT image in Fig. 8-34 shows the articulation of the femoral head with the acetabulum of the os coxa. It is similar to the line drawing in Fig. 8-16. The humeral head articulates at the periphery of the socket, leaving the acetabular fossa in the center. The gluteal muscles are evident in the posterior region. The piriformis and obturator internus are deep lateral rotator muscles. Anteriorly, the femoral artery and vein are in the femoral triangle.

The transverse CT image in Fig. 8-35 is similar to the one in Fig. 8-34 but is slightly inferior and intersects the greater trochanter of the femur. Again, note that the humeral head articulates at the periphery of the acetabulum, leaving an acetabular fossa in the center.

The transverse CT image in Fig. 8-36 shows the lateral and medial condyles of the femur with the intercondylar fossa between them. This space contains the anterior and posterior cruciate ligaments. Anteriorly, the patella articulates with the patellar surface of the femur.

FIG. 8-34. Transverse CT image through the acetabulum.

FIG. 8-35. Transverse CT image through the greater trochanter of the femur.

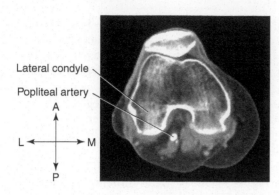

Lateral condyle

Popliteal artery

FIG. 8-36. Transverse CT image through the femoral condyles.

Important Anatomical Relationships in the Lower Extremity

- In the femoral triangle, the sequence of structures, from lateral to medial, is the femoral nerve, femoral artery, and femoral vein (see Fig. 8-5).
- The boundaries of the femoral triangle are the sartorius muscle laterally and the adductor longus muscle medially (see Fig. 8-5).
- The floor of the femoral triangle is formed by the iliopsoas and pectineus muscles (see Fig. 8-5).
- The quadriceps femoris muscle group occupies the anterior compartment of the thigh (see Figs. 8-12 and 8-13).
- The biceps femoris is the most lateral of the hamstring muscles, and the semimembranosus is the most medial (see Figs. 8-12 and 8-13).
- The gastrocnemius muscle is the most superficial muscle in the posterior compartment of the leg (see Figs. 8-8, 8-14, and 8-15).
- The soleus muscle is deep to the gastrocnemius muscle in the leg (see Figs. 8-8 and 8-15).
- The fibula on the lateral side and the tibia on the medial side of the leg are connected by an interosseous membrane (see Figs. 8-8 and 8-15).
- The tibialis anterior and tibialis posterior muscles are anterior and posterior to the interosseous membrane, respectively (see Figs. 8-8 and 8-15).
- The upper boundaries of the popliteal fossa are the biceps femoris muscle on the lateral side and the semitendinosus muscle on the medial side. The lower boundaries are the diverging heads of the gastrocnemius muscle. The plantaris muscle also contributes to the boundary on the lateral side (see Fig. 8-9).
- In the popliteal fossa, the sequence, from lateral to medial, is the sciatic nerve, popliteal vein, and popliteal artery (see Fig. 8-9).
- In the popliteal fossa, the sciatic nerve divides into its two terminal branches, the common peroneal nerve and the tibial nerve (see Fig. 8-9).
- The gluteus medius is the most superior of the three gluteus muscles (see Figs. 8-17 to 8-19).

- The head of the femur articulates with the acetabulum of the os coxa to form the hip joint (see Figs. 8-17 to 8-20).
- The obturator foramen is closed by the obturator internus and obturator externus muscles (see Figs. 8-19 and 8-20).
- Fibrocartilaginous pads called menisci are interposed between the condyles of the femur and the tibial plateaus in the knee joint (see Figs. 8-23 to 8-25).
- The talus articulates with the distal tibia superiorly, with the calcaneus inferiorly, with the distal fibula laterally, and with the navicular anteriorly (see Figs. 8-26 to 8-29).
- The anterior and posterior subtalar articulations are separated by a tarsal sinus (see Fig. 8-29).
- The sustentaculum tali is the most medial portion of the calcaneus (see Fig. 8-26).

Summary

- Two os coxae make up the pelvic girdle. In the child, each os coxa consists of an ilium, an ischium, and a pubis.
- The muscles in the gluteal region are the tensor fasciae latae, gluteus maximus, gluteus medius, gluteus minimus, piriformis, obturator externus, obturator internus, gemellus, and quadratus femoris.
- The only bone in the thigh is the femur.
- The muscles associated with the thigh are divided into three compartments: the anterior compartment has the quadriceps femoris, iliopsoas, and sartorius muscles; the medial compartment has the adductor longus, adductor brevis, adductor magnus, pectineus, and gracilis muscles; the posterior compartment has the biceps femoris, semimembranosus, and semitendinosus muscles.
- The femoral artery is the major blood supply to the thigh. It is accompanied by a femoral vein. The great saphenous vein is a superficial vein in the thigh.
- Two major nerves provide innervation to the muscles in the thigh. The femoral nerve innervates the anterior muscles, and the sciatic nerve innervates the posterior muscles.
- The inguinal ligament, sartorius muscle, and adductor longus muscle form the three sides of the femoral triangle. The iliopsoas and pectineus muscles form the floor. From lateral to medial, the structures within the triangle are the femoral nerve, femoral artery, and femoral vein.
- The bones in the leg are the tibia on the medial side and the fibula on the lateral side.
- The muscles of the leg are separated into anterior, lateral, and posterior compartments: the anterior compartment has the tibialis anterior muscle and the extensor muscles; the small lateral compartment contains the peroneus longus and peroneus brevis muscles; the large posterior compartment contains the gastrocnemius, soleus, plantaris, tibialis posterior, flexor digitorum longus, flexor hallucis longus, and popliteus muscles.
- Arterial blood supply to the leg is provided by the anterior tibial, posterior tibial, and peroneal arteries. Corresponding

veins accompany the arteries. The great saphenous and small saphenous veins are superficial on the medial and lateral sides, respectively.

- The tibial nerve provides innervation for the posterior muscle compartment of the leg; the deep peroneal nerve innervates the anterior muscle compartment; and the superficial peroneal nerve innervates the lateral muscle compartment.

- The popliteal fossa is a diamond-shaped region posterior to the knee joint. The hamstring and gastrocnemius muscles form the margin of the region, which contains the popliteal artery, popliteal vein, tibial nerve, and common peroneal nerve.

- The ankle (tarsus) contains the calcaneus, talus, cuboid, navicular, lateral cuneiform, intermediate cuneiform, and lateral cuneiform bones. Five metatarsals are located in the instep of the foot, and 14 phalanges make up the toes.

- The multiaxial ball-and-socket hip joint is formed by the articulation of the head of the femur in the acetabulum of the os coxa. The concavity of the acetabulum is deepened by the acetabular labrum around the margin, and the head of the femur is held in place by the ligamentum teres femoris.

- The joint capsule of the hip joint extends from the margin of the acetabulum to the neck of the femur near the trochanter. It is reinforced by the iliofemoral, pubofemoral, and ischiofemoral ligaments.

- Muscles in the gluteal region and thigh surround the hip joint and stabilize it. Sections in the region of the hip joint show the femoral artery, femoral vein, femoral nerve, and sciatic nerve.

- The osseous components of the knee joint are the femur, tibia, and patella. The rounded condyles of the femur articulate with the flat tibial plateaus. The patella fits between the condyles of the femur anteriorly.

- The fibrous capsule of the knee joint is strengthened by five extracapsular ligaments. These are the medial (tibial) collateral, lateral (fibular) collateral, patellar, oblique popliteal, and arcuate popliteal ligaments.

- Intracapsular anterior and posterior cruciate ligaments extend from the femur to the tibia to help stabilize the knee joint.

- Fibrocartilaginous pads called *menisci* are interposed between the femoral condyles and tibial plateaus. The lateral and medial menisci are connected by a transverse ligament.

- Muscular support for the knee is provided by the quadriceps femoris, hamstrings, sartorius, gracilis, and gastrocnemius muscles.

- Neurovascular structures in the region of the knee joint include the popliteal artery and vein, tibial nerve, and common peroneal nerve.

- The talocrural joint, or ankle, consists of the articulations of the tibia and fibula with the talus. In addition, three facets of the talus articulate with the calcaneus.

- The fibrous joint capsule of the talocrural articulation is strengthened by the lateral (fibular) and medial (tibial or deltoid) ligaments.

- The joint capsule of the talocalcaneal, or subtalar, articulation is distinct from the talocrural capsule.

- Musculotendinous support for the ankle is divided into lateral, medial, and posterior groups. The thickest and strongest tendon in the body is the calcaneal tendon in the posterior compartment.

• REVIEW QUESTIONS •

1. What bones make up the pelvic girdle?
2. What superficial muscle is the most lateral in the gluteal region?
3. What muscle is superior to the gemelli muscles in the deep gluteal region? What muscle is inferior to the gemelli muscles?
4. What muscles make up the quadriceps femoris muscle group? The hamstring muscle group?
5. Which muscles are located in the medial muscle compartment of the thigh?
6. What vein begins in the foot and ascends through the leg and thigh in the superficial fascia on the medial side?
7. What are the two terminal branches of the sciatic nerve?
8. What forms the lateral margin of the femoral triangle? The medial margin?
9. What is contained in the femoral triangle, from lateral to medial?
10. What two bones are in the leg and which one is lateral?
11. What three structures combine to separate the muscles of the leg into anterior and posterior compartments?
12. In general, what is the primary function of the muscles in the anterior compartment of the leg? Posterior compartment? Lateral compartment?
13. What two superficial muscles in the posterior compartment of the leg form most of the contour of the calf of the leg?
14. What nerve supplies innervation for all the muscles in the posterior compartment of the leg? Where is it located?
15. What muscles form the margins of the popliteal fossa?
16. Name the seven tarsal bones.
17. What is the intracapsular ligament associated with the hip (coxal) joint?
18. What is the nonarticular space in the center of the acetabulum called?
19. Name the intracapsular ligaments associated with the knee joint.
20. Name the five extracapsular ligaments associated with the knee joint.
21. What portion of the talus articulates with the tibia?
22. What two ligaments reinforce the fibrous capsule of the talocrural joint?
23. What space in the talocalcaneal joint contains an interosseous ligament?
24. What is the thickest and strongest tendon in the body?

• CHAPTER QUIZ •

Name the Following:

1. The bones that comprise the pelvic girdle
2. The most inferior muscle in the deep gluteal region
3. The two large articulating surfaces on the distal femur
4. The superficial, long, straplike muscle of the anterior thigh
5. The most lateral of the hamstring muscles
6. The nerve that supplies innervation to the sartorius and quadriceps femoris
7. The ligament that extends from the fovea capitis to the acetabular fossa
8. The most superficial muscle in the calf of the leg
9. The bone that forms a distal articulation with the tibia
10. The bone that forms a subtalar articulation with the talus

True/False:

1. The muscles in the posterior muscle compartment of the thigh are collectively called the *hamstring muscles*.
2. From lateral to medial, the neurovascular structures in the femoral triangle are the femoral artery, the femoral nerve, and the femoral vein.
3. The tendons of the gastrocnemius muscle extend over two joints; therefore the muscle affects both the knee and the ankle.
4. The muscles in the anterior compartment of the leg function principally to dorsiflex the foot and extend the toes.
5. The transverse acetabular ligament thickens the anterior portion of the fibrous capsule of the coxal joint.
6. The oblique popliteal and arcuate popliteal ligaments are intracapsular ligaments of the knee and function to connect the femur to the tibia.
7. The fibrocartilaginous pads between the femoral condyles and the tibial plateaus are connected on the posterior margin by the transverse ligament.
8. The ankle joint is called the *talocrural joint*.
9. The trochlea of the talus articulates with the fibula.
10. The ligament that reinforces the fibrous capsule of the ankle on the medial side is divided into four parts: the anterior tibiotalar ligament, the posterior tibiotalar ligament, the tibiocalcaneal ligament, and the tibionavicular ligament.

Answers to the Review Questions and Chapter Quiz questions can be found at http://evolve.elsevier.com/Applegate/SAlearning/

Suggested Readings

Applegate E: *The anatomy and physiology learning system*, ed 3, St Louis, 2006, WB Saunders/Elsevier.

Bo WJ et al: *Basic atlas of sectional anatomy with correlated imaging*, ed 4, St Louis, 2007, WB Saunders/Elsevier.

Dean D, Herbener TE: *Cross-sectional human anatomy*, Philadelphia, 2000, Lippincott, Williams & Wilkins.

Drake R, Vogl W, Mitchell AW: *Gray's anatomy for students*, St Louis, 2005, Mosby/Elsevier.

Ellis H, Logan B, Dixon A: *Human sectional anatomy: atlas of body sections-CT and MRI images*, ed 2, Boston, 1999, Butterworth-Heinemann.

Kelley R, Petersen C: *Sectional anatomy for imaging professionals*, ed 2, St Louis, 2007, Mosby/Elsevier.

Moore KL: *Clinically oriented anatomy*, ed 5, Philadelphia, 2005, Lippincott, Williams & Wilkins.

Spitzer VM, Whitlock DG: *National library of medicine atlas of the visible human male*, Sudbury, Mass, 1998, Jones & Bartlett.

Thibodeau G, Patton K: *Anatomy and physiology*, ed 6, St Louis, 2007, Mosby/Elsevier.

Weir J, Abrahams PH: *Imaging atlas of human anatomy*, ed 3, St Louis, 2003, Mosby/Elsevier.

Glossary

abdomen Area between the thorax and the pelvis; the belly

abdominal cavity Superior portion of the abdominopelvic cavity; contains the stomach, liver, spleen, pancreas, gallbladder, and most of the small and large intestines

abdominopelvic cavity Portion of the ventral body cavity that is inferior to the diaphragm; can be subdivided into an upper abdominal cavity and a lower pelvic cavity

abducens nerve Cranial nerve VI

abduction Movement of a body part away from the axis, or midline, of the body or one of its parts

abscess Localized accumulation of pus

absorption Taking up of substances by the skin or other tissues of the body

acetabular labrum Rim of fibrocartilage around the margin of the acetabulum

acetabulum Cup-shaped depression on the lateral surface of the os coxa (hipbone) in which the head of the femur fits

Achilles tendon Calcaneal tendon; combined tendon of the gastrocnemius and soleus muscles

acidity State of being acidic; the acid content of a fluid; the opposite of alkalinity

acromion process Flattened portion of bone at the lateral end of the spine of the scapula; most prominent point of the shoulder

acute Disease state that has a sudden onset or a short duration; the opposite of chronic

adduction Movement of a body part toward the axis, or midline, of the body or one of its parts

adductor brevis One of the muscles that adducts the thigh; lies deep to the adductor longus but anterior to the adductor magnus

adductor longus One of the muscles that adducts the thigh; the most anterior muscle of the adductor group

adductor magnus One of the muscles that adducts the thigh; the largest and the most posterior muscle of the adductor group

adenoids Pharyngeal tonsils; enlargement of the pharyngeal tonsils as a result of chronic inflammation

adhere To stick, to bind, or to hold fast

adipose Type of connective tissue containing large quantities of fat; fatty tissue

adjoin To be in contact with or to lie next to

adrenal Gland located on the superior pole of each kidney; also called the *suprarenal gland*

afferent Carrying a nerve impulse or fluid toward an area or an organ

aggregation An accumulation or clump

ala (pl. alae) Winglike structure

alkalinity State of being alkaline or basic; the alkaline content of a fluid; the opposite of acidity

alveolus Small, hollow area or cavity (e.g., the socket of a tooth or an air sac in the lungs)

amylase An enzyme that splits starches into smaller molecules called *disaccharides*

anastomose Opening one into another; generally pertains to blood vessels or lymphatics

anastomosis The connection, or union, of tubular structures (e.g., in blood vessels or lymphatics)

anatomy A study of the structure of the body and the relation of the parts to each other

anesthesia A partial or total loss of sensation

aneurysm A saclike bulge in a blood vessel, usually an artery, as a result of a weakening of the vessel wall

annular Relating to a ring-shaped or circular structure

antagonistic Working in opposition to each other; frequently pertains to muscle action or drugs

anteflexion A displacement characterized by the bending forward of the superior portion of an organ

anterior To the front of the body; ventral

anterolateral In front and to one side of the body

anteroposterior Directed from the front to the back

anterosuperior To the front and the superior (above) part of the body

anteversion Leaning forward (tilting) of an organ as a whole, without bending

antrum Nearly closed cavity or chamber

anulus fibrosus Fibrous outer part of the intervertebral disc

aorta Main trunk of the systemic arterial circulation

aperture Hole or opening

apex Pointed end of a conical structure

aponeurosis White, fibrous sheet composed of closely packed collagenous fibers; serves as a connection between a muscle and its attachment; a broad, flat sheet of tendon

appendage Structure attached to the body

appendicular Relating to an appendix or an appendage

aqueduct Canal or passageway, especially used for the conduction of fluid

aqueduct of Sylvius Channel through the midbrain that connects the third and fourth ventricles; also called the *cerebral aqueduct*

aqueous humor Watery, clear solution that fills the anterior cavity of the eye

arachnoid Thin, cobweb-appearing layer of the meninges located between the dura and the pia mater

arbor vitae cerebelli Treelike branching arrangement of white matter in the cerebellum

arcuate artery Artery between the interlobar and interlobular arteries in the kidney; forms an arch between the cortex and the medulla of the kidney

267

areola   Pigmented area of skin around the nipple of the breast

artery   Blood vessel that carries blood away from the heart

articular   Referring to an articulation or a joint

articulate   To join or to connect by means of a joint

articulation   Joint; a place of contact between bones

aryepiglottic fold   Membranous tissue in the larynx that attaches the arytenoid cartilage to the border of the epiglottis

arytenoid cartilages   Pair of small pyramidal cartilages located in the posterior region of the larynx

ascites   Accumulation of serous fluid in the peritoneal cavity

atrial   Relating to an atrium, especially in the heart

atrioventricular   Relating both to an atrium and a ventricle of the heart

atrium (pl. atria)   Upper chambers of the heart, which receive blood from the veins

auditory   Relating to the sense of hearing

auricle   External portion of the ear; also, the pouchlike projections from the atria of the heart

autonomic nervous system   Division of the nervous system that transmits impulses from the brain and spinal cord to the visceral effectors, such as smooth muscles, glands, or cardiac muscle

axial   Forming an axis; relating to the head, the neck, and the trunk of the body, as distinguished from the extremities

axilla (pl. axillae)   Region where the arm meets the chest; commonly called the *armpit*

axillary artery   Artery that arises from the subclavian artery and passes through the axilla

axon   Process of a neuron that carries the nerve impulse away from the cell body; the efferent process of a neuron

azygos vein   Unpaired vein that drains the thoracic wall and empties into the superior vena cava

baroreceptor   Sensory nerve ending that responds to changes in blood pressure; also called *pressoreceptor*

Bartholin's glands   Paired female accessory reproductive glands, one on either side of the vaginal orifice, that open by a duct into the vestibule; also called the *greater vestibular glands*

basal ganglia   Clusters of gray matter located within the white matter of each cerebral hemisphere; also called *cerebral nuclei*

basilar artery   Artery in the pontine cistern that receives blood from the vertebral arteries and carries this blood into the circle of Willis at the base of the brain

basilic vein   Superficial vein located on the medial side of the arm

biceps brachii   Muscle of the arm that has two heads of origin and flexes the forearm

bicipital groove   Groove on the proximal humerus for the tendon of the long head of the biceps brachii muscle

biconvex   Having a protruding surface on both sides

bicuspid valve   Left atrioventricular valve with two cusps or flaps; also called the *mitral valve*

bifid   Divided into two parts (e.g., the spinous processes of the cervical vertebrae)

bifurcate   To divide or separate into two parts

bile   Secretion of the liver that is stored in the gallbladder and aids in the digestion of fats

bipolar   Having two poles; relating to both ends of a cell

brachial   Relating to the arm

brachialis muscle   Muscle in the arm that flexes the forearm

brachiocephalic artery   Most anterior branch of the aortic arch; provides blood to the arm and head on the right side

brachioradialis muscle   Muscle in the arm that flexes the forearm

brachium (pl. brachia)   Region between the shoulder and the elbow; the arm

brainstem   Portion of the brain that connects the cerebrum and spinal cord; consists of the midbrain, the pons, and the medulla oblongata

bronchial   Relating to the bronchi

bronchopulmonary   Relating to the bronchi and the lungs

bronchus (pl. bronchi)   Either of the two branches of the trachea; further subdivides into secondary and tertiary branches and conveys air to and from the lungs

buccal   Relating to the cheek and/or the mouth

buccinator muscle   Muscle in the cheek

bulbospongiosus muscle   One of the muscles of the perineum

bulbourethral glands   Small, paired accessory glands of the male reproductive system; also called *Cowper's glands*

bulbus oculi   Eyeball

bursa (pl. bursae)   Sac, or pouch, of synovial fluid located at friction points, especially in the region of the joints

buttock   One of two fleshy masses formed by the gluteal muscles on the posterior surface of the lower trunk

calcaneofibular   Relating to the calcaneus and the fibula

calcaneus   Tarsal bone that is commonly called the *heel bone*

calvaria   Upper part of the skull

canaliculus (pl. canaliculi)   Small channel or canal

capitulum   Small, rounded eminence or articular extremity of a bone; rounded surface on the distal humerus that articulates with the radius; also called the *capitellum*

carcinoma   Malignant tumor that originates in epithelial cells

cardiac   Relating to the heart; relating to the esophageal entrance to the stomach

carina   Ridge formed at the bifurcation of the trachea into the two mainstem bronchi

carotid   Relating to the major arteries of the neck

carpal   Relating to the bones in the wrist

cartilage   Tough, nonvascular type of connective tissue with chondrin in the matrix

cartilaginous   Consisting of cartilage

cauda equina   Collection of spinal nerves that extends beyond the conus medullaris at the distal end of the spinal cord

caudal   Relating to the tail

caudate nucleus   Mass of gray matter located adjacent to the lateral ventricles in the cerebrum

caval   Relating to the superior or inferior vena cava

cavernous sinus Space, or cavity, on either side of the dorsum sellae of the sphenoid bone

cecum Blind pouch, or cul-de-sac, at the beginning of the large intestine and inferior to the ileocecal valve

celiac trunk First major branch from the abdominal aorta; divides into the common hepatic, left gastric, and splenic arteries

cephalic Relating to the head or superior in position

cerebellar Relating to the cerebellum portion of the brain

cerebellomedullary cistern Subarachnoid cistern between the cerebellum and the medulla oblongata; also called the *cisterna magna*

cerebellum Portion of the brain that is posteroinferior to the cerebrum and functions in the coordination of movements

cerebral aqueduct Channel between the third and fourth ventricles in the brain; passes through the midbrain and contains cerebrospinal fluid; also called the *aqueduct of Sylvius*

cerebrospinal fluid Fluid produced by the choroid plexus of the ventricles that circulates through the ventricles of the brain and in the subarachnoid space around the brain

cerebrum Largest part of the brain, consists of two hemispheres

cervical Relating to the neck

cervix Neck-shaped structure; often used to denote the narrow, neck region of the uterus

chemoreceptor Nerve ending or sense organ that is sensitive to chemical stimuli

chiasma X-shaped crossing; the optic chiasma is the X-shaped crossing of the optic nerves

chiasmatic cistern Subarachnoid space in the region of the optic chiasma; contains cerebrospinal fluid

choana (pl. choanae) Funnel-shaped opening, especially the opening of the nasal cavity into the nasopharynx; also called the *internal nares*

chordae tendineae Stringlike or chordlike structures that extend between the papillary muscles and the flaps of the atrioventricular valves in the ventricles of the heart

choroid Middle or vascular layer of the eyeball

choroid plexus Specialized vascular structures that produce cerebrospinal fluid in the ventricles of the brain

chronic Slowly progressive disease that persists over a long period; the opposite of acute

cilium (pl. cilia) Microscopic, hairlike projection from the cell surface for cell locomotion or to move substances across the cell surface

circulus arteriosus cerebri Circle of anastomosing arteries at the base of the brain; also called the *circle of Willis*

circumcision Surgical removal of the prepuce or foreskin from the glans penis

circumduction Circular movement of a part in which the distal end of the bone moves in a circle, whereas the proximal end remains relatively stable

circumflex Relating to arched structures

circumflex artery Branch of the left coronary artery located in the left arterioventricular sulcus

cistern Enclosed space or reservoir for body fluids, especially areas of the subarachnoid space that act as reservoirs for cerebrospinal fluid

cisterna ambiens Subarachnoid space at the posterior end of the corpus callosum; also called the *superior cistern* or the *cistern of the great cerebral vein*

cisterna chyli Dilation at the beginning of the thoracic duct in the abdomen

cisterna magna Subarachnoid cistern located between the cerebellum and the medulla oblongata; also called the *cerebellomedullary cistern*

claustrum Thin layer of gray matter on the lateral margin of the external capsule of the brain

clavicle Bone that extends from the sternum to the acromion process of the scapula and forms the anterior portion of the pectoral girdle; collarbone

cleft palate Condition characterized by a fissure in the palate, or roof of the mouth, because the palatine processes of the two maxillae did not unite before birth

clitoris Small, erectile organ at the anterior end of the vulva in the female; homologous to the penis in the male

coccygeus muscle Smaller of the two muscles in the anal region of the pelvic floor

coccyx Three or four fused bones at the distal end of the vertebral column, commonly called the *tailbone*

cochlea Spiral cavity in the inner ear that contains the essential organ of hearing

coitus Sexual intercourse or copulation

collateral circulation Secondary or alternate path of blood flow through anastomosing vessels

colliculus (pl. colliculi) Small, round elevation found in the dorsal portion of the midbrain

colon Portion of the large intestine that extends between the cecum and the rectum; divided into ascending, transverse, descending, and sigmoid regions

concave Characterized by having a hollow or depressed shape

concha (pl. conchae) Scroll- or shell-shaped bone found in the nasal cavity; also called a *turbinate*

condyle Rounded prominence at the end of a bone for articulation with another bone

confluence of sinuses Junction of venous sinuses in the dura mater in the region of the internal occipital protuberance

congenital Present at birth

conjunctiva Delicate mucous membrane that lines the eyelids and covers the exposed surface of the outer layer of the eyeball

connective tissue Most abundant tissue of the four basic tissue types; it binds and supports

constrict To make narrow or to reduce in size

contraction Shortening of a muscle or an increase in tension in a muscle

conus medullaris Tapered distal end of the spinal cord

convex Having a rounded or bulging surface

convoluted Twisted, coiled, or rolled

Cooper's ligament Suspensory ligament of the breast

copulation Sexual intercourse, coitus

coracobrachialis Muscle that flexes and adducts the arm

coracoid process Thick, curved process at the superior border of the scapula

cornea Transparent anterior portion of the outer layer of the eyeball

corniculate cartilage Pair of small cartilages in the larynx

coronal plane   Plane parallel to the long axis of the body that divides the body into anterior and posterior portions; also called the *frontal plane*

coronary arteries (left and **right)**   First branches from the ascending aorta; located at the level of the aortic semilunar valve; they supply blood to the heart wall

coronary sinus   Thin-walled venous dilation on the posterior surface of the heart; drains into the right atrium

coronoid process   Certain processes of bones, such as the coronoid process of the mandible

corpora quadrigemina   Four bodies that form the dorsal part of the midbrain

corpus (pl. corpora)   Body, or main portion, of a structure

corpus callosum   Large band of white fibers that connects the two cerebral hemispheres

corpus spongiosum   Ventral column of erectile tissue that surrounds the urethra in the penis

corpus cavernosum   Either of the two dorsal columns of erectile tissue in the penis

cortex   Outer layer of an organ; the outer layer of gray matter of the cerebrum

costal   Pertaining to the ribs

Cowper's gland   Accessory gland of the male reproductive system; also called *bulbourethral gland*

coxa (pl. coxae)   Hipbone, or os coxa

cranial cavity   One of the divisions of the dorsal body cavity; contains the brain

cranium   Bones of the skull that enclose the brain

cremaster muscle   Extension of the internal oblique muscle found in the spermatic cord that contracts to elevate the testes

crest   Bony ridge

cribriform plate   Flat region on either side of the crista galli of the ethmoid bone, perforated by many small holes called *olfactory foramina*

cricoid cartilage   Most inferior cartilage of the larynx

crista terminalis   Ridge that separates the sinus venarum and pectinate regions of the right atrium

cruciate   Overlapping, or crossing, such as the cruciate ligaments of the knee

crus (pl. crura)   Derived from the Latin word for leg; slender, tapered portion of a muscle or organ, such as the crus of the diaphragm or the crura of the penis

cubital   Relating to the forearm; *cubitus* refers to the elbow joint, and the *cubital fossa* is the depression on the anterior surface of the elbow joint

cul-de-sac   Blind-ended pouch or sac

cuneiform   Wedge shaped; three of the tarsal bones

cusp   Triangular piece of an atrioventricular valve in the heart; an elevation or projection on a tooth

cutaneous   Pertaining to the skin

cystic duct   Duct from the gallbladder

dartos   Muscle in the subcutaneous tissue of the scrotum

decussation   Crossing over to the other side, especially in nerve tracts; if bilateral, then forms an X shape

degeneration   Deterioration or breakdown of tissues

delineate   To mark boundaries

deltoid   Superficial muscle over the shoulder; abducts the arm

demarcation   Marking of boundaries; delineation

detrusor muscle   Smooth muscle in the wall of the urinary bladder

diaphragma sellae   Extension of the dura mater over the sella turcica of the sphenoid bone

diaphragmatic   Relating to the diaphragm

diencephalon   Portion of the brain surrounded by the cerebral hemispheres that encloses the third ventricle; principal components are the thalamus and hypothalamus

digastric   Muscle in the floor of the oral cavity

dilation   Enlarged or swollen area, usually used in reference to a tubular structure, opening, or cavity

dilate   To expand, to enlarge, or to swell

dislocation   Displacement of a part from normal position, usually used in reference to bone in joints

dissect   To cut apart or to separate tissues or organs in the study of anatomy

distal   Directional term for something located away from a point of reference, such as the center, the midline, the point of attachment, or the point of origin; opposite of proximal

distensible   Capable of being stretched

diverge   To spread apart from a common point

diverticulum (pl. diverticula)   Pouch, or sac, protruding from the wall of a tubular organ

dopamine   Compound produced primarily in the substantia nigra of the cerebral peduncles of the midbrain, diminished in some disease states such as parkinsonism

dorsal   Directional term relating to the back or posterior surface of a structure

dorsal root ganglion   Enlargement in the dorsal root of spinal nerves that contains the cell bodies of afferent neurons

dorsum   Back or posterior surface of a structure

duct   Tube or channel, usually for carrying secretions

duct of Wirsung   Pancreatic duct

ductus arteriosus   Channel or vessel between the pulmonary artery and the aorta in the fetus that allows blood to bypass the lungs in fetal circulation

ductus deferens   Tube or channel that conveys sperm from the epididymis to the ejaculatory duct in the male

duodenum   First part of the small intestine

dura mater   Outer, tough covering around the brain and spinal cord; the outer layer of the meninges

echogenic   Tissues that produce echoes

ectopic   Located outside the normal place

edema   Swelling caused by an abnormal accumulation of interstitial fluid

efferent   Carrying a nerve impulse or fluid away from an area or an organ

ejaculatory duct   Tube that transports sperm from the vas deferens to the prostatic urethra

embryo   Developing human, from the time of conception to the end of the eighth week of development

eminence   Elevated area or prominence, especially used in reference to regions on bones

encircle   To surround

endocardium   Innermost layer of the heart, composed of endothelium

endocrine   Glands that secrete their products, called *hormones*, directly into the bloodstream; a ductless gland

endometrium   Mucous membrane that makes up the inner layer of the uterine wall

endosteum   Membranous lining of bone cavities

endothelium   Thin layer of simple squamous epithelium that lines the heart, blood vessels, and lymphatics

enzyme   Protein secreted by the body that acts as a catalyst to speed up chemical reactions in the body

epicardium   Visceral or innermost layer of the serous pericardium, which is in contact with the heart and forms the outermost layer of the heart wall

epicondyle   Projection above or on a condyle

epicranium   Scalp; structures that cover the skull, including the muscle, the aponeurosis, and the skin

epididymis   Comma-shaped structure on the posterior surface of the testis; site of sperm maturation

epidural   Located above or on the dura mater

epigastric region   Upper, middle abdominal region, directly superior to the umbilical region

epiglottic   Relating to the epiglottis

epiglottis   Leaf-shaped piece of cartilage that covers the trachea during swallowing to prevent food from blocking the airway

epiploic   Relating to the omentum

epiploic appendages   Bodies of fat along the taeniae coli of the large intestine

epiploic foramen   Opening along the right margin of the lesser omentum that allows access to the omental bursa; also called the *foramen of Winslow*

epithalamus   Small area of the diencephalon above the thalamus

epithelium   Nonvascular layer of cells that lines body cavities and covers the exterior surface of the body; one of the four main types of tissue in the body

equilibrium   State of balance

erectile tissue   Tissue that becomes rigid when filled with blood

erector   Muscle that can raise a structure or cause it to become erect

erector spinae   Intermediate layer of intrinsic muscles associated with the vertebral column; includes the iliocostalis, the longissimus, and the spinalis muscles

esophagus   Muscular passageway that takes food from the pharynx to the stomach

estrogens   Term for female sex hormones that maintain secondary sex characteristics

ethmoid   Bone resembling a sieve because of its many foramina that is located behind the nose

eustachian tube   Tube that connects the middle ear to the nasopharynx; auditory tube

eversion   Movement of turning a joint outward (e.g., eversion of the foot)

evert   To turn outward

excretory   Relating to excretion

exocrine   Glands that secrete their products to a surface via ducts

expel   To force outward

extension   Act of increasing the angle at a joint; the opposite of flexion

extensor   Muscle that increases the angle between bones at a joint

extensor carpi radialis   Lateral muscle of the forearm that extends the hand

extensor carpi ulnaris   Medial muscle of the forearm that extends the hand

extracapsular   Located outside a capsule

extradural   Located outside the dura mater

extrapelvic   Located outside the pelvic cavity

extremity   Limb or appendage of the body

extrinsic   Located on the outside of the structure acted upon

facet   Very smooth bone surface for articulation with another structure

facial   Relating to the face; cranial nerve VII

falciform ligament   Fold of peritoneum extending from the diaphragm and the anterior abdominal wall to the surface of the liver, between the two major lobes

fallopian tube   Duct that carries the ova from the ovary to the uterus; also called the *uterine tube* or the *oviduct*

falx cerebelli   Triangular extension of the cranial dura mater located between the two lobes of the cerebellum

falx cerebri   Fold of cranial dura mater that extends into the longitudinal fissure between the two cerebral hemispheres

fascia   Loose connective tissue, located under the skin, or a fibrous membrane that covers and separates muscles

fauces   Opening from the oral cavity into the oropharynx

femoral   Relating to the femur or the thigh

femur   Large bone of the thigh

fetus   Developing offspring in the uterus from the beginning of the third month of development until birth

fibrocartilage   Cartilage that contains a large number of collagenous fibers

fibromuscular   Denotes a tissue that is both muscular and fibrous

fibroserous   Denotes a tissue that is both serous and fibrous

fibrous   Composed of fibers of connective tissue

fibula   Smaller and more lateral bone of the leg

fimbriae   Fingerlike projections that surround the openings of the uterine tubes

fissure   Slit, cleft, or groove

flaccid   Muscles without tone; flabby

flexion   Act of decreasing the angle at a joint; the opposite of extension

flexor   Muscle that decreases the angle between bones at a joint

flexor carpi radialis   Lateral muscle of the forearm that flexes the hand

flexor carpi ulnaris   Medial muscle of the forearm that flexes the hand

flexure   Bend or turn

follicle   Mass of cells containing a cavity; small depression in the skin from which the hair emerges

foramen (pl. foramina)   Hole or opening

foramen of Magendie   Medial opening in the fourth ventricle through which cerebrospinal fluid enters the subarachnoid space; also called the *median aperture*

foramen magnum   Large hole in the occipital bone through which the spinal cord passes

foramen of Monro   Opening from the lateral ventricle into the third ventricle; also called the *interventricular foramen*

foramina of Luschka   Two lateral openings in the fourth ventricle through which cerebrospinal fluid enters the subarachnoid space; also called *lateral apertures*

fornix (pl. fornices)   Arched structure, or the space created by such a structure (e.g., the fornix of the vagina)

fossa (pl. fossae)   Pit or shallow depression

fovea   Small depression

frenulum   Small fold of mucous membrane that connects two parts and limits movement (e.g., the lingual frenulum on the underside of the tongue)

frontal   Relating to the forehead

frontal plane   Plane parallel to the long axis of the body that divides the body into anterior and posterior portions; also called the *coronal plane*

frontalis muscle   Muscle that wrinkles the forehead

fundus   Part of a hollow organ that is farthest from, above, or opposite its opening

galea aponeurotica   Broad, flat tendon that connects the frontalis muscle with the occipitalis muscle; a part of the scalp; also called the *epicranial aponeurosis*

gallbladder   Oblong sac located on the visceral surface of the liver that stores bile

ganglion (pl. ganglia)   Group of nerve cell bodies located outside the brain and spinal cord

gaster   Refers to the belly

gastric   Relating to the stomach

gastrocnemius   Muscle of the posterior region of the leg that plantarflexes the foot

gastrocolic   Relating to the stomach and large intestine

gastroduodenal   Relating to the stomach and the duodenum

gastroepiploic   Relating to the stomach and the omentum

gastroesophageal   Relating to the stomach and the esophagus

gastrohepatic   Relating to the stomach and the liver

gastrointestinal   Relating to the stomach and the intestines (gastroenteric)

gastrosplenic   Relating to the stomach and the spleen

gemellus (pl. gemelli)   Means twins; two muscles deep to the gluteal muscles that laterally rotate and abduct the thigh

geniohyoid   One of the muscles that acts on the hyoid bone

genital   Relating to reproduction

genitalia   Reproductive organs

genitourinary   Relating to the genital system and the urinary system; also called *urogenital*

genu   Any structure that resembles a flexed knee (e.g., genu of the corpus callosum)

gingiva   The gum; mucous membrane that surrounds the alveolar process and the neck of the tooth

glans penis   Caplike extension of the corpus spongiosum at the distal tip of the penis

glenohumeral   Relating to the glenoid fossa of the scapula and to the humerus

glenoid   Relating to an articular depression or socket of a joint (e.g., glenoid fossa of the scapula)

glenoid labrum   Rim of fibrocartilage around the margin of the glenoid fossa

globus pallidus   Medial region of gray matter in the lentiform nucleus

glossopharyngeal   Relating to the tongue and the pharynx

glottis   Vocal apparatus in the larynx, consisting of the vocal folds and the rima glottidis between them

gluteal   Relating to the buttocks

gluteus maximus   Large, fleshy muscle that forms the prominent portion of the buttocks

gluteus medius   Broad, thick muscle situated on the outer surface of the pelvis

gluteus minimus   Smallest and deepest muscle of the three gluteal muscles

gonad   Primary reproductive organ; the ovary in the female and the testes in the male

gonadal   Refers to the gonad

graafian follicle   Fluid-filled follicle that contains an immature ovum and its surrounding estrogen-secreting cells; also called a *vesicular ovarian follicle*

gracilis   Straplike muscle located on the medial surface of the thigh that functions in adduction of the thigh

gyrus (pl. gyri)   Rounded elevations on the surface of the brain

hallucis muscles   Muscles that work on the big toe (e.g., the adductor hallucis)

hallux   Big toe

hamate   One of the bones of the wrist (carpals)

hemidiaphragm   Half or one dome of the diaphragm

hemorrhage   Profuse bleeding

hepatic   Relating to the liver

hepatoduodenal   Relating to the liver and the duodenum

hepatogastric   Relating to the liver and the stomach

hepatorenal   Relating to the liver and the kidney

hernia   Protrusion of an organ through an abnormal opening

hiatus   Opening or aperture

hilum   Region where vessels and nerves enter and leave an organ

homologous   Organs that are alike in structure or origin

hormones   Substances secreted by endocrine glands that are released into the blood, causing a response in the target organ

humeral   Relating to the humerus

humeroradial   Relating to the humerus and the radius

humeroscapular   Relating to the humerus and the scapula

humeroulnar   Relating to the humerus and the ulna

humerus   Bone of the arm between the shoulder and the elbow

hyaline cartilage   Gelatinous material with a glassy appearance found in many extracellular areas

hyoid   U-shaped bone found in the neck; serves as an anchor for the tongue

hypertrophy   Increase in the bulk or size of a tissue without cell division

hypochondriac region   Abdominal region located superiorly and laterally, near the ribs, on either side of the epigastric region

hypogastric region   Lower, middle abdominal region located directly inferior to the umbilical region

hypoglossal   Located beneath the tongue

hypopharynx   Below the pharynx

hypophysis   Endocrine gland located under the brain; also called the *pituitary gland*

hypothalamus   Portion of the diencephalon located inferior to the thalamus; also forms the floor of the third ventricle

ileocecal   Relating to the ileum and the cecum

ileum   Third, or distal, part of the small intestine

iliac   Relating to the ilium of the os coxa

iliacus   Muscle that lines the ilium of the os coxa

iliofemoral   Relating to the ilium and the femur

iliopsoas   Muscle that results from the joining of the iliacus and the psoas muscles, located in the upper thigh

iliotibial   Relating to the ilium and the tibia

ilium   Superior, broad portion of the os coxa

incisura angularis   Notch, or indentation, between the body and the pylorus of the stomach

incus   One of three ossicles of the ear; small, anvil-shaped bone of the middle ear located between the malleus and the stapes

inferiorly   Located below or inferior to another structure

infraglenoid   Located below the glenoid fossa of the scapula bone

infraglottic   Located below the glottis

infrahyoid   Located below the hyoid bone

infraorbital   Located below the orbit of the eye

infrapubic   Located below the pubis

infraspinatus muscle   Muscle located below the spine of the scapula

infraspinous   Located below the spinous process (e.g., the infraspinous fossa located under the spine of the scapula)

infrasternal   Located below the sternum

infundibulum   Funnel-shaped structure (e.g., the infundibulum of the pituitary gland or the infundibulum of the uterine tube)

inguinal   Refers to the groin

innervation   Nerve or nerves that supply an area

innominate artery   First and most anterior arterial branch off the aorta; also called the *brachiocephalic artery*

inspiration   Act of breathing in, inhalation

insula   Hidden lobe of the brain, deep to the temporal lobe; also called the *island of Reil*

interatrial   Located between the two atria

interclavicular   Located between the two clavicles

intercondylar   Located between two condyles

intercostal   Located between adjacent ribs

intercristal   Located between two crests

interiliac   Located between the two ilia

intermuscular   Located between muscles

interosseous   Connecting or lying between bones

interpeduncular   Located between the two cerebral peduncles

interposed   Located between two structures

intertubercular   Located between two tubercles

interventricular   Located between two ventricles

interventricular foramen   Opening between a lateral ventricle and the third ventricle; also called the *foramen of Monro*

intervertebral   Located between two vertebrae

intestine   Portion of the gastrointestinal tract that extends from the stomach to the anus

intracapsular   Located within a capsule

intracranial   Located within the skull

intramuscular   Located within a muscle

intrathoracic   Located within the thorax

inversion   Turning inside out or reversing the normal relationship between organs; turning the sole of the foot medially; the opposite of eversion

iris   Colored portion of the eye, a circle of smooth muscles that controls the size of the pupil

ischiocavernosus   Muscles of the perineum

ischiofemoral   Relating to the ischium and the femur

ischiopubic   Relating to the ischium and the pubis

ischium   Lowest and most posterior portion of the ox coxa

island of Reil   Hidden lobe of the brain, deep to the temporal lobe; also called the *insula*

isthmus   Narrow band of tissue that connects two larger parts or a narrow passageway between two larger cavities

jejunum   Middle portion of the small intestine, located between the duodenum and the ileum

jugular   Relating to the neck; structures located in the neck

labia majora   Two large folds of fat-filled tissue that are lateral to the labia minora

labia minora   Two narrow folds of tissue that enclose or delineate the vestibule in the female

labrum   Lip or edge

laceration   Jagged tear in tissues

lacerum   Foramen resembling a jagged tear

lacrimal   Relating to tears

lactiferous   Secreting or carrying milk

lamina (pl. laminae)   Thin layer or flat plate

laryngeal   Relating to the larynx

laryngopharynx   Lowest part of the pharynx, located posterior to the larynx, that leads into the esophagus

larynx   Voice box, organ of voice production that contains the vocal folds

lateral   Located away from the center

latissimus dorsi   Broad superficial muscle of the back

lenticular nucleus, lentiform nucleus   Mass of gray matter, lateral to the internal capsule, that is part of the basal ganglia

leptomeninges   Collective term relating to the arachnoid and pia mater

levator ani muscle   Muscle of the pelvic floor

levator costarum muscle   Muscle that raises the ribs

lienorenal   Relating to the spleen and the kidney; also called *splenorenal*

ligament   Band of fibrous tissue that connects bone

ligamenta flava   Short bands of elastic fibers that connect the laminae of adjacent vertebrae

ligamentum arteriosum   Band of tissue that represents the remnant of the ductus arteriosus from the fetal circulation

ligamentum nuchae   Supraspinous and interspinous ligaments from C7 to the occipital bone

linea alba   White line, a narrow band of the anterior aponeurosis, between the two rectus abdominis muscles, in the middle of the abdomen, from the xiphoid process to the pubic symphysis

linea aspera   Long ridge on the posterior surface of the femur

lingual   Referring to the tongue

lobule   Small lobe

longitudinal fissure   Fissure of the brain that separates the cerebrum into two cerebral hemispheres

lordosis   Abnormally exaggerated lumbar curvature; swayback

lumbar region   Abdominal region on either side of the umbilical region

lumbosacral   Relating to the lumbar region of the spine and the sacrum

lumen   Open space in the interior of a tubular structure

lymph   Clear or yellowish fluid derived from the interstitial fluid that is contained in the lymph vessels

lymphatic   Relating to lymph, lymph nodes, or lymph vessels

lymphoid   Referring to or resembling lymph or lymphatic tissue

malignant   Refers to a disease that resists treatment and tends to be fatal; frequently pertains to tumors that have the properties of uncontrolled growth and dissemination

malleolus   Projections on either side of the ankle; one is located on the tibia, the other on the fibula

malleus   One of the three ear ossicles in the middle ear; the ossicle located next to the tympanic membrane and shaped like a hammer or mallet

mammary   Referring to the breasts

mammillary bodies   Rounded structures located at the base of the hypothalamus

mandible   Bone of the lower jaw

manubrium   Means *handle;* refers to the superior part of the sternum

masseter   Muscle that acts to close the jaw, a muscle of mastication

mastication   Process of chewing

mastoid   Projection on the temporal bone located posterior to the ear

maxilla (pl. maxillae)   Bones that form the upper jaw

maxillary   Relating to the upper jaw

meatus   Channel or opening

medial   Toward the middle or median plane of a body or organ

median   Centrally located

mediastinal   Relating to the mediastinum

mediastinum (pl. mediastina)   Central region of the thoracic cavity

medulla   Inner part of an organ

medulla oblongata   Inferior-most part of the brainstem; extends from the pons to the spinal cord and is continuous with the spinal cord at the foramen magnum

melanin   Dark pigment found in the skin, the hair, and the iris of the eye

meninges   Membranes that cover the brain and the spinal cord

meningitis   Inflammation of the meninges

meniscus (pl. menisci)   Crescent-shaped structure; frequently refers to the pad of fibrocartilage found in certain joints (e.g., the knee)

menopause   Normal termination of the menstrual cycle

mesenteric   Relating to the mesentery

mesentery   Double layer of peritoneum that is attached to the intestines and to the body wall

mesocolon   Fold of peritoneum that attaches the colon to the posterior wall of the abdomen

mesovarium   Fold of peritoneum that attaches the ovary to the posterior layer of the broad ligament

metacarpals   Bones located in the hand, between the carpals and the phalanges

metastasis   Spread of disease from its starting point to a distant point

metatarsals   Bones of the foot, between the tarsals and phalanges

midbrain   Part of the brain located between the pons and the diencephalon; also called the *mesencephalon*

midsagittal   Plane that divides the body into equal right and left sides

mitral valve   Valve located between the left atrium and the left ventricle; also called the *bicuspid valve*

mnemonic   Relating to or assisting the memory

molar   Posterior tooth that grinds food

mons pubis   Prominence created by a pad of fat over the symphysis pubis in the female

morphology   Study of the form or structure of living organisms

motility   Ability to move

mucoid   Resembles mucus

mucosa   Mucous membrane that lines a cavity opening to the exterior; consists of epithelium and lamina propria

mucous   Relating to, consisting of, or producing mucus

mucus   Viscous secretions produced by specialized membranes (mucous membranes)

multiaxial   Having many axes

musculature   System of muscles in the body or in a body part

myelin   Fatty substance that surrounds and insulates the axon of some nerve cells

mylohyoid   One of the muscles associated with the hyoid bone, located in the neck

myocardium   Muscular layer of the heart

myometrium   Muscular layer of the uterus

naris (pl. nares)   One of the external openings of the nose; also called *nostril*

nasal   Relating to the nose

nasolacrimal   Relating to the nose and the lacrimal bones

nasopharynx   Superior part of the pharynx, located above the level of the soft palate, posterior to the nasal cavity

navel   Umbilicus; depressed area where the umbilical cord was attached

navicular   Anterior bone of the ankle or tarsus

neural   Relating to the nervous system

neurons   Nerve cells; the basic structural unit of the nervous system

neurovascular   Relating to the nervous and vascular systems

neutralize   To render ineffective or to make neutral

nodules   Small nodes

nuchal   Relating to the back or the nape of the neck

nucleus pulposus   Inner, soft core of an intervertebral disc

oblique   Slanting or sloping direction; deviating from the perpendicular or horizontal

obturator externus   One of the muscles that closes the obturator foramen; one of the lateral rotators of the thigh

obturator internus   One of the muscles that closes the obturator foramen and is part of the lateral pelvic wall; one of the lateral rotators of the thigh

occipital   Relating to the back of the head

ocular   Relating to the eye

oculomotor   Cranial nerve III, innervates muscles that affect eye movement

odontoid   Shaped like a tooth; process on the second cervical vertebra, also called the *dens*

olecranon Curved process on the ulna that forms the point of the elbow

olfactory Relating to the sense of smell; cranial nerve I

omentum (pl. omenta) Fold of peritoneum in the abdominal cavity, usually associated with the stomach

omohyoid One of the infrahyoid muscles

oocyte Immature cell in the ovary that, after undergoing meiosis, produces an ovum

ophthalmic Pertaining to the eye

optic Cranial nerve II; refers to the eye, vision, or properties of light

optimum Most suitable or favorable conditions

orbicularis Circular muscle

orbicularis oculi Circular muscle around the eye

orbicularis oris Circular muscle around the mouth

orbit Cavity in the skull that contains the eyeball; called the *eye socket*

orbital Relating to the orbit

organ of Corti Sensory receptors for hearing, located in the inner ear; also called the *spiral organ of Corti*

orifice Opening or aperture

oropharynx Middle portion of the pharynx, directly posterior to the oral cavity; extends from the soft palate to the hyoid bone

os Mouth or opening, such as the os of the cervix; may also refer to bone, such as os coxa

osseous Consisting of bone

ossicle Small bone; auditory ossicles are three small bones (malleus, incus, stapes) in the middle ear (see individual definitions for each ossicle)

ossification Formation of bone

ovarian Relating to the ovary

ovary Female gonad that produces ova, estrogens, and progesterone

oviduct Slender tube that extends from the uterus to the region of the ovary; also called the *uterine tube* or the *fallopian tube*

ovulation Rupture of a mature ovarian follicle with the release of a secondary oocyte into the pelvic cavity

ovum (pl. ova) Female gamete or germ cell; egg cell

oxytocin Hormone produced in the hypothalamus and stored in the posterior pituitary, stimulates smooth muscle contractions in the pregnant uterus and ejection of milk from the breasts

pacemaker Structure that establishes a basic rhythmic pattern; sinoatrial node in the heart

palate Roof of the mouth, separates the oral and the nasal cavities

palatine Relating to the roof of the mouth

palmar Relating to the palm of the hand

palpate To examine by touch or by feel

palpebra (pl. palpebrae) Eyelid

pampiniform plexus In the male, a plexus of veins from the testicle and epididymis that is included in the spermatic cord; in the female, a plexus of ovarian veins in the broad ligament

pancreatic Relating to the pancreas

papillary muscles Conical projections of myocardium on the inner surface of the ventricles

papilledema Swelling of the optic nerve as a result of increased intracranial pressure

paranasal Located adjacent to or near the nose

parasagittal plane Vertical plane that divides the body into unequal right and left portions; does not pass through the midline

parasympathetic Refers to the part of the autonomic nervous system that is concerned with conserving and restoring energy

parathyroid gland One of four small glands embedded on the posterior surface of the thyroid gland

paraurethral glands Pair of small, mucus-secreting glands associated with the orifice of the urethra in the female; also called *Skene's glands*

parenchyma Characteristic or functional tissue of an organ or gland

parietal Pertaining to the outer wall of a body cavity

parotid Largest of the salivary glands

parturition Act of giving birth; childbirth; delivery

patella Flattened bone in front of the knee; also called the *kneecap*

pectinate Comb shaped; region of the atria of the heart with comb-shaped muscular ridges

pectineus muscle One of the muscles that adducts and flexes the thigh

pectoral Relating to the chest or thorax

pedicle Stem or stalk; a short process that connects the body with the lamina of a vertebra

peduncle Stalk or ropelike mass of nerve fibers that connects one part of the brain to another

pelvic Relating to the pelvis

pelvis Basinlike skeletal structure that acts as an attachment for the lower extremity and contains viscera; a funnel-shaped region, such as the pelvis of the kidney

pendulous Drooping or sagging

penile Relating to the penis

penis Male copulatory organ and organ of urinary excretion

pericardium Membranous sac that encloses the heart

perineal Relating to the perineum

perineum Region bounded by the pubis, coccyx, and thighs; clinically, the perineum is the region between the anus and the external genitalia

periosteum Connective tissue membrane that covers bone

periphery Area away from the center; outer surface of the body

peritoneal Relating to the peritoneum

peritoneum Serous membrane of the abdominal cavity

peroneal Relating to the fibula or lateral portion of the leg

peroneus muscles Group of muscles that originate on the fibula and function to evert the foot

petrosal Relating to the petrous portion of the temporal bone

phalanx (pl. phalanges) Bone of the finger or toe

pharyngeal Relating to the pharynx

pharynx Musculomembranous cavity or tube posterior to the nasal, oral, and laryngeal cavities

phonation Production of sound

phrenic Relating to the diaphragm

pia mater Delicate membrane, the innermost layer of meninges around the brain

piriform Pear shaped

piriformis muscle One of the muscles that laterally rotates the thigh, located in the greater sciatic notch

plantar   Relating to the sole of the foot

plantar flexion   Flexion at the ankle that bends the foot downward toward the sole of the foot

plantaris muscle   One of the leg muscles that plantarflexes the foot

platysma   Thin muscle in the superficial fascia of the anterior neck region that contracts to depress the lower jaw and to wrinkle the skin of the neck

pleura   Serous membrane that covers the lungs and lines the walls of the chest cavity

pleural   Relating to the pleura

plexus   Network of blood vessels, lymphatic vessels, or nerves

pons   Central part of the brainstem, located between the cerebral peduncles and the medulla oblongata

pontine   Relating to the pons

popliteal   Relating to the back of the knee

popliteus muscle   Small muscle on the medial side of the back of the knee that flexes and medially rotates the leg

porta   Entrance or door; the region where blood vessels, nerves, lymphatic vessels, and ducts enter and leave an organ

porta hepatis   Fissure on the visceral surface of the liver through which the hepatic portal vein, the hepatic artery, and the hepatic ducts pass

posterior   Nearer to or toward the back of the body; dorsal

prepuce   Loose fold of skin that covers the glans penis; also called the *foreskin*

progesterone   Hormone produced by the corpus luteum in the ovary; it functions to prepare the lining of the uterus for implantation of a fertilized ovum

prolactin   Hormone produced in the anterior pituitary gland that stimulates the production of milk

prolapse   To fall or to slip down; the inferior displacement of an organ or part of an organ from its normal position

promontory   Projection or elevation

pronate   To place in a face-down position; to turn the hand so that the palm is turned downward or backward

proprioception   Sense of body position and movement as a result of information received from sense receptors in the muscles and tendons

prostate   Accessory gland in the male reproductive system, located inferior to the urinary bladder

proximal   Located nearest the center, midline, point of attachment, or point of origin; opposite of distal

psoas muscle   Large muscle mass, located on either side of the lumbar vertebrae, that flexes and medially rotates the thigh

pterygoid   Wing shaped; refers to the pterygoid processes on the sphenoid bone and the pterygoid muscles

ptosis   Drooping or sagging

pubic   Relating to the pubis

pubis   Pubic bone or the region over the pubic bone

pudendal   Relating to the genital area

pudendum   External genital organs, especially in the female; also called the *vulva*

pulmonary   Relating to the lungs

Purkinje fibers   Conduction myofibers of the heart; specialized cells that are part of the conduction system of the heart

putamen   Lateral portion of the lentiform nucleus, a region of gray matter in the cerebrum

pyloric   Relating to the pylorus

pylorus   Distal portion of the stomach; the opening between the stomach and the duodenum

pyramidal   Relating to or having the shape of a pyramid

quadrant   One of four sections; used to designate regions of the abdomen

quadrate   Having four sides, such as the quadrate lobe of the liver

quadratus lumborum   One of the muscles of the posterior abdominal wall, lateral to the psoas muscles

quadriceps femoris   Muscle mass of the anterior thigh; consists of four muscles

radial   Relating to the radius, a bone in the forearm; diverging in various directions from a central point

radiograph   Processed photographic film used in radiography

radius   Lateral bone in the forearm

ramus (pl. rami)   Branch; a branch of an artery, vein, or nerve

raphe   Ridge or line that marks the union of two similar structures

receptor   Sensory end-organ; it receives a stimulus and converts it into a nerve impulse

rectouterine pouch   Peritoneal space between the rectum and uterus; also called the *cul-de-sac* or *pouch of Douglas*

rectovesical pouch   Peritoneal space between the rectum and the urinary bladder

rectum   Terminal portion of the intestinal tract; section of intestine that extends from the sigmoid colon to the anus

rectus   Straight; used to describe some muscles that run a straight course, such as the rectus abdominis muscle and the rectus muscles of the eye

reflux   Backward flow

renal   Pertaining to the kidney

respiration   Physical and chemical processes by which an individual acquires oxygen and releases carbon dioxide

respiratory   Pertaining to respiration

retina   Innermost layer of the eyeball; part of the eye that contains the visual receptors

retinaculum   Bandlike ligament found in the wrist and the ankle

retinal   Relating to the retina

retromammary   Located behind or deep to the mammary gland

retroperitoneal   Located behind the peritoneum

retropharyngeal   Located behind or dorsal to the pharynx

retroversion   Backward tilt of an organ

rima   Slitlike opening

rima glottidis   Slitlike opening between the true vocal folds

rima vestibuli   Slitlike opening between the vestibular, or false, vocal folds

rotation   Circular motion around an axis

rotator   Muscle that rotates a part

ruga (pl. rugae)   Fold or wrinkle; gastric rugae are folds in the lining of the stomach

rupture   To break or to tear apart; hernia

sac   Anatomical structure that resembles a bag or pouch

saccule   Small sac

sacral   Relating to the sacrum

sacroiliac   Relating to both the sacrum and the ilium (e.g., the sacroiliac joint)

sacrum   Curved, triangular bone made up of five fused vertebrae that are inferior to the lumbar vertebrae and are wedged between the two hipbones

sagittal plane   Vertical plane that divides the body into right and left portions

salivary   Relating to saliva; salivary glands produce saliva

saphenous   Relating to either of two long, superficial veins in the leg, the great (long) saphenous vein and the small (short) saphenous vein; the great (long) saphenous vein is the longest vein in the body

sartorius   Long, straplike muscle that courses obliquely across the anterior thigh and flexes the thigh and leg

scalene muscles   Group of muscles associated with the first and second ribs

scalp   Skin that covers the cranium

scapula (pl. scapulae)   Part of the pectoral girdle that provides the attachment for the upper extremity; also called the *shoulder blade*

scapular   Relating to the scapula

sciatic   Relating to the hip or ischium, such as the sciatic nerve

sclera   Outermost layer of the eyeball

scrotum   Pouch or sac that encloses the testes and the proximal portion of the spermatic cord

sebaceous   Relating to a fatty or oily substance called *sebum*

sella turcica   Depression on the upper surface of the sphenoid bone that marks the location of the pituitary gland

semimembranosus   One of the hamstring muscles located in the thigh

seminal   Relating to semen; seminal vesicles are paired glands, posterior and inferior to the bladder in the male, that secrete a component of semen into the ejaculatory duct

seminiferous tubules   Tightly coiled ducts, located in the testes, where spermatozoa are produced

semitendinosus   One of the hamstring muscles located in the thigh

septal   Relating to a septum

septum (pl. septa)   Wall or partition

septum pellucidum   Thin partition between the two lateral ventricles in the brain

sigmoid   Crooked, or having an S shape; the sigmoid colon is the S-shaped portion of the colon, between the descending colon and the rectum

sinoatrial node   Portion of the conduction system of the heart that initiates and establishes the rhythm of the heartbeat; also called the *pacemaker* or the *S-node*

sinus   Air-filled cavity in a cranial bone; a dilated channel for the passage of blood or lymph

sinusoid   Like a sinus; venous channels in some organs, such as the liver and spleen

skeletal   Relating to the skeleton or bone

skullcap   Top portion of the cranium; also called the *calvaria*

soleus   Muscle in the calf of the leg, deep to the gastrocnemius muscle; it plantarflexes the foot

somatic   Pertaining to the body or the soma

sperm   Spermatozoa; mature male gametes or germ cells

spermatic cord   Supporting structure of the male reproductive system that contains the vas deferens, blood vessels, lymphatics, cremaster muscle, and connective tissue

spermatogenesis   Formation of spermatozoa

spermatozoon (pl. spermatozoa)   Mature male gamete or germ cell; sperm

sphenoethmoidal   Relating to both the sphenoid bone and the ethmoid bone

sphenoidal   Relating to the sphenoid bone

sphincter   Circular muscle that closes an opening when it contracts

spinal   Relating to a spine; relating to the vertebral column

spine   Short projection of bone, a spinous process; the vertebral column

splenic   Relating to the spleen

squama (pl. squamae)   Thin, flat portion of the temporal bone; squamous region of the temporal bone

squamous   Flat or scaly

stapes   One of three ear ossicles in the middle ear; attached to the oval window

stasis   Cessation of or halt in the normal flow of fluids

Stensen's duct   Duct from the parotid gland that empties into the oral cavity; also called the *parotid duct*

sternal   Relating to the sternum

sternum   Long, flat bone that forms the anterior portion of the thoracic cage; also called the *breastbone*

stroma (pl. stromata)   Supporting or connective tissue framework of an organ, as opposed to its functional part, the parenchyma

styloid process   Long, pointed process on the temporal bone

substantia nigra   Region of deeply pigmented cells in the cerebral peduncles

sulcus (pl. sulci)   Groove or furrow

superficial   On, or near, the surface; shallow, such as a superficial wound

superior   Located higher, or toward the head; the upper surface of an organ

supination   Act of lying on the back; rotation of the forearm so that the palm of the hand is forward or upward

supinator   Muscle that supinates the forearm

supine   Lying on the back

sura   Calf of the leg

sutures   Immovable joints that unite bones of the skull

sympathetic   One of the two divisions of the autonomic nervous system

symphysis   Slightly movable joint that has a pad of fibrocartilage between the opposing bones, such as the symphysis pubis

synapse   Junction or region of communication between nerve cells

synovial joints   Freely movable articulations characterized by a membrane that secretes a fluid for lubrication of the joint

systemic   Relating to, or affecting, the entire body

tailbone   Coccyx

talus   One of the tarsal bones that articulates with the tibia and fibula to form the ankle joint

tarsal   Relating to the bones that form the heel, ankle, and instep of the foot

tarsus   Collective term for the seven bones that form the heel, ankle, and instep of the foot

temporal   Relating to the bone that forms the temple or side of the head

temporalis   Muscle of mastication that extends from the temporal bone to the mandible

tendinous   Having the nature of or relating to a tendon

tendon   Cord of dense, fibrous connective tissue that attaches muscle to bone

tensor fasciae latae   Superficial muscle of the lateral thigh; muscle that flexes and abducts the thigh

tentorium cerebelli   Extension of dura mater that acts as a partition between the cerebrum and the cerebellum

teres major and minor   Muscles associated with movement of the shoulder joint

testicular   Relating to the testes

testis (pl. testes)   Male gonad that produces spermatozoa and the male hormone testosterone; also called the *testicle*

thalamic   Relating to the thalamus

thalamus (pl. thalami)   Oval mass of gray matter, located on either side of the third ventricle in the cerebrum; primarily functions as a relay center for sensory impulses

thigh   Proximal portion of the lower extremity, located between the hip and the knee

thoracic   Relating to the thorax or chest

thorax   Upper part of the body, between the neck and the diaphragm; the chest

thrombus   Blood clot in an unbroken blood vessel, located at its point of formation, usually within a vein

thymus   Lymphoid structure, located in the mediastinum posterior to the sternum; plays a role in the development of the immune system

thyroid   Bilobed endocrine gland, located on either side of the trachea, that functions in the regulation of the body's metabolism

tibia   Long bone in the thigh

tibial   Relating to the tibia

tibialis anterior   Muscle along the anterior surface of the tibia

tonsil   Small mass of lymphoid tissue embedded in mucous membrane

tortuous   Twisted

trabecula (pl. trabeculae)   Supporting cord of connective tissue

trabeculae carneae   Muscular bands or ridges of myocardium on the inner surface of the ventricles of the heart

trachea   Passageway for air between the larynx and the bronchi, also called the *windpipe*

tracheal   Relating to the trachea

transected   Cut across

transverse   Term indicating horizontal or crosswise direction

transversospinalis muscles   Deep layer of intrinsic muscles associated with the vertebral column; includes the semispinalis, the multifidus, and the rotatores

trapezius   Superficial muscle of the upper back

traverse   To navigate, cross, bridge, or span

triceps brachii   Large muscle with three heads, located on the posterior surface of the arm that functions to extend the arm at the elbow

tricuspid   Having three cusps, the valve between the right atrium and the right ventricle

trigeminal   Cranial nerve V

trigone   Triangular area on the floor of the bladder marked by the openings for the two ureters and the urethra

trochanter   One of two large prominences on the proximal femur

trochlea   Any pulleylike structure or surface

trochlear   Cranial nerve IV

tubercle   Rounded elevation on a bone

tuberosity   Rounded projection from a bone

tunic   Layer or coating

turbinate   Shaped like a scroll; a bone that is shaped like a scroll or conch shell; one of the nasal conchae

ulna   Medial bone of the forearm

ulnar   Relating to the ulna

umbilical   Relating to the umbilicus or navel

umbilicus   Region on the abdomen that marks the former attachment of the umbilical cord; also called the *navel*

uncinate   Shaped like a hook; an extension or region of the pancreas

uniaxial   Allows movement along one axis, such as a hinge joint

unmyelinated   Does not possess myelin, a fatty sheath; refers to nerve axons

ureter   Tubular structure that conveys urine from the renal pelvis to the urinary bladder

urethra   Tubular structure that conveys urine from the urinary bladder to the exterior

urogenital   Relating to both the urinary (renal) system and the genital (reproductive) system; also called *genitourinary*

uterus   Hollow, muscular organ in the female pelvis that is the site of menstruation, implantation of the fertilized egg, and the development of the embryo and fetus; also called the *womb*

utricle   Part of the membranous labyrinth, located in the vestibule of the inner ear, that contains sense receptors for static equilibrium

uvula   Fleshy projection at the posterior end of the soft palate

vagina   Muscular tube that extends from the vestibule to the cervix of the uterus in the female

vaginal   Relating to the vagina

vagus   Cranial nerve X

vallecula   Shallow groove; the groove between the epiglottis and the root of the tongue

vas (pl. vasa)   Channel or duct that conveys a liquid

vascular   Pertaining to or containing vessels

vasculature   Blood vessels of an organ

vastus muscles   Part of the quadriceps femoris group of muscles on the anterior thigh   vastus lateralis, vastus intermedius, and vastus medialis

vein   Vessel that carries blood toward the heart

vena (pl. venae)   Latin term for vein

venous   Relating to veins

ventral   Pertaining to the front or anterior side of the body; opposite of dorsal

ventricle   Chamber or cavity, especially in the heart or brain

ventricular   Pertaining to a ventricle

vermiform   Shaped like a worm, such as the vermiform appendix

vermis   Latin term for worm; the central part of the cerebellum that connects the two cerebellar hemispheres

vertebra (pl. vertebrae)   One of the bones that form the spinal column, or backbone

vertebral   Relating to the vertebrae

vesicle   Small pouch or sac that contains liquid

vestibule   Chamber or space, such as the vestibule of the larynx or vestibule of the inner ear

vestibulocochlear   Cranial nerve VIII; functions in the sense of hearing and equilibrium

villus (pl. villi)   Small, hairlike projection from the surface of a membrane

viscera   Organs inside the ventral body cavity

visceral   Relating to the viscera

vitreous body   Soft, gelatinous substance that fills the posterior portion of the eyeball, between the lens and the retina

vomer   Bone of the face that forms the lower portion of the nasal septum

vulva   Collective term for the external genitalia of the female; also called the *pudendum*

Wharton's duct   Duct of the submandibular salivary gland; also called the *submandibular duct*

Wharton's jelly   Homogeneous intercellular substance of the umbilical cord; also called *mucous connective tissue*

xiphoid   Shaped like a sword; the distal portion of the sternum

zygomatic   Relating to the cheekbone or the zygomatic bone, such as the zygomatic process or the zygomatic arch

zygomatic bone   Cheekbone; also called *zygoma*

zygote   Fertilized egg; single cell, resulting from the union of male and female gametes

Combining Forms

Many anatomical and medical terms are made up of combinations of word roots, or combining forms, together with prefixes or suffixes. Some of the more commonly used word roots and combining forms and their definitions are listed here, along with examples of their uses in a word and their definitions.

Ab– away from; *abduct*—to take away from

Abdomino– abdomen; *abdominopelvic cavity*—the portion of the ventral body cavity that includes the abdomen and the pelvis

Acro– extremity; *acromion process*—the extremity or extreme end of the spine of the scapula

Ad– toward; *adduct*—to move toward the axis of the body

Alb– white; *linea alba*—vertical white line in the center of the abdomen

Alveol– cavity, socket; *alveolus*—air cavity in the lung

Ante– before; *antecubital*-region in front of the elbow

Antero– in front, ventral; *anterolateral*—located in front and to one side

Atrio– relating to an atrium of the heart; *atrioventricular valve*—valve between an atrium and a ventricle

Bi– two; *biceps brachii*—muscle in the arm with two heads

Brachi– arm; *brachial artery*—the principal artery in the arm

Bronch– relating to the bronchi; *bronchoscopy*—direct visual examination of the bronchi

Capit– relating to the head; *capitulum*—a head-shaped eminence on a bone

Cardi– relating to the heart; *cardiology*—study of the heart and its diseases

Cephal– head; *cephalad*—toward the head

Cerebello– relating to the cerebellum; *cerebellomedullary*—relating to the cerebellum and the medulla oblongata

Cerebro– brain; *cerebrospinal fluid*—fluid that circulates around the brain and spinal cord

Chondr– cartilage; *hypochondriac region*—abdominal region below the cartilage of the ribs

Coraco– relating to the coracoid process of the scapula; *coracoacromial ligament*—ligament between the coracoid and acromion processes of the scapula

Cor–, Coron– crown; *coronary arteries*—arteries that form a crown, or circle, around the base of the heart and supply blood to the heart muscle

Cost– rib; *costal cartilage*—the cartilage that connects the ribs to the sternum

Crani– skull; *craniotomy*—surgical opening of the skull

Cysti– sac or bladder; *cystic duct*—duct from the gallbladder

Dorso–, Dorsi– denotes a relationship to the dorsal or the posterior surface; *dorsolateral*—on the posterior surface and to one side

Duodeno– denotes a relationship to the first part of the small intestine; *duodenojejunal flexure*—turn at the junction of the duodenum and the jejunum

Dura– hard or tough; *dura mater*—outer, tough membrane that covers the brain and the spinal cord

Ecto– outside; *ectopic pregnancy*—pregnancy or gestation outside the uterus

Endo– inside; *endocardium*—membrane that lines the inside of the heart wall

Epi– above or upon; *epidural*—above the dura mater

Ex–, Exo–, Extra– out or away from; *extrinsic muscles*—muscles outside the structure being acted upon

Fibro– denotes fibers; *fibrocartilage*—cartilage with an abundance of white fibers in the matrix

Gastr– stomach; *gastritis*—inflammation of the stomach

Gingiv– gum; *gingivitis*—inflammation of the gums

Glosso– tongue; *glossopharyngeal nerve*—nerve that provides innervation for the tongue

Hepat– liver; *hepatitis*—inflammation of the liver

Hyper– beyond or excessive; *hypertrophy*—excessive growth of a tissue

Hypo– under, below, deficient; *hypoglossal*—below the tongue

Hyster– uterus; *hysterectomy*—surgical removal of the uterus

Ileo– ileum; *ileocecal valve*—junction of the ileum and the cecum

Ilio– ilium; *iliosacral*—pertaining to both the ilium and the sacrum

Infra– beneath; *infraorbital foramen*—foramen below the orbit of the eye

Inter– among or between; *intercostal muscles*—the muscles between the ribs

Intra– within or inside; *intracranial pressure*—pressure inside the cranium

Labi– lip; *glenoid labrum*—rim or lip of fibrocartilage around the margin of the glenoid fossa

Laryngo– relates to the larynx; *laryngopharynx*—the portion of the pharynx in the region of the larynx

281

Lieno– relates to the spleen; *lienorenal ligament*—peritoneal ligament between the spleen and the kidney

Lingua– tongue; *lingual frenulum*—fold of tissue that anchors the tongue to the floor of the mouth

Lumb– lower back, loin; *lumbar vertebrae*—vertebrae in the lower back region

Mening– membrane; *meningitis*—inflammation of the membranes around the brain and spinal cord

Meta– after or beyond; *metacarpals*—bones of the hand, beyond the wrist

Metr– uterus; *endometrium*—lining of the uterus

Mid– located in the middle; *midsagittal*—sagittal section in the middle, divides into equal right and left portions

Musculo– muscular system; *musculoskeletal*—pertains to both the muscular system and the skeletal system

Myo– muscle; *myocardium*—muscle in the heart wall

Naso– referring to the nose; *nasolacrimal duct*—duct that drains tears into the nasal cavity

Nephro– kidney; *nephron*—basic functional unit of the kidney

Neuro– nerve; *neuromuscular*—pertaining to both nerves and muscle

Oculo– eye; *oculomotor*—nerve that transmits impulses to the muscles of the eye

Odont– tooth; *odontoid process*—toothlike process on the second cervical vertebra

Oo– egg; *oocyte*—egg cell

Ophthalm– eye; *ophthalmology*—study of the eye and its diseases

Orchid– testicle; *cryptorchidism*—failure of the testicle to descend into the scrotum

Oro– mouth; *oropharynx*—region of the pharynx posterior to the cavity of the mouth

Oss–, osseo–, osteo– bone; *osseous*—containing bone

Palpebr– eyelid; *levator palpebrae superioris*—muscle that raises the upper eyelid

Para– adjacent, alongside, or deviation from normal; *parasagittal section*—a sagittal section that is not in the midline

Pariet– relates to the wall of a cavity; *parietal peritoneum*—layer of peritoneum that lines the wall of the abdominal cavity

Patho– disease; *pathology*—study of disease mechanisms

Peri– around; *pericardium*—membrane around the heart

Phon– voice, sound; *phonation*—the production of sound

Phren– diaphragm; *phrenic nerve*—nerve that stimulates the diaphragm

Postero– a direction toward the back of the body; *posterolateral*—toward the sides on the back of the body

Pre– before, either in time or in space; *prenatal*—before birth

Pulmon– lung; *pulmonary*—relating to the lungs

Quadr–, quadri– of or relating to the number four; *quadriceps femoris*—muscle group that contains four muscles

Radio– relating to radiation; *radiograph*—picture formed by radiation

Radio– relating to the radius; *radioulnar joint*—articulation between the radius and the ulna

Recto– relating to the rectum; *rectouterine pouch*—pouch or cul-de-sac between the rectum and the uterus

Retro– situated behind or backward; *retroperitoneal*—located behind the peritoneum

Sacr–, sacri– relating to the sacrum; *sacroiliac*—relating to both the sacrum and the ilium

Semi– denoting half or partial; *semicircular canals*—canals that are shaped like half of a circle

Spheno– relating to the sphenoid bone; *sphenoethmoidal*—relates to both the sphenoid bone and the ethmoid bone

Sterno– relating to the sternum; *sternopericardial ligament*—membranous ligament located between the sternum and the pericardium

Stylo– relating to the styloid process of the temporal bone; *stylomastoid foramen*—foramen located between the styloid process and the mastoid

Sub– below or less than; *submandibular*—below the mandible

Supero– relating to superior; *superomedial*—in a direction that is superior and medial to the reference

Super–, supra– meaning above or too much; *supraspinatus muscle*—muscle above the spine of the scapula

Trans– across, through, or beyond; *transected*—cut through

Tri– three; *trigone*—a triangular region, marked by three openings, on the floor of the urinary bladder

Utero– relating to the uterus; *uterovesical pouch*—peritoneal pouch between the uterus and the urinary bladder

Vas– vessel or duct; *cerebrovascular*—pertaining to the blood vessels of the brain

Vertebro– relating to the vertebrae; *vertebrosternal ribs*—ribs that are attached to the vertebrae and the sternum

Vesico– relating to the urinary bladder; *vesicoprostatic*—relating to the urinary bladder and the prostate gland

Viscer– organ; *visceral peritoneum*—peritoneum that covers the abdominal organs

Eponyms

Eponyms are names of diseases, structures, or procedures that include the name of an individual. The current trend is to avoid, or at least to discourage, the use of eponyms because they are nondescriptive and often vague. However, eponyms are still used in many places, and this list has been prepared to help you relate common eponyms to the preferred terminology. For convenience, the eponyms are listed alphabetically by the name of the person associated with them.

Eponym	Preferred Terminology
Achilles tendon	calcaneal tendon
Adam's apple	thyroid cartilage
Addison's place	transpyloric plane
Alcock's canal	pudendal canal
Auerbach's plexus	myenteric plexus
Bartholin's duct	major sublingual duct
Bartholin's gland	greater vestibular gland
Bauhin's valve	ileocecal valve
Bellini, ducts of	collecting ducts in the kidney
Bertin's columns	renal columns of the kidney
Bigelow's ligament	iliofemoral ligament
Billroth's cords	red pulp cords in the spleen
Botallo's duct	ligamentum arteriosum
Bourgery's ligament	oblique popliteal ligament
Bowman's capsule	glomerular capsule
Buck's fascia	deep fascia of the penis
Cooper's ligament	suspensory ligament of the breast
Corti, organ of	spiral organ of Corti
Cowper's gland	bulbourethral gland
Douglas, pouch of	rectouterine pouch
Eustachian tube	auditory tube
Fallopian tube	uterine tube
Galen, vein of	great cerebral vein
Graafian follicle	vesicular ovarian follicle
Highmore, antrum of	maxillary sinus
His, bundle of	atrioventricular (AV) bundle
Hunter's canal	adductor canal or subsartorial canal
Koch's node	sinoatrial node
Leydig's cells	interstitial cells of the testis
Lieberkühn, crypt of	intestinal gland

Eponym	Preferred Terminology
Louis, angle of	sternal angle
Luschka, foramen of	lateral aperture
Magendie, foramen of	median aperture
Malpighian corpuscle	renal corpuscle
Monro, foramen of	interventricular foramen
Montgomery, glands of	sebaceous glands of the areola
Oddi, sphincter of	hepatopancreatic sphincter
Peyer's patches	aggregated lymphatic follicles
Poupart's ligament	inguinal ligament
Purkinje fibers	conduction myofibers
Reil, island of	insula
Rivinus, duct of	lesser sublingual duct
Rolando, fissure of	central fissure (sulcus)
Rosenmüller, fossa of	pharyngeal recess
Schlemm, canal of	scleral venous sinus
Sertoli's cells	sustentacular cells of the testis
Skene's gland	paraurethral gland
Spieghelian lobe	caudate lobe of the liver
Stensen's duct	parotid duct
Sylvius, aqueduct of	cerebral aqueduct
Sylvius, fissure of	lateral cerebral fissure
Treitz, ligament of	suspensory muscle of the duodenum
Vater, ampulla of	hepatopancreatic ampulla
Wharton's duct	submandibular duct
Wharton's jelly	mucous connective tissue
Willis, circle of	cerebral arterial circle
Winslow, foramen of	epiploic foramen
Wirsung, duct of	pancreatic duct
Wormian bones	sutural bones

Answers to Quick Check Boxes

Chapter 1

1.1 sagittal planes and frontal (coronal) planes
1.2 transverse plane
1.3 distal
1.4 superior
1.5 cranial cavity and spinal cavity
1.6 mediastinum
1.7 umbilicus
1.8 epigastric, umbilical, and hypogastric
1.9 meninges
1.10 pericardium
1.11 visceral peritoneum
1.12 appendicular
1.13 axial

Chapter 2

2.1 T1 (first thoracic vertebra)
2.2 diaphragm
2.3 sternal angle
2.4 jugular notch
2.5 second through seventh ribs
2.6 ribs 8, 9, and 10
2.7 cartilage of ribs 8, 9, and 10
2.8 body and transverse processes
2.9 12
2.10 intercostal muscles
2.11 levator costarum
2.12 scapula and clavicle
2.13 pectoralis major
2.14 trapezius and latissimus dorsi
2.15 deltoid
2.16 supraspinatus, infraspinatus, subscapularis, and teres minor
2.17 right pleural cavity, left pleural cavity, and mediastinum
2.18 visceral pleura
2.19 a capillary layer of serous fluid for lubrication
2.20 root of the lung
2.21 (a) right; (b) left; (c) right; (d) right
2.22 sternal angle and intervertebral disk between the fourth and fifth vertebrae
2.23 heart
2.24 apex of the heart
2.25 left ventricle
2.26 pectinate muscle
2.27 tricuspid (right atrioventricular) valve
2.28 circumflex artery and anterior intervertebral artery
2.29 atrioventricular (AV) node
2.30 brachiocephalic artery
2.31 superior vena cava
2.32 immediately superior to the aortic semilunar valve in the ascending aorta
2.33 trachea
2.34 pulmonary artery
2.35 pericardium and left atrium
2.36 right—azygos vein; middle—thoracic duct; left—descending aorta
2.37 anterior scalene and middle scalene
2.38 axillary lymph nodes
2.39 thyroid gland
2.40 internal jugular vein
2.41 right common carotid artery and right subclavian artery
2.42 left subclavian artery
2.43 left brachiocephalic vein
2.44 superior vena cava
2.45 right pulmonary artery
2.46 pulmonary trunk
2.47 right ventricle
2.48 right pulmonary artery
2.49 tricuspid valve
2.50 esophagus
2.51 left side
2.52 left atrium

Chapter 3

3.1 diaphragm
3.2 linea alba
3.3 transpyloric plane
3.4 horizontal transumbilical plane and vertical median plane
3.5 five lumbar vertebrae
3.6 L2
3.7 caval hiatus for the superior vena cava
3.8 rectus abdominis
3.9 psoas muscle
3.10 celiac trunk, superior mesenteric artery, and inferior mesenteric artery
3.11 suprarenal, renal, and gonadal arteries
3.12 right and left common iliac arteries
3.13 passes through the caval hiatus of the diaphragm at the T8 vertebral level

3.14 right and left common iliac veins

3.15 right and left lumbar veins, right gonadal vein, right and left renal veins, right suprarenal vein, right inferior phrenic vein, right and left hepatic veins

3.16 the splenic vein is anterior to the SMA, and the left renal vein is posterior to the SMA, between the SMA and the aorta

3.17 mesentery is peritoneum that encloses the intestine and attaches it to the posterior abdominal wall; omentum is peritoneum associated with the stomach

3.18 retroperitoneal

3.19 falciform ligament

3.20 porta hepatis

3.21 hepatic artery and hepatic portal vein; hepatic artery has the higher oxygen content

3.22 quadrate lobe

3.23 T10

3.24 fundus

3.25 greater omentum

3.26 duodenum

3.27 jejunum and ileum

3.28 ascending colon, descending colon, and rectum

3.29 cecum

3.30 left hypochondriac region

3.31 splenic vein and superior mesenteric vein join to form the hepatic portal vein

3.32 diaphragm, quadratus lumborum, and psoas

3.33 suprarenal gland

3.34 left hepatic vein

3.35 caudate lobe

3.36 the hepatic arteries and hepatic ducts are anterior to the portal vein; hepatic ducts are to the right of the hepatic arteries

3.37 quadrate lobe of the liver

3.38 gastroduodenal artery

3.39 second part of the duodenum

3.40 right lobe of the liver

3.41 second part of the duodenum

3.42 first part is superior to the pancreatic head and third part is inferior

3.43 right side

3.44 aorta is to the left of the IVC

3.45 left renal vein passes horizontally across (or anterior to) the aorta and posterior to the SMA, just inferior to where the SMA branches from the aorta

3.46 the spleen is posterior to the stomach and superior to the left kidney

3.47 right lobe of the liver, spleen, and both kidneys

3.48 psoas muscle

3.49 splenic artery and splenic vein

3.50 stomach

Chapter 4

4.1 pelvic brim

4.2 ilium to form the sacroiliac joint

4.3 ilium, ischium, and pubis

4.4 acetabulum

4.5 obturator internus

4.6 piriformis

4.7 levator ani and coccygeus

4.8 transversus perinea

4.9 internal iliac veins

4.10 pudendal nerve

4.11 rectum and seminal vesicles

4.12 prostate gland

4.13 two openings for the ureters and one for the internal urethral orifice

4.14 prostatic urethra

4.15 broad ligament

4.16 anteriorly

4.17 cervix

4.18 posterior fornix

4.19 pudendum

4.20 paraurethral glands and greater vestibular glands

4.21 tunica albuginea

4.22 spermatic cord

4.23 prostate gland

4.24 corpus cavernosum

4.25 bulb

4.26 common iliac veins

4.27 rectouterine pouch

4.28 cervix of the uterus

4.29 uterus

4.30 vesicouterine space

4.31 ductus deferens

4.32 prostatic urethra

4.33 bulbospongiosus muscle

4.34 seminal vesicles

4.35 crura of corpus cavernosum

Chapter 5

5.1 parietal and temporal bones

5.2 frontalis and occipitalis muscles

5.3 mandible and vomer bones

5.4 maxillary sinuses

5.5 sphenoid sinus

5.6 foramen magnum

5.7 cranial nerve VII (facial nerve)

5.8 temporalis muscle is most superior; innervated by cranial nerve V (trigeminal nerve)

5.9 parotid gland

5.10 corpus callosum

5.11 thalamus

5.12 midbrain, pons, medulla oblongata; midbrain is most superior

5.13 cerebellar peduncles

5.14 cerebral aqueduct (aqueduct of Sylvius)

5.15 third ventricle

5.16 in the subarachnoid space between the arachnoid and the pia mater

5.17 falx cerebri

5.18 internal carotid arteries and vertebral arteries

5.19 sigmoid sinus
5.20 cranial nerve X (vagus nerve)
5.21 oculomotor (III), trochlear (IV), abducens (VI), and the ophthalmic and maxillary branches of the trigeminal (V)
5.22 optic foramen
5.23 central artery of the retina
5.24 upper lateral margin
5.25 body of the caudate nucleus
5.26 third ventricle
5.27 great cerebral vein
5.28 cerebral aqueduct (aqueduct of Sylvius)
5.29 tentorium cerebelli
5.30 basilar artery
5.31 anterior
5.32 external auditory meatus
5.33 submandibular gland
5.34 nasopharynx
5.35 middle cerebellar peduncle
5.36 middle cerebral artery
5.37 masseter
5.38 middle meatus

Chapter 6

6.1 vertebral foramen
6.2 intervertebral foramina
6.3 transverse foramina
6.4 costal facets for articulation with the ribs
6.5 sacroiliac joint
6.6 nucleus pulposus
6.7 cervical and lumbar regions
6.8 thoracic and sacral curvatures
6.9 anterior and posterior longitudinal ligaments
6.10 ligamentum nuchae
6.11 erector spinae muscles
6.12 the dura mater around the brain has two layers, and the dura mater around the spinal cord has only one layer
6.13 conus medullaris
6.14 cervical enlargement and lumbosacral enlargement
6.15 31 pairs
6.16 phrenic nerve
6.17 sacral plexus
6.18 seven cervical vertebrae
6.19 sternocleidomastoid muscle
6.20 common carotid artery, internal jugular vein, and vagus nerve
6.21 nasopharynx
6.22 oropharynx
6.23 rima glottides
6.24 esophagus
6.25 parathyroid glands
6.26 thyroid gland
6.27 the internal jugular vein is lateral to the common carotid artery
6.28 at the bifurcation of the common carotid artery
6.29 in the transverse foramina of the cervical vertebrae

6.30 vagus nerve
6.31 cervical plexus
6.32 masseter
6.33 the external jugular vein is lateral to the muscle, and the internal jugular vein is medial to the muscle
6.34 brachial plexus
6.35 nasopharynx

Chapter 7

7.1 30 (humerus, radius, ulna, 8 carpals, 5 metacarpals, 14 phalanges)
7.2 move the scapula
7.3 humerus
7.4 scapula and subscapularis muscle
7.5 axillary artery and vein
7.6 extend the forearm at the elbow
7.7 biceps brachii
7.8 median nerve and ulnar nerve
7.9 anterior side of the elbow joint
7.10 radial artery
7.11 median cubital vein
7.12 radius, ulna, and the interosseous membrane between the two bones
7.13 flex the hand and fingers
7.14 radial artery and ulnar artery
7.15 median nerve
7.16 flexor retinaculum
7.17 median nerve
7.18 coracobrachialis
7.19 basilic vein
7.20 biceps brachii and brachialis muscles
7.21 radial artery
7.22 basilic vein
7.23 synovial membrane, joint capsule, articular cartilage, joint cavity with synovial fluid
7.24 acromion and coracoid processes of the scapula and the coracoacromial ligament between them
7.25 transverse humeral ligament, coracohumeral ligament, and glenohumeral ligament
7.26 inferiorly because there is little support in that direction
7.27 tendon for the long head of the biceps brachii muscle
7.28 supraspinatus muscle
7.29 pronation and supination
7.30 humeroulnar and humeroradial articulations
7.31 medial (ulnar) and lateral (radial) collateral ligaments
7.32 trochlear notch of the ulna and the trochlea of the humerus
7.33 brachialis and biceps brachii muscles; biceps brachii is superficial
7.34 head of the radius and the capitulum of the humerus

Chapter 8

8.1 two os coxae
8.2 iliac crest superiorly and lower margin of the gluteus maximus muscle inferiorly

8.3 tensor fasciae latae

8.4 piriformis

8.5 femur

8.6 vastus lateralis, vastus medialis, vastus intermedius, and rectus femoris

8.7 adduct the thigh

8.8 biceps femoris

8.9 femoral artery

8.10 femoral nerve and sciatic nerve

8.11 inguinal ligament, adductor longus muscle, and sartorius muscle

8.12 tibia and fibula

8.13 dorsiflexion of the foot and extension of the toes

8.14 gastrocnemius and soleus muscles

8.15 posterior tibial artery and tibial nerve

8.16 behind the knee

8.17 diverging tendons of the hamstring muscles and the lateral and medial heads of the gastrocnemius muscle

8.18 calcaneus

8.19 five metatarsals

8.20 big (or great) toe

8.21 gracilis muscle

8.22 in proximal regions, the sartorius muscle is in the anterior compartment; however, as it descends, it crosses obliquely, and in distal regions, it is on the medial side with the gracilis

8.23 lateral and medial condyles of the tibia and the head of the fibula

8.24 tibialis anterior and extensor digitorum longus muscles

8.25 acetabulum of the os coxa and head of the femur

8.26 fovea capitis femoris

8.27 transverse acetabular ligament

8.28 synovial membrane

8.29 iliofemoral, pubofemoral, and ischiofemoral ligaments

8.30 femoral nerve and sciatic nerve

8.31 piriformis muscle

8.32 piriformis muscle is superior, gemellus muscle is in the middle, and quadratus femoris is inferior

8.33 obturator externus and obturator internus muscles

8.34 gracilis muscle

8.35 hyaline cartilage

8.36 between the femoral condyles and the tibial plateaus

8.37 anterior and posterior cruciate ligaments

8.38 move the leg at the knee joint

8.39 patellar ligament

8.40 anterior and posterior cruciate ligaments

8.41 trochlea of the talus with the distal tibia, talus with the lateral malleolus of the fibula, and talus with the medial malleolus of the tibia

8.42 three facets of the talus articulate with the calcaneus

8.43 tendocalcaneus (Achilles tendon)